STRAIGHT FROM THE GUT

Living with Crohn's Disease and Ulcerative Colitis

Cliff Kalibjian

D1412576

O'REILLY®

Beijing • Cambridge • Farnham • Köln • Paris • Sebastopol • Taipei • Tokyo

Straight from the Gut: Living with Crohn's Disease and Ulcerative Colitis
by Cliff Kalibjian

Published by O'Reilly & Associates, Inc., 1005 Gravenstein Hwy North, Sebastopol, CA 95472.

Editor: Nancy Keene

Production Editor: Tom Dorsaneo

Cover Designer: Kristen Throop

Printing History: May 2003. First Edition

Library of Congress Cataloging-in-Publication Data:

Kalibjian, Cliff, 1969–.
 Straight from the gut : living with Crohn's disease and ulcerative colitis / Cliff Kalibjian.— 1st ed.
  p. cm.—(Patient-centered guides)
 Includes bibliographical references and index.
 ISBN 0-596-50005-X
 1. Ulcerative colitis—Popular works. 2. Crohn's disease—Popular works. I. Title. II. Series.

RC862.C63K35 2003
616.3'447—dc21   2003048279

[M]

To my parents, Ralph and Lillian Kalibjian,
for all their love, care, and support

Table of Contents

Preface

I'LL NEVER FORGET THE DAY in seventh-grade science class when we were learning about the seven warning signs of cancer. One of them was "a change in bowel or bladder habits." Being the curious student I was, I raised my hand and asked what this meant. My teacher very matter-of-factly explained that this could mean many things, but typically blood in the stool was a major sign of cancer. I was shocked by this answer, as never in my twelve years of life did I ever even consider that something like that could happen. I quickly dismissed the unpleasant image in my mind and never thought about it again. That is, until one year later.

It was December 1982, and I had to rush to the bathroom. I previously had had diarrhea only one other time in my life that I could remember. To my horror, though, as I stood up, the color in the toilet bowl was not brown. It was something between a mahogany and cranberry color. My 13-year-old mind immediately jumped to the dreaded conclusion that I had cancer.

I kept my secret for a few days, hoping everything would magically clear up. But it didn't. Finally, I broke down and told my parents. We immediately saw my pediatrician, who referred us to a nearby university hospital. Within a couple of weeks of that first day of bloody diarrhea, I had a diagnosis. But it wasn't cancer. It was instead a chronic disease called ulcerative colitis. Neither my family nor I had ever heard of this disorder or its close cousin, Crohn's disease (as it was later diagnosed). But we would soon be experts.

There were many challenges living with a chronic illness during junior high and high school. My years in college were even more demanding as I faced living with Crohn's away from home for the first time. However, by this time in my life, I had the courage to seek out others with inflammatory bowel disease (IBD, which includes both Crohn's disease and ulcerative colitis) through support groups sponsored by the Crohn's and Colitis Foundation of America (CCFA). What a relief it was to know that there were others going though similar experiences. And how comforting it was to know that others were feeling the exact same things I was feeling. Finally, I didn't feel so quite alone.

Despite my health problems, I somehow managed to graduate from college. However, after college my health really began to deteriorate. Healthy time between flares became shorter and shorter. Flares became more severe and lasted longer. Hospitalization became routine. At times I couldn't eat for many weeks if I was on intravenous or nose tube feedings. I was trapped in a vicious cycle, and I couldn't seem to find my way out.

I tried everything. No medications worked except prednisone. I read and researched both conventional and alternative medicine. I tried every diet and many, many different natural treatments, including mind–body therapies. Yet I still continued in the same pattern.

Of course, all along I knew I had one other choice. But it was one I was desperately avoiding at all costs. Because Crohn's disease only was affecting my colon, I could have my entire colon removed and have a very good chance of being healthy again. The cost, however, was that I'd have a permanent ileostomy, which would mean I'd have to wear a bag on my lower abdomen for the rest of my life to collect intestinal waste products. I really felt this choice was fine for other people, but not for me.

But I was running out of options. I had been on high amounts of prednisone for over twelve years, and sensed I couldn't take much more before permanent damage set in. I knew many people with ileostomies, and most were healthy and could do whatever they wanted. What was I waiting for?

In January 1999, I had the surgery. It was rough, but I recovered. Within a few months, I was well and no longer required any medication. For the first time in my adult life, I was actually healthy. I almost didn't know what to do with myself after having been sick for so many years. Yes, it did take a while to adapt to living with the bag, but having an ileostomy has truly given me my life back. For this, I will always be thankful.

Why I wrote this book

Even as a teenager, I felt I would someday write a book on Crohn's disease and ulcerative colitis. Despite all the pain and suffering, I had a sense there might be a higher purpose for everything I was going through. I thought that perhaps one day my experience might enable me to help others dealing with similar issues. Over the years, I also amassed a lot of knowledge as I struggled to find my own answers through research. I also got to know many people with IBD through my role as a support group facilitator. I thought it would be wonderful to combine all the latest research, hundreds of practical coping tips, and dozens of people's stories into one totally comprehensive book. And thanks to a subsidiary of O'Reilly and Associates— Patient-Centered Guides—my dream of writing a book to help people with IBD became reality.

What this book offers

This book is not my autobiography. Instead, it is a compilation of the latest research on Crohn's disease and ulcerative colitis. My goal was to take technical information and explain it in easy-to-understand language. Woven among the facts are hundreds of personal vignettes from dozens of people touched by IBD. These stories are the heart and soul of the book. *Straight from the Gut* would not have been complete without each and every one of them. I think readers will appreciate the different viewpoints and the myriad of emotions shared. My hope is that readers will come away knowing that they are indeed not alone on their journey in this world with IBD.

All the stories in the book are true and are from real people. However, all names have been changed to protect the privacy of interviewees. The book also offers countless practical coping tips for people with Crohn's disease and ulcerative colitis.

This book is not a substitute for seeking advice from your physician. On the contrary, professional medical care is essential for anyone with IBD. My hope, though, is that this book—in combination with your medical team—will help empower you to make the most educated decisions regarding your health care.

How this book is organized

This book is organized so you can read it straight through or just read the chapter currently of most interest to you. If you are not familiar with IBD, however, I suggest you read Chapter 1, *Introduction to IBD,* and Chapter 2, *Signs and Symptoms,* to gain a better understanding of Crohn's disease and ulcerative colitis.

Subsequent chapters cover every major topic related to IBD. Some, such as diagnostic procedures, medications, working well with your doctor, effects of the disease on relationships, insurance issues, the emotional impact of the illness, and living well with IBD are subjects almost every person with Crohn's or colitis faces at one time or another. Other chapters cover more specialized topics, such as complications, surgical treatments, diet and complementary medicine, alternative forms of feeding, hospitalization, living with an ostomy, coping with prednisone, pregnancy, and the disease's effect on children and teens. Every chapter is a blend of facts, tips, and personal stories to help you manage your life with IBD.

At the end of the book, I've included a comprehensive resource appendix that lists many different organizations, books, tapes, and web sites that may be of interest to you.

IBD tends to affect both men and women equally. Unfortunately, the English language doesn't have a standard gender-neutral singular pronoun. As a result, it was decided to alternate between masculine and feminine pronouns throughout the book. Although not everyone is used to this style, it helps prevent the favoring of one gender over the other and ultimately allows everyone to feel more included.

Acknowledgments

I am extremely grateful for all the people in my life who have enabled me to write this book. First, I wish to thank members of my immediate family for their never-ending love and support through all the years of Crohn's: my parents, Ralph and Lillian Kalibjian; my sister, Sharrese DeKock; my brother-in-law, Pieter DeKock; my niece, Bianca DeKock; my nephew, Tanner DeKock; my brother, Jeff Kalibjian; and my sister-in-law, Renée C. Lyons, MD.

A special thank-you goes out to Barry Barsamian and Aram Mashlakian, two terrific people who have provided me with much friendship and support through all the healthy and not-so-healthy times.

Straight from the Gut would not exist if hadn't been for my life-long friend Mitch Patenaude. There was never a time I did not know Mitch, as we lived next door to each other from the time we were babies. He was the person who suggested I contact Patient-Centered Guides about writing a book on IBD. Thank you, Mitch, for directing me to this opportunity of a lifetime.

I also wish to thank my supervisor, Kelly Doughty, for allowing me to have a flexible work schedule during the times I needed to meet deadlines for this book. I would not have been able to write *Straight from the Gut* if not for his flexibility and support.

I will always be grateful for Nancy Keene, my editor. Her wisdom, instinct, and guidance—which have truly been priceless—are reflected in every chapter. Thank you as well to Linda Lamb, Deanna Blevins, and everyone else at Patient-Centered Guides who worked behind the scenes to produce *Straight from the Gut*.

Over 30 people very generously took time out of their busy schedules to review portions of this book for content, tone, and accuracy. I was blessed to have a wonderful mix of reviewers who provided such insightful feedback. Some of them also took additional time to talk to me on the phone and answer last-minute emails when I had further questions. Thanks so much to the following individuals: James Allison, MD; Jeffrey Aron, MD; Jennifer Basurto, MSW, LCSW; Tami Blaj; Charles O. Elson, MD; Teresa Evans; Nancy A. Feldman-Saylor, LCSW; Carol Gerstein; Sheila Gustaveson; Jo Ann Hattner, MPH, RD; Melvin B. Heyman, MD, MPH; John Huffman; Pyng Lee, MS, RD; Sandy Green Lobdell, RN, CWOCN; Edward V. Loftus, Jr., MD; Priscilla Minn, MSW; Shelby Z. Modell; William D. Modell; Joe Moynihan; Terry Neifing, LCSW; Donald Palmer, MD, FACS; Julie Perry; Janet Rao; Suzanne Rosenthal; Marta Rottman; Arlyn Serber; Lisa Smythe; Rand L. Stephens, JD; Jonathan Terdiman, MD; Martha Turchyn, MD; and Tracey Wallen-Ortiz.

Over 40 people graciously volunteered to share their personal stories regarding IBD. Some of these people have been my IBD buddies for many years, and others are now new friends. I enjoyed talking to each and every one of you. Your stories moved my heart, and they will move the hearts of the many, many people with IBD who read this book. Thanks so much to the following people: Ernestine Bach, Tami Blaj, Stephanie Chipman, Barbara De Marco, Carrie Emerson-Price, Sirarpi Feredjian-Aivazian, Carol Ford, Kim Gallaway, Sheila Gustaveson, Patty Haykin, Heather, Marjorie M. Helm, Diana Hendin, John Huffman, Jill Irwin, Jenny, Indu Johal, Joanne M. Klotz, Pamela C. Lee, Nancy Lisser, Rebekah Lucier, Russ Lucier, Samantha Lucier, Tom Manley, Connie McLennan, Thomas McLennan, Martha M. Moon, Ernie Moor, Donald Palmer, MD, FACS, Carolyn Paredes, Alissa Picker, Janet Rao, Breda Rolle, Marta Rottman, Arlyn Serber, Lisa Smythe, Joella Trupin, Cynthia Aleene Van Lammeren, Byron O. Young, and those who wish to remain anonymous.

Another thanks to Nancy Keene. One story in Chapter 9, *Working with Your Doctor,* was taken from her book, *Working with Your Doctor: Getting the Healthcare You Deserve* (O'Reilly & Associates, 1998). In addition, some material from Chapter 15, *Children and Teens,* and Chapter 17, *Emotions and Coping,* was adapted from her book, *Childhood Leukemia: A Guide for Families, Friends, and Caregivers* (O'Reilly & Associates, 2002). Lastly, thanks to the authors of *Childhood Cancer Survivors: A Practical Guide to Your Future* (O'Reilly & Associates, 2000)—Nancy Keene, Wendy Hobbie, and Kathy Ruccione. Some material from Chapter 16, *Record-Keeping, Insurance, Employment, and Disability* was adapted from their text.

—Cliff Kalibjian

CHAPTER 1

Introduction to IBD

INFLAMMATORY BOWEL DISEASE (IBD) is a general term used to describe chronic inflammation (consisting of redness, swelling, and ulceration) in the digestive tract. The two major forms of IBD, Crohn's disease and ulcerative colitis, are generally characterized by pain, diarrhea, bleeding, fatigue, and weight loss. IBD has a wide range of severity, with some cases quite mild and others very disabling. Although theories abound, no one knows the cause of IBD. And worse, no one knows its cure.

This chapter provides you with important background information on IBD. It begins with a section that describes the normal function and structure of the digestive tract. It then takes a brief look at Crohn's disease and ulcerative colitis and explains how these conditions differ. Next it describes the history of IBD, who gets it, and where it occurs around the world. Finally, it discusses various theories about what causes IBD.

The normal digestive tract

The digestive tract, also known as either the alimentary or gastrointestinal (GI) tract, extends from mouth to anus. The term "gut" is also used to describe this hollow tube that runs from one end of your body to the other. The major purpose of the GI tract is to break down food into small, simple components. Portions of the digested food are then absorbed into your bloodstream, providing the materials and energy your body needs to live and function properly.

Although they're not part of the GI tract, other organs such as the liver and pancreas are part of the body's digestive system. The liver contributes a product called bile that aids in the digestion of fats. The pancreas produces a variety of digestive enzymes that help break down complex food components into simpler ones.

Digestion begins in the mouth. Your teeth mechanically grind your food into small pieces while chemicals in your saliva begin the breakdown of starches (breads, cereals) into sugars. After swallowing, the food goes down your esophagus—the tube that connects your mouth to your stomach.

When the food reaches your stomach, strong acids help reduce the level of harmful bacteria, as well as begin the breakdown of protein foods (meat, eggs) into smaller parts. The muscles in the stomach churn the food until it turns into a soft pulp.

The semidigested food then moves into the small intestine, also known as the small bowel. The small intestine, coiled in the center of your abdomen, is about 20 feet long. This is where digestion of carbohydrates, fats, and proteins is completed. Nutrients are absorbed by the cells that line the small bowel, passed into small blood vessels, and then carried to the rest of the body.

The three parts of the small intestine are the duodenum, jejunum, and the ileum. Digestive fluids from the pancreas and liver empty into the first part of the small intestine, the 10-inch-long duodenum. The 10-foot long jejunum, the middle section, is where the absorption of most nutrients takes place. The ileum—also about 10 feet long—is responsible for the absorption of bile salts and vitamin B_{12}.

What the body can't digest or absorb in the small intestine moves on to the large intestine, also known as the colon. It is about 4 to 5 feet long and significantly wider than the small intestine. Virtually no digestion takes place in the colon, but absorption of water and certain minerals, such as sodium, occur here. The colon also stores food waste products until you eliminate them through your anus.

The colon is divided into different segments. The first part is the cecum, a 2.5-inch-long cul-de-sac that is found below the end of the ileum. The next part of the large intestine is called the ascending colon, because it extends upward on the right side of the abdomen. The transverse colon is the next piece that, after making a 90-degree turn from the ascending colon, extends across the abdomen, just below the rib cage. The following section is called the descending colon, because it courses down the left side of the abdomen. Next comes the sigmoid colon, named after its S-shape. Last comes the rectum, which is the holding area for stool at the end of your colon. When it fills up, you become aware of the need to eliminate.

Crohn's disease at a glance

Crohn's disease is a chronic disorder of the GI tract that is usually diagnosed in children and young adults, although it can develop at any age. It's typically characterized by abdominal pain, diarrhea, fever, fatigue, and weight loss. Crohn's can occur anywhere in the GI tract from mouth to anus, but inflammation is usually found in the small intestine and/or large intestine.

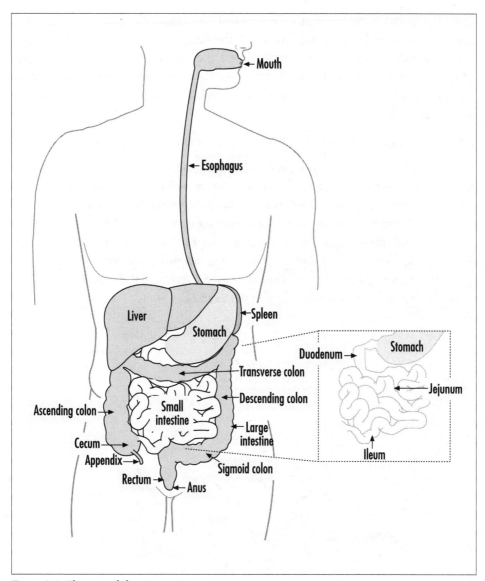

Figure 1-1. The normal digestive tract

One major hallmark of Crohn's is that inflammation can occur in segments throughout the GI tract. Inflamed areas of intestine often have areas of healthy tissue between them. Crohn's disease affects all three layers of the bowel, which include the mucosa (innermost lining), the muscular layers, and the serosa (outermost layer).

Crohn's is occasionally referred to as regional enteritis (inflammation of the small intestine) or regional ileitis (inflammation of the ileum). Other terms used to describe Crohn's reflect the area of the GI tract where the disease is present. For example, Crohn's colitis is Crohn's disease that only occurs in the colon. The most common type of Crohn's is sometimes called ileocecal Crohn's, because the ileum and cecum are the areas affected.

Jamie, now 41 years old, describes her early experience with Crohn's disease:

> I had been experiencing painful cramping, diarrhea, fevers, and even blood in my stool for about two years before my diagnosis of Crohn's at age 30. My inflammation was fairly typical in that I had it in the end of small intestine and beginning of my colon. When I was finally diagnosed, I was rather shocked that I had a chronic illness. I had never heard of Crohn's. I was hoping that once we knew what was wrong with me, I could just have some surgery and it would be over. But such is not the case with this disease.

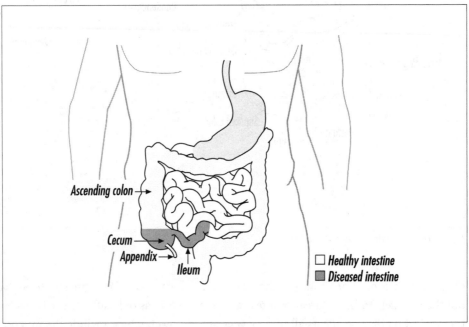

Figure 1-2. Ileocecal Crohn's disease

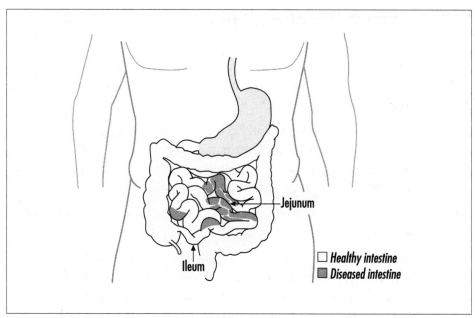

Figure 1-3. Small-bowel Crohn's disease

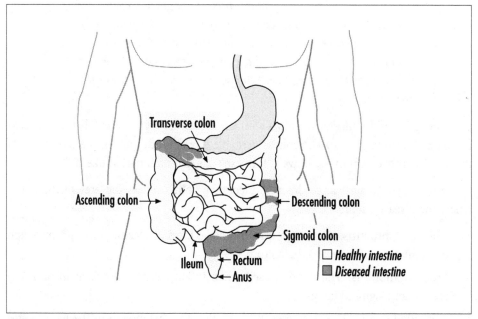

Figure 1-4. Crohn's colitis

Ulcerative colitis at a glance

Ulcerative colitis occurs only in the colon. As its name accurately describes, the disease involves colitis (inflammation in the colon) that is ulcerated (like a sore). Like Crohn's, it's generally a disease of children and young adults. People often experience abdominal pain, fatigue, weight loss, and bloody diarrhea.

Unlike Crohn's, ulcerative colitis only affects the innermost lining of the large intestine. Because its inflammation occurs in a continuous stretch, there are no segments of healthy intestine between inflamed areas. Inflammation is generally present in the rectal area and spreads upward toward the small intestine.

Carla, who's had ulcerative colitis for over 30 years, describes her experience when she was diagnosed as a teenager:

> *My ulcerative colitis began quite suddenly at the age of 14. Within one or two weeks, I literally went from a healthy girl having one or two bowel movements a day to a very sick, dehydrated girl having bloody diarrhea ten to fourteen times a day. I wound up in the hospital, and they were immediately able to diagnose my problem as ulcerative colitis. I saved my records from my original diagnosis and they say that my inflammation was in my rectum and spread up my colon about fourteen centimeters. That doesn't seem like much inflammation, but it sure caused a lot of problems and really wiped me out. I don't even remember being scared at the time—I was just too weak to care.*

Some people confuse ulcerative colitis with irritable bowel syndrome (also called spastic colon or, erroneously, spastic colitis). Irritable bowel syndrome (IBS) is a disorder of the physical movement of the bowels. It doesn't cause inflammation like IBD.

Other terms you may hear to describe ulcerative colitis reflect the area of the colon where the disease occurs.

- **Ulcerative proctitis.** This is the least extensive form of ulcerative colitis, in which inflammation is limited to the rectum.

- **Proctosigmoiditis.** This term is used when inflammation is present in both the rectum and sigmoid colon.

- **Left-sided colitis.** This describes inflammation that extends from the rectum and then up the entire left side of the colon. It stops at the beginning of the transverse colon.

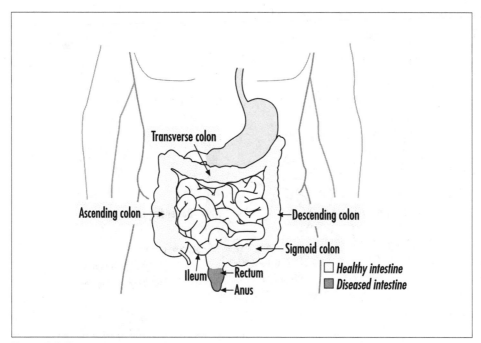

Figure 1-5. Proctitis

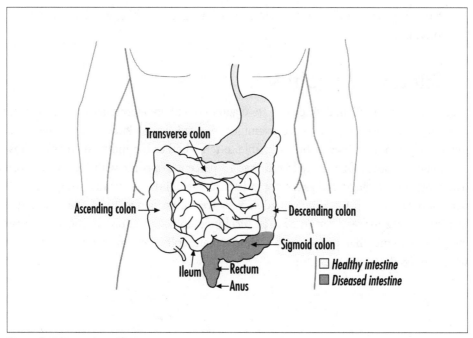

Figure 1-6. Proctosigmoiditis

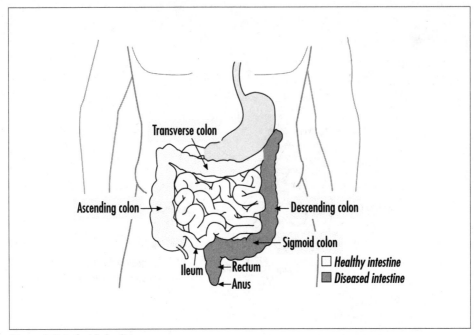

Figure 1-7. Left-sided colitis

- Pancolitis. This is the most severe form of ulcerative colitis, in which the entire colon is inflamed.

Indeterminate colitis

Some people with IBD in their colons are diagnosed with indeterminate colitis. In these cases, a pathologist (a doctor who examines diseased tissue) knows the diagnosis is inflammatory bowel disease, but is unable to tell whether the individual has Crohn's or ulcerative colitis. One study found that 13 percent of people with IBD who never had surgery were diagnosed as having indeterminate colitis.[1] The same study found 4 percent of those with IBD who've had surgery were classified as such. Over time, the disease usually makes itself known as ulcerative colitis or Crohn's. The study just mentioned found that people with indeterminate colitis are most often diagnosed with Crohn's disease in the future.

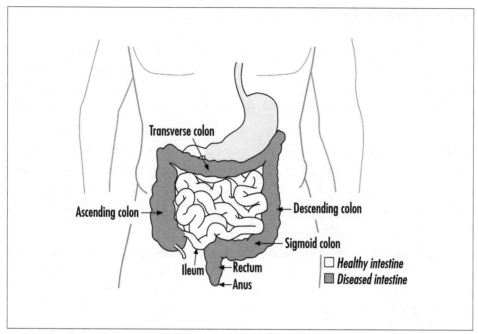

Figure 1-8. Pancolitis

The history of IBD

Reports of illnesses involving bowel problems with symptoms similar to IBD (such as diarrhea with or without blood) can be traced back thousands of years.[2] However, not until the second half of the nineteenth century did inflammation in either the colon or small intestine attract any serious attention. There are at least two reasons why this is so. First, because diagnostic technologies were limited, not until this point in history could these kinds of diseases be differentiated from other illnesses. Second, it's also possible that, for whatever reason, IBD was uncommon before this time.

The term "ulcerative colitis" has been used since 1888. The name Crohn became associated with regional ileitis because of a paper Burrill Crohn published with two other colleagues in 1932 (although other researchers had described the syndrome earlier). Until 1959, Crohn's disease was thought to occur only in the small intestine, and the notion of Crohn's in the colon was not accepted in the United States until the mid-1960s.

Who gets IBD

Epidemiology is the study of the "who" and "where" of a particular disease. Epidemiologists look at what kinds of risk factors are common to the people who develop certain disorders. For example, when researchers are studying an illness, they consider factors such as age, gender, genes, socioeconomic status, race, occupation, diet, lifestyle, and geographic residence.

Epidemiologists also examine what may cause a disease and how to prevent it. A clear example is black lung disease. The only people who get this disease are those who were exposed to coal dust while working in coal mines for many years. Thus, epidemiologists can have a high degree of certainty about what causes this disease, because it only affects a specific population.

IBD presents a much more challenging case for epidemiologists, because few known risk factors are directly linked to it, nor is there a specific group of people who always (or almost always) develop it. To make matters even more complicated, the following features of IBD make epidemiologic studies very difficult.

- IBD is not a disease that doctors are required to report to any governmental agency, so the true number of those affected is unknown.
- IBD frequently has a gradual onset, and making a diagnosis sometimes takes months or even years. Thus, environmental causes are hard to pinpoint.
- IBD is often challenging to diagnose. Doctors sometimes have difficulty distinguishing between Crohn's and ulcerative colitis, and between IBD and other intestinal disorders.

Fortunately, research on the epidemiology of IBD has provided clues to help people understand the mystery of Crohn's disease and ulcerative colitis.

IBD in the United States

No one really knows the exact number of people with IBD, especially in countries such as the United States, where detailed medical records are not kept in one centralized location for epidemiologists to study. In the United States, statistical data on people with IBD are mostly based on information provided from hospitals. The problem is that many people with IBD are never hospitalized, and they simply seek treatment from their physician on an outpatient basis. These people are not officially counted, because Crohn's and ulcerative colitis are not diseases that doctors are required to report to any government agency.

The Crohn's and Colitis Foundation of America (CCFA) currently estimates that there are about 1 million Americans with IBD, half with Crohn's and half with ulcerative colitis.[3] In addition, the National Institute of Diabetes, Digestive, and Kidney Diseases (NIDDK), a division of the National Institutes of Health (NIH), estimated in 1987 that the number of individuals afflicted with IBD in the United States was somewhere between 300,000 and 500,000, resulting in approximately 100,000 hospitalizations that year (64 percent of them for Crohn's).[4]

IBD in other parts of the world

The geography of IBD is fascinating, because it occurs mostly in the developed world. The highest rates are found in North America (except Central America), northern Europe (including Great Britain), and Israel.

Moderate rates of IBD occur in central and southern Europe, South Africa, and Australia, whereas in most of South America, most of Africa, and Asia, IBD appears to be quite rare.[5] Exceptions in Asia are Japan and South Korea, where the rate of new cases, particularly of ulcerative colitis, has increased in recent years.[6,7]

The spread of IBD

Some researchers are concerned about how the rate of new cases of IBD has changed over time. For example, in one major long-term study conducted in the United States, researchers found that the rate of new cases of both Crohn's and ulcerative colitis steadily increased from the 1940s through the 1970s, but then stabilized. However, they found that the total number of Crohn's cases has been increasing faster than the total number of ulcerative colitis ones.[8,9] Indeed, the general consensus is that although rates of ulcerative colitis have stabilized, rates of Crohn's are still increasing.[10]

As for other parts of the world, one study from Israel found that the total number of Crohn's cases more than doubled from 1987 to 1997, prompting the researchers to conclude that rates there are approaching those of Europe and North America.[11] And in Japan, although the number of new cases is still relatively low, the rate has increased greatly over the past 25 years compared to Western countries.[12]

Other epidemiological data on IBD

Epidemiologists study more than just the numbers of people and where they live. The following sections take a brief look at some of the other factors that may be associated with IBD.

Age

Both forms of IBD are chronic diseases of young adults, because most cases are diagnosed when people are in their teens or twenties. However, some studies have found that after a drop in new cases from about age 25 to 50, a second but smaller peak occurs between the ages of 50 and 80 for either one or both forms of IBD.[13]

The following is the experience of David, who was diagnosed with Crohn's in his 50s:

> I'm one of those people who was diagnosed at an older age. I didn't get Crohn's till I was 51. Since most of the information I read at the time said that it was a disease of young people, I wondered why I would develop it at my age. It was especially surprising since I was previously in great shape and the picture of health—I was a marathon runner! I remember reading one thing that said if IBD is diagnosed in older people that it tends to be milder. Nothing could be further than the truth in my case. I had one of the most severe cases that my doctor ever saw. Fortunately, I'm doing much better now. But even now when certain problems develop, it's hard to know whether it's the Crohn's causing the problem, or just old age.

Sex

The general consensus is that there are no major sex-related differences when it comes to having IBD. Some researchers, however, have reported that women may have a somewhat greater risk of developing Crohn's, whereas men may have a slightly increased chance of getting ulcerative colitis.[14]

Race/Ethnicity

Because IBD is found mostly in North America and Europe, it seems natural to assume that Caucasians would have the highest rates of Crohn's and ulcerative colitis. However, studies examining IBD among ethnic groups in the United States have revealed some interesting findings. These studies have found that African-Americans and Caucasians have about the same annual hospitalization rates and rates of newly diagnosed cases per year.[15,16] However, when looking at the total number of cases in both groups (not just new cases), the proportion of Caucasians with IBD is still about 1.5 times that of African-Americans with IBD.[17]

Also of interest from these studies is that Asians and Hispanics were found to have very low rates of IBD (for hospitalization, new cases per year, and total number of cases).

Sarah, a woman of Indian descent who has lived most of her life in England and the Unites States, shares her experience of IBD:

> I've had Crohn's since I was a young teen. Over the first twenty years, I maybe heard of a few other Indian people who had the disease. What's so strange is that in the last six months, I've come across four or five more. I don't know if it's really that more people of Indian descent are suddenly developing it. Perhaps before people didn't talk about it, but now they are. My family talks about Crohn's pretty openly. I often hear my mom telling others I have it and I am often asked to talk to others who have it, especially if they are newly diagnosed.

Research indicates that IBD is about three to five times more common in Jewish people than in non-Jews.[18] It also appears that Ashkenazi Jews (those from central and eastern Europe and their descendants) are at higher risk than other Jewish people. However, rates of IBD in Ashkenazi Jews vary depending on where they live. Those who live in the United States and northern Europe have higher rates than those living in Israel, suggesting that environmental factors may play a role in the development of the disease.

The following is Jamie's reaction to hearing that IBD was more common among people of her ancestry:

> As a Jewish woman, I was surprised to hear that IBD is so many times more common in Ashkenazi Jews. Before I had Crohn's, I had never even heard of the disease—and I certainly had known many Jewish people. But since I've been diagnosed, I'm running into people with Crohn's and ulcerative colitis all over the place—including many Jews. It's funny how that works.

Geography

Interestingly, geographic latitude may have an influence on the risk of developing IBD. One group of researchers reported that both ulcerative colitis and Crohn's disease are more common in northern parts of the United States than in southern areas.[19] Another study found similar findings in Europe: Rates of ulcerative colitis were 40 percent higher in the northern portions of Europe than the southern areas, whereas rates of Crohn's disease were 80 percent higher in the more northerly latitudes.[20]

Smoking

The relationship between cigarette smoking and IBD is very puzzling. Research suggests that smoking may protect people from developing ulcerative colitis but may increase one's chances of developing Crohn's.[21] Another interesting finding is that ex-smokers are about 1.7 times more likely to develop ulcerative colitis than those who have never smoked.[22]

Ellen, who was diagnosed with ulcerative colitis at almost age 50, describes how she developed the disease after she kicked the smoking habit:

> I quit smoking in 1979, and was diagnosed with ulcerative colitis in 1981. I actually began developing symptoms even sooner—so it probably started around a year after I quit. I had never heard of any connection between smoking and ulcerative colitis until recently. It was certainly surprising to hear that smoking may help ulcerative colitis—I suppose that was about the only thing it was good for. But there really must have been some connection in my case since it did develop so soon after I had stopped.

No one should ever start or resume smoking to treat his ulcerative colitis. The hazardous effects of smoking are well established, and they are the last thing that anyone—including people with ulcerative colitis—needs.

Causes of IBD

No one really knows what causes IBD. However, there is no shortage of theories on this topic. IBD is a complex disease that probably arises from a confluence of many different factors—there doesn't have to be just one cause. Although research on Crohn's disease and ulcerative colitis often gets lumped together, the causes of each are probably not identical, though you might expect at least some overlap. To complicate the issue even further, it's possible there may be different subtypes of both Crohn's and ulcerative colitis—and each subtype may result from different combinations of various factors. What follows is a brief and basic description of some of the most popular thinking on the causes of IBD.

Genetics

Evidence of a genetic factor in IBD is very convincing. Researchers have studied the rates of ulcerative colitis and Crohn's in identical and fraternal twins. One study found that if one identical twin developed Crohn's, the other twin developed the disease approximately 60 percent of the time.[23] But if one twin developed ulcerative colitis, the other one only came down with the disorder in about 20 percent of the cases. Among fraternal twins in this study, if one twin had Crohn's, the other twin never developed the illness. Yet with ulcerative colitis, both twins developed the disease in about 5 percent of cases. These data strongly suggest a genetic factor in IBD, with hereditary factors playing a stronger role in Crohn's than in ulcerative colitis.

Research on families also suggests a hereditary component to IBD. Although it's rare for both a husband and wife to have it, about 5 to 10 percent of people with IBD have a first-degree relative (sibling, parent, or child) with either ulcerative colitis or Crohn's.[24]

IBD runs in Susie's family:

> I was diagnosed with ulcerative colitis almost fifteen years ago, but have probably had it for about twenty. I was familiar with IBD because my dad had Crohn's disease. I don't think it affected me too much growing up. It was just part of our family life and I dealt with it.
>
> However, as a mother with IBD, I do worry about its effect on my children. What's worse is that I worry that I may have passed this on to my children. I know any time my daughter has diarrhea, a part of me gets scared. Of course it's not unusual for kids to have diarrhea from time to time. But it's hard not to be concerned when IBD runs in your family.

Unlike some traits (such as blood type) or illnesses (such as sickle cell anemia) that have a simple pattern of inheritance, the genetics of IBD are much more complicated. Currently, researchers are working to better understand the genetics behind IBD. They presently think that certain areas of chromosomes 6, 12, 14, and 16 are strongly associated with susceptibility to IBD.[25] Indeed, in 2001 researchers discovered a specific defect in a gene called NOD2 (also known as CARD15), which is located on chromosome 16. This defect occurs twice as frequently in people with Crohn's than those without the disease.[26]

Infectious

Although no definitive microbe has been identified as a cause of IBD, some researchers theorize that certain types of bacteria may play at least some role in precipitating the disease.

More evidence exists linking an infectious cause to Crohn's than to ulcerative colitis. For example, Crohn's very closely resembles intestinal tuberculosis as well as another bacterial illness called Johne's disease (found in ruminants such as cattle). Interestingly, the same bacterium that causes Johne's disease in cattle—*Mycobacterium paratuberculosis*—has occasionally been identified in some people with Crohn's disease. However, this bacterium is not found in all people with Crohn's, and it is also found in those without the disease. Nevertheless, some researchers report that genetic material from this bacterium has been found in the tissues of a higher proportion of Crohn's patients than in those who don't have the illness.[27] Another piece of evidence supporting this link is that drugs that kill this particular strain of bacteria have occasionally shown some promising results in people with Crohn's.[28] However, the results of studies haven't been consistent. *Mycobacterium paratuberculosis'* role in causing Crohn's is thus a controversial subject. Currently, most IBD experts don't feel it plays a significant role—if any—in the development of Crohn's.

Some researchers have suggested that Crohn's may be due in part to the measles virus, especially if exposure occurs in utero or early in life. One study, for example, found that people born during measles epidemics had significantly higher rates of Crohn's.[29] Other groups of researchers, however, have not found an IBD–measles link.[30] Today, most leading experts do not believe there is a connection between IBD and measles.

The immune system

The immune system is believed to play a critical role in both Crohn's disease and ulcerative colitis. Many researchers believe IBD is a result of an abnormal immune response in people genetically predisposed toward the disease to something in the environment that's normally harmless. Scientists studying IBD have suggested that bacteria in the intestine are likely culprits. This is currently the major, prevailing theory as to what causes IBD, as data from experimental research strongly support this hypothesis.

Why would people with IBD have an abnormal immune response to bacteria present in the bowel? No one knows for sure, but it could have something to do with a leaky gut. Some researchers believe that people with Crohn's may have a defective intestinal barrier that makes the bowel more permeable (things can pass through more easily) to foreign substances. Thus, bacteria and toxins that are normally kept away can penetrate into intestinal tissue, activating an inflammatory response.[31] In fact, another study found that intestinal permeability was the best predictor of relapse in people with Crohn's.[32]

Some scientists studying IBD hypothesize that ulcerative colitis and Crohn's are autoimmune diseases, meaning that the immune system attacks part of the body (in this case, the intestine) as if it were foreign tissue. In this process, the body forms antibodies against itself, much like it would form them against bacteria or viruses if they were invading the body. Some evidence suggests that autoimmunity is a more significant factor in ulcerative colitis than in Crohn's.[33] However, other researchers have not found any indication that IBD—either ulcerative colitis or Crohn's—is an autoimmune disorder.[34] Most researchers today agree that Crohn's and colitis are probably not autoimmune diseases. Future research will eventually clarify in more detail the relationship between the immune system and IBD.

Psychosomatic

The term "psychosomatic" has almost become a dirty word in some circles, because some people take it to mean that a disease is "just" in one's mind or "only" caused by emotional distress. Understandably, calling ulcerative colitis or Crohn's disease a psychosomatic illness might anger a person with IBD if he were using this definition. Crohn's disease and ulcerative colitis are real diseases that are in people's gastrointestinal tracts, not their minds. The inflammation is there, and the pathology is real.

Researchers today do not believe emotional factors cause Crohn's disease or ulcerative colitis. People with IBD living before the 1960s, however, were not so fortunate. Prior to this time, the predominating view was that IBD—particularly ulcerative colitis—was a psychosomatic illness. Unfortunately, it was during this time that the term "psychosomatic" earned its bad reputation, because it implied an illness was caused either by dysfunctional personality or by mental conflicts.

No evidence links developing ulcerative colitis or Crohn's to emotional or psychological states. Research has not ruled out emotional stress as playing at least some role in the exacerbation of IBD in people who already have it. However, as pointed out by some researchers, most studies finding an association between psychiatric factors and IBD have serious flaws in their research design.[35] IBD itself is a major stressor. Thus, it wouldn't be surprising to find those affected with the disorder are more stressed and anxious when compared with the general population.

Marcy, who's been dealing with IBD for over twenty years, shares her opinions on the connection between stress and her disease:

> When I was first diagnosed, my doctor told me that stress had
> nothing to do with my illness. In my case, I don't think stress caused
> my Crohn's, but I have certainly seen over the years how stress can

aggravate it. For me, it's only been certain kinds of stress—namely
work-related—that have caused me problems. When I took on a
stressful job, I had quite an active case for as long as I held that
position—seven years. When I finally retired, within six months, I got
everything back under control. For whatever reason, family stress has
never affected my Crohn's. I'd also agree that the disease itself, in
addition to people not understanding it, caused a lot of stress in my
life as well. But when it came to exacerbating my disease, I know my
job-related stress was always a factor. During my five years of
retirement I've remained prednisone free.

For a more information on the emotional factors associated with IBD and how to effectively deal with them, see Chapter 17, *Emotions and Coping.*

Diet

It would seem reasonable to think that a disease of the gastrointestinal tract might have something to do with the food put into it. Indeed, some researchers suggest that the differences in rates of IBD around the world, and the increased rates in people who have moved to Westernized countries from areas where IBD is rare, could be accounted for by diet.[36]

So, does a Western diet of refined carbohydrates (white flour, white sugar) and processed fats (hydrogenated oils) cause IBD? Or does diet not make any difference in the development of Crohn's and ulcerative colitis? The honest answer is that there isn't conclusive proof for either position. One major problem is that studies on diet are very difficult to conduct. First of all, people are sometimes not able to recall with great accuracy what they ate months or years before their diagnosis. Another issue is determining at what point the pre-illness diet is important. The onset of IBD is often gradual, so would you need to look back several years? Or just to the period before diagnosis? Or as far back as when a person was a small child? No one knows, yet this is probably important, because people's diets may change over time. Lastly, a person often self-treats before diagnosis by either avoiding certain foods or consuming more of others in an effort to control symptoms. Thus, just because consumption of certain foods is associated with IBD doesn't mean they cause the disease—they can just as easily be a result of it. Hopefully, researchers will design better studies to properly ascertain what role diet plays in the development of IBD.

People with IBD can have a difficult time trying to figure out what's best for them to eat, as explained by Marcy, who's had Crohn's in her colon for many years:

> I really haven't been able to correlate what I eat to the flaring of my disease. With the exception of foods such as popcorn and nuts that do irritate my colon, everything else seems to agree with me. Of course, during a severe flare-up, just about anything causes diarrhea. But for the most part, I tolerate most foods. In the past, people have told me to avoid dairy products but they agree with me just fine. I also have no problems with most fruits or vegetables. I guess the right diet just depends upon the individual.

For information on how diet can affect IBD, see Chapter 7, *Diet and Complementary Therapies*.

Some of the factors listed earlier may play at least some role in the development of IBD, but there may be other factors, too, that no one has yet discovered. Much more work needs to be done to unravel the mystery of IBD. Fortunately, research on Crohn's disease and ulcerative colitis continues to progress.

Craig, who developed IBD about twenty years ago, sums up why he thinks he got the disease:

> I really don't know why I developed IBD. However, I suspect that it probably wasn't just one thing. I obviously had some sort of genetic predisposition to it or else I wouldn't have developed it at all. One doctor said it could have been triggered by some bacteria or virus to which my immune system—for some reason—had a bad reaction. I don't know if it was a coincidence, but there was a lot of stress going on in my life at and before the time of my diagnosis. Also, my diet wasn't too good either at that point in my life. In retrospect, I suspect these factors may have played a role in weakening my immune system, and maybe that's partly why its reaction to the bacteria or virus got out of control. At that point, I guess the inflammatory reaction took on a life of its own, which then led to my developing IBD. I know there's no way I can prove this, but it's just my own theory. It seems like people think it has to be one thing that causes it, but I believe many factors came together to produce IBD in my body.

CHAPTER 2

Signs and Symptoms

DOCTORS USE SIGNS AND SYMPTOMS to help diagnose disease and to evaluate how well treatments are working. A sign is something you or your physician can objectively observe. For example, a sign of IBD is the presence of blood in the stool, because it is either seen by the eye or revealed by a test. A symptom is something you subjectively experience. A common symptom of IBD, for instance, is pain in the abdominal area. It's something only you feel and no one else can objectively measure.

This chapter begins by examining the pathology of ulcerative colitis and Crohn's disease. Next it shows how the structural changes associated with IBD result in the digestive dysfunction that people with Crohn's and colitis know all too well. It then describes the signs and symptoms of both diseases and how they impact people's lives.

The pathology of IBD

The term "pathology" refers to the structural and functional changes that a disease can cause. IBD involves inflammation in the GI tract that alters both the structure and function of the bowel. However, the pathologies of Crohn's disease and ulcerative colitis are different.

Structural changes in ulcerative colitis

Ulcerative colitis almost always involves inflammation in the rectum. Depending on the extent of the disease, inflammation spreads in an uninterrupted pattern toward the small bowel.

Inflammation is confined to the innermost layer (the mucosa) of the colon. The lining of the mucosa is ulcerated and often swollen, with sores that frequently leak blood and pus. Crypt abscesses, another characteristic feature of ulcerative colitis, are pit-like depressions in the mucosa that are filled with pus. Over time, inflammation can wear away portions of the inner lining of the bowel. The result is the development of pseudopolyps, which are islands of relatively normal intestinal lining that stand out around the surrounding, worn-away mucosa.

Structural changes in Crohn's disease

Crohn's disease can occur anywhere in the GI tract. Approximately half of the people with Crohn's have it in both the small and large intestine. About 25 percent of affected people have it only in the small bowel, and 20 percent have it only their colon. A small number of people may develop the disease in the upper GI tract, such as in their esophagus or stomach, but this is rare.

Crohn's inflammation penetrates through the entire thickness of the bowel. As a result, deep ulcers (beyond the mucosal layer) may form. The bowel can also thicken and swell, causing the lumen (the hollow space where intestinal contents pass) to narrow, particularly in the small intestine. The combination of a swollen intestinal lining and deep ulcers results in a cobblestone appearance that is characteristic of Crohn's. In addition, because inflammation literally eats away through all layers of the bowel, fistulas—tubelike connections between the intestine and other organs— are much more likely to form.

Crohn's disease sometimes involves inflammation of the rectal area. It presents in a patchy pattern: Diseased areas of the gut are interspersed with healthy segments. Crypt abscesses can occur but are not as common as in ulcerative colitis. Instead, a more characteristic feature of Crohn's is the presence of granulomas, distinctive-looking collections of specific types of inflammatory cells. Approximately half of people with Crohn's develop granulomas.

Functional changes in ulcerative colitis

The pathological features just mentioned describe some of the structural changes that occur in the gut as IBD and its associated inflammation develop. As these structural changes in the bowel occur, proper functioning of the intestine is affected. In ulcerative colitis, for example, the inflamed mucosa prevents the colon from properly absorbing fluids. This can result in diarrhea. In addition, when an abundance of unabsorbed fluids reaches an inflamed rectal area, urgent need to defecate can result as well. Prolonged inflammation can also cause increased peristaltic contractions (muscular movements that push contents through the GI tract) in the colon. These are often experienced as pain and cramping.

Functional changes in Crohn's disease

The structural changes that occur in Crohn's disease also alter function. For instance, if swelling of the small intestine narrows the lumen, partially digested food may have a difficult time passing through the bowel. This in turn can lead to bloating, pain, nausea, and vomiting. Also, if certain areas of the small intestine are inflamed, the bowel cannot perform its normal job of absorbing nutrients into the bloodstream. If the inflammation persists, malnutrition can result. Lastly, if a fistula forms between the bowel and another organ, such as the bladder or vagina, normal body functions can be seriously affected. For more information on fistulas, see Chapter 4, *Complications*.

Signs and symptoms of ulcerative colitis

The signs and symptoms of ulcerative colitis vary depending on the location and severity of the inflammation. For example, people with just a few centimeters of mild inflammation in their rectums (proctitis) do not have the same experience as those with severe pancolitis (total colon involvement).

The following sections describe the most common signs and symptoms associated with ulcerative colitis.

Diarrhea

Diarrhea is probably the most common symptom experienced by people with ulcerative colitis. If the colonic mucosa is inflamed, the colon often cannot properly reabsorb fluids back into the rest of the body. Because the disease process can also throw the normal peristaltic contractions (referring to the wavelike motions that propel intestinal contents through the gut) out of whack, it's not surprising that people with ulcerative colitis often develop diarrhea.

Denise, who's had ulcerative colitis for several years, shares how chronic diarrhea has affected her life:

> *I have had to deal with diarrhea throughout the course of my illness. Perhaps the worst time though was a six-week period when I was first diagnosed. I was going to the bathroom ten, fifteen, even twenty times a day. I could have just stayed in the bathroom all day long. The biggest problem for me was dealing with the lack of control in my life. How could I ever plan or commit to things if I couldn't control the diarrhea? It was scary. Fortunately for me, even though I still have the disease and sometimes have to deal with diarrhea, it hasn't ever been as bad as it was during those six weeks. My fears have lessened over time, but it's something I still think about.*

Constipation

People with ulcerative colitis sometimes develop constipation, especially if inflammation is limited to the anal area. Because the rest of the colon is functioning normally, the stool is not watery as it approaches the end of the GI tract. Although there is generally no blockage, the inflammation in the anal region makes it difficult for the stool to pass out of the body. Thus, the stool can back up above the anus, and constipation can result.

In some cases, people may experience both diarrhea and constipation. It sounds paradoxical, but if only the anal/rectal area is inflamed an individual may experience frequent, low-volume stools (sometimes consisting of mostly blood and pus) that can be perceived as diarrhea. Yet if a large volume of stool is backed up higher in the colon, the person may also feel constipated.

Anemia

Anemia is a condition in which the blood's ability to deliver oxygen around the body is impaired, usually by a reduced number of red blood cells. Red blood cells are made in the bone marrow and generally live for about 120 days. They contain hemoglobin, which carries oxygen to your body's cells. Hemoglobin contains an iron atom, which easily bonds to oxygen from the air you breathe. As it flows through the bloodstream, hemoglobin delivers the oxygen to other cells of your body so they can perform their normal tasks.

In people with ulcerative colitis, anemia is usually caused by a bleeding colon. When the mucosal layer of the colon is inflamed, sores on its surface tend to ooze both blood and pus. When the stool passes through the colon, blood and pus can easily rub off on or mix with the feces. If the inflammation is in the rectal area, it's not uncommon to see bright red blood in the toilet after defecation. If the worst inflammation is present further up the colon, the blood is not generally as noticeable. In either case, the blood loss can add up and lead to an increased heart rate, fatigue, shortness of breath, lightheadedness, and a pale complexion—all indications of anemia.

The bloody stools associated with ulcerative colitis often provoke fear and anxiety in some people. Denise describes her feelings when dealing with this problem:

> *I've experienced quite a bit of bleeding over the course of my*
> *ulcerative colitis. And it's not just when I have diarrhea. I'll often have*
> *blood even when my stools are otherwise regular and normally*

*formed. In the beginning, it was something that was very anxiety
provoking for me. The bright red blood in the toilet is something that
is very startling. In time, I've just sort of gotten used to it, but still,
there's always that fear in the back of your mind. I do make a point to
get my blood checked to make sure everything is okay. I've been lucky
that despite all the blood I see in my stool, I'm actually not anemic.*

Anemia can also result from the toxic effects of widespread, severe inflammation. Inflammatory cells produce chemicals that circulate around the body. If enough of these are present in the bloodstream, they can suppress the production of new red blood cells in the bone marrow. Because red blood cells only live for about 120 days, anemia can occur if inflammation is present for an extended period. Over time, the body can't produce enough new red blood cells to replace the ones that have naturally died off.

Urgency

Another common symptom of ulcerative colitis is a feeling of urgency to evacuate the bowels. This urgent feeling does not always indicate an upcoming bowel movement. Often it's a false urgency, meaning the person runs to the bathroom feeling he really needs to go, but then only eliminates a tiny amount of stool, some blood, some pus, and/or some "wet" gas. What makes this even more frustrating is that this kind of urgency is often painful, and the minor elimination often does not fully relieve the feeling of needing "to go." A term sometimes used for this painful, false urge phenomenon is "tenesmus." It's usually a result of severe inflammation and spasms in the rectum.

The number of runs a person makes to the bathroom each day is generally proportional to the severity of the disease. If you're going to the toilet ten or twenty times a day, you probably have severe inflammation in your colon. Fewer trips a day to the bathroom suggest milder disease, but a minority of people who have only four or five bowel movements a day can be quite ill. If you have urgency that wakes you up in the middle of the night, it's often another indicator of severe disease.

Carla, who's had ulcerative colitis since she was a young teenager, shares her experience:

*Urgency has always been a challenging problem during flares, but
like everything else in life, I've learned to deal with it. There are
simply times when I have very little time to get to the bathroom. On
more than one occasion I have had accidents, both at home and in*

public. After an incident at school one time, I was determined to carry on. So I went to the store and bought the largest size of overnight training pants for little kids. I'm a small woman, so they fit just right. I only had to wear them for a short time, but it was the perfect solution to get me through that difficult time. My colitis may derail me occasionally, but overall I don't let it interfere with what I want to do.

Pain and cramping

The pain and cramping associated with ulcerative colitis is often one of the most difficult symptoms. Typically, pain is felt in the lower left part of the abdomen. If the whole colon is inflamed, however, you can experience pain in almost any part of the abdominal area. Although the pain can be severe, it's generally not constant (except in extreme cases) and is usually relieved at least partially with bowel movements and/or the passing of gas.

Carla, who has dealt with ulcerative colitis for most of her life, has had varied experiences with pain:

> *I suppose I've been fortunate compared to others with ulcerative colitis. For most of the course of my illness, I never really experienced much in the way of pain, even when I had severe flares and hospitalizations. But this all changed recently. The pain with my last flare was just the worst thing this time. At times, I felt that there was nothing I could do other than to curl up in agony and pray for it to stop. I tried my best to breathe through it, but ultimately it required contacting my doctor so we could adjust my medications. As we got the disease under control, the pain gradually diminished. I'm happy to say that I'm pain-free today, but it was still a terrible thing to have to go through.*

Systemic issues

The signs and symptoms of ulcerative colitis are also sometimes systemic (affecting the whole body). Even if inflammation is localized, it can produce chemicals that enter the bloodstream and are then spread throughout the body. For example, fever is a natural result of inflammation, and most people experience the fatigue and malaise associated with it. Appetite may also be reduced—not only because of the inflammatory chemicals but because food itself may irritate the colon and further aggravate the inflammatory response. Less food means less energy—which means more fatigue and also weight loss. With one symptom leading to another, it's easy to see how the disease can quickly get out of control. Other systemic complications that can occur with ulcerative colitis are covered in Chapter 4. For more information on coping with the symptoms of ulcerative colitis, see Chapter 17, *Emotions and Coping*.

Signs and symptoms of Crohn's disease

Signs and symptoms of Crohn's vary depending on the severity of the disease, just as in ulcerative colitis. Moreover, Crohn's can occur in any part of the GI tract, and therefore signs and symptoms also vary based on what areas of the gastrointestinal tract are affected.

Diarrhea

Diarrhea is a common symptom in many people with Crohn's, except in cases where only the small bowel is involved. If the colon is unaffected, it can properly regulate the fluid content of the stool. In people with significant colonic inflammation, however, diarrhea is often just as severe as in those with ulcerative colitis.

Jamie, a 41-year-old with Crohn's, describes the difficulties she's faced with managing her diarrhea:

> *I've gone through a lot of toilet paper over the years thanks to my diarrhea. Probably the most difficult part is how inconvenient and embarrassing it can be. At work, it often occupies my thoughts. I try to not make it obvious that I'm going back and forth, but it's not always easy. I find myself asking, "How am I going to get to and from the bathroom this time without everyone noticing that I have to go again?"*

Constipation

Constipation is also a problem for some people with Crohn's disease. As with ulcerative colitis, if inflammation is most severe in the anal area—and the rest of the colon is mostly spared—stool can get backed up above the area because an inflamed anal region makes it difficult to eliminate the feces from the body. Individuals with Crohn's may also experience significant narrowing of the lumen (particularly in the small bowel) that can also slow down the passage of contents through the intestinal tract, thus contributing to constipation.

Craig, who had a severe case of Crohn's for many years, explains:

> I struggled with constipation in addition to diarrhea for a long time. For years, I'd often get some pretty bad inflammation in my rectal area. Although I'd run to the bathroom several times a day, I'd seldom pass any significant amount of stool. Instead, it would just be one of those "wet farts," as I call them. It was really frustrating, because I could feel how I was getting backed up and constipated; yet nothing would really come out. When this first happened, I found it strange that I could have constipation as a symptom of this disease. You usually only hear about the diarrhea. But my doctor said that it sometimes happens.

Anemia

Anemia, as discussed earlier in this chapter, is a condition in which the delivery of oxygen to your body's cells is insufficient. It's usually due to a reduced number of red blood cells in your bloodstream. Crohn's primarily causes anemia through an inflammatory process. As in ulcerative colitis, inflammatory cells created during Crohn's flares release chemicals that can suppress the bone marrow's production of new red blood cells. If inflammation persists for an extended period, the body can't create enough new red blood cells to replace ones that naturally die after their 120-day life span.

Anemia can also occur because of a bleeding bowel. Although bloody stools are not as common in Crohn's as in ulcerative colitis, they do happen. If you have Crohn's in the rectum or left side of the colon, bloody bowel movements often occur. Even if your inflammation is further up in your GI tract and you don't see blood in your stool, the bleeding may be occult (hidden).

Craig, who was diagnosed with Crohn's twenty years ago, explains how the blood loss associated with his disease affected him:

> I lost quite a bit of blood during the years my disease was so active. As a result, there were periods when my hemoglobin swung up and down quite dramatically. It would often fall quickly to 7 or 8, climb slowly back up to 14, and then fall again to 7. My doctor once commented that it was like watching the stock market!
>
> The resulting anemia was always difficult for me to deal with. It seems like I would spend so much time trying to get back into shape

when it was slowly moving up. Then, when it started dropping fast,
I would lose all my physical conditioning that I worked so hard for. I
experienced breathlessness, rapid heart rate, and fatigue with just the
simplest activities. It seemed so unfair. I would spend months
achieving a certain level of cardiovascular fitness, and then I could
lose it all in a matter of a week or two once I flared up and started
bleeding.

Urgency

Urgency is common in Crohn's disease but occurs less frequently than in ulcerative colitis. This is because a higher proportion of people with Crohn's don't have inflammation in the lower colon and rectal area. But for those who do, all the same information applies that was mentioned in the urgency section for ulcerative colitis, discussed earlier in this chapter.

Jamie, who has Crohn's in both her colon and small intestine, explains how this condition has affected her life:

> *I've had a few accidents over the years. Sometimes you just can't*
> *make it to the bathroom in time. Unfortunately, this makes it difficult*
> *when you want to plan things. I always have to be thinking, "Will*
> *there be a bathroom nearby?"*

Pain and cramping

Crohn's disease often causes two different types of pain. The first is similar to that experienced by those with ulcerative colitis. It's often described as a crampy type of discomfort. It can be mild or intense, depending on how inflamed the bowel is. If the intestine is severely diseased, it can go into spasms as a result of increased peristaltic contractions. This can leave a person in quite an uncomfortable situation. Fortunately, this type of pain is usually not constant and is at least somewhat relieved through bowel movements and the passing of gas. Because most people with Crohn's have inflammation in the ileocecal region, the most common area of pain is frequently in the lower right portion of the abdomen. However, pain can be felt any place in the abdominal region depending on where the disease strikes.

A second type of pain involves the narrowing of the lumen. This phenomenon is typical of small-bowel Crohn's. Normal peristaltic action tries to move intestinal contents, but only a portion can pass through a narrowed area, creating pressure. If a segment of small intestine is completely blocked, the pain becomes extremely sharp and excruciating. This type of pain can be relentless. It only passes once the blockage re-opens and pressure is relieved. If you experience such pain, it's best to get to the nearest emergency room right away.

Brenda, a mother of two young children, provides an interesting perspective on the pain of IBD:

> I've experienced terrible pain with my Crohn's. How terrible, you ask? I had both my children at home with no drugs, and that was literally a field day compared to my worst Crohn's pain. In a way, the pain is similar to labor, but what makes it so much worse is that there are no breaks—it's just like one long contraction.

Nausea and vomiting

Nausea and vomiting are significant problems for people with Crohn's, especially when partial or complete blockages occur in the small intestine. If GI contents are unable to pass through, the bowel moves them back toward the stomach. The stomach may then expel the partially digested food in order to relieve the pressure caused by the blockage, so the person vomits.

Brenda, who has Crohn's, tells how she was stricken with nausea while away from home:

> It's amazing how the body knows how to protect itself. Just before my surgery I was in Bali attending a wedding. I had difficulty eating anything on this trip. I thought there was some spice in all the food that didn't agree with me since it made me so nauseous that I could barely eat. However, when I asked other people if the spice bothered them, they said, "What spice? The food tastes fine." But it did not taste fine to me. When I got home, my doctor said that sometimes when you're so sick and your body knows it can't handle food, it will alter your taste buds such that the taste of food will make you nauseous and unable to eat.

Malabsorption

Malabsorption is often a significant problem for people with Crohn's in their small intestine. Inflammation can cause the small bowel to have difficulty absorbing nutrients into the bloodstream. Malnutrition can therefore result.

Brenda has had problems over the years digesting her food:

> *Although I wasn't tested for various nutrient deficiencies, I know I must have had some degree of malabsorption with my Crohn's. I knew this because food would just go right through my system very quickly. When it came to certain vegetables, it was especially obvious since their appearance didn't change much from the time they went in to when they came out! I'm sure I became deficient in many nutrients. But interestingly, the one test they did do was for vitamin B_{12}. And that test was normal.*

Systemic issues

Crohn's disease can also affect your body systemically. As inflammatory chemicals enter the bloodstream and permeate the body, fever, loss of appetite, and fatigue can occur. These in turn will lead to weight loss and even more fatigue.

Jamie, who was diagnosed with Crohn's at age 30, shares her feelings on how systemic symptoms affect her life:

> *Fevers, fatigue, weight loss—I have had them all. I'm not sure which comes first but they all seem to go together and feed upon each other. The fatigue has especially hit me hard. There are times when it's so extreme that it feels as though every cell and every fiber of my body is exhausted. I've had extended periods where I don't even have energy to walk my dogs. Instead, I have to get a friend or family member to come and walk them. The same goes for doing basic housework or yard work. Preparing meals is often difficult during these times, too, but it sometimes doesn't matter since even the thought of eating something is unappealing. When I'm recovering from a really bad flare-up, I've often had to rest after taking a shower. Fortunately, it's not like this all of the time, but when it is, it's really frustrating because you can't really get out and do the things you want to do.*
>
> *On another level, dealing with my Crohn's symptoms brings up issues for the bigger picture. I don't like to think that my Crohn's symptoms should control my life, but realistically, it forces me to think about bigger life choices. Should I have a family? How would this impact my children if I had them? On the one hand, it doesn't seem right that I should have to make these decisions based on this disease.*

Yet there's the physical reality that I deal with every day, and unfortunately I have limitations that come with it. I'm not saying I or anyone else with IBD should give up their dreams—not in the least! We can all still achieve and accomplish a lot. But IBD and its accompanying symptoms have made me take a good look on where I stand with major life choices.

CHAPTER 3

Diagnostic Procedures

A DIAGNOSIS IS SOMETIMES DESCRIBED AS the art of identifying a disease. Physicians identify illnesses by looking at signs and symptoms. If a person comes in and says she has abdominal pain and bloody diarrhea, these indications possibly suggest she has IBD. In almost all cases, however, what the individual feels and observes is not enough to make a diagnosis. To gather more information, medical tests are necessary.

Doctors have a number of tools available to diagnose Crohn's disease and ulcerative colitis. These same tools are also used after diagnosis to identify IBD flare-ups or to assess your condition between recurrences of your disease.

This chapter explains the process used to diagnose IBD. It covers blood and stool tests and then explains imaging and endoscopic examinations. Throughout the chapter, people with IBD share how they dealt with diagnostic tests and procedures.

Problems getting a diagnosis

Ulcerative colitis and Crohn's disease are sometimes difficult to diagnose. As a result, people may go months or years without knowing what they have. This usually happens when the symptoms of IBD are mistaken for those of other disorders. For instance, irritable bowel syndrome (IBS) is a bowel problem that can also bring about abdominal aches and diarrhea, but it doesn't cause inflammation as IBD does. At other times, women or their doctors may mistakenly assume that lower abdominal cramping is caused by a gynecological problem instead of IBD. Also, some healthcare providers tell symptomatic individuals that they're just under a lot of stress.

Gina explains what happened to her when she was in high school:

> *It took about two years for me to get a diagnosis. In high school,*
> *I started having pains in my abdomen that would come and go. After*
> *several more months, I began to experience nausea and vomiting.*
> *When I'd eat, it would frequently either hurt or come right back up.*
> *I started getting thin. My doctor told me that my condition was*

probably due to stress. My parents were having problems, so I thought he might be right. So he gave me anti-anxiety pills. For a long time, I really thought this was all in my head. I began thinking that somehow I was doing this to myself.

Finally it reached a point where my mother stepped in and insisted that I be referred to a gastroenterologist. By this time I was extremely thin and could barely keep down anything. I was worried that maybe I was anorexic. But they did some tests and found out I had Crohn's.

Those years were a really tough time. I wish we had insisted on a referral sooner but sometimes you don't think to question your doctor's judgment.

It also took Jamie two years to find out she had IBD:

I had Crohn's at least two years before it was officially diagnosed. During this time I intermittently had various symptoms such as cramping, fever, and vomiting. Twice, it got so bad that I went to the emergency room. However, both times I was told that I had a severe case of the flu. My doctor did blood tests that showed I was anemic, but he said it was normal for women my age to have low hemoglobin.

When I was finally diagnosed, it was no relief. The word chronic stuck in my mind, suggesting there was no easy fix. However, it was validating. I know my body, and I know when something is wrong with it. Of course, I didn't want to find out that I have some strange disease, but I still wanted proof that it was not just the flu or something all in my head.

Crohn's and ulcerative colitis can develop gradually. Some people don't make it a priority to go to the doctor if they are not experiencing any dramatic changes in their health. Instead, they adapt to their slowly developing symptoms, or attribute them to other problems.

Ulcerative colitis and Crohn's disease are also hard for doctors to identify, because the symptoms sometimes begin outside of the intestine, such as in the joints or eyes. Fatigue is also another symptom that may develop months before bowel symptoms do.

Some people with IBD are diagnosed very quickly. This usually happens when blood is present in the stool. This sign is generally taken quite seriously, because doctors immediately want to know its cause.

Denise describes how her ulcerative colitis was diagnosed:

> *My very first symptom actually was arthritis with pain in my collarbone and sternum. If it had just stayed this way with no other symptoms, I'm sure it would have been a long time till they figured out I had ulcerative colitis. However, they gave me some non-steroidal anti-inflammatory drugs and I soon started having blood in my stools. We immediately stopped the drugs, but I kept having the bleeding. My doctor was concerned so I had a colonoscopy. They were able to diagnose the ulcerative colitis right away.*

Blood tests

Blood tests by themselves can't identify whether you have Crohn's disease or ulcerative colitis. However, they can give you and your doctor information that is helpful in determining what's going on in your body. Also, if you already know you have IBD, blood tests are often helpful in diagnosing a flare-up of your illness and its impact on your body. Your doctor may choose to order a variety of different blood tests; the following ones are some of the most common.

Complete blood count (CBC)

A CBC measures components of your blood. The test supplies information about your red blood cells, including how many you have and their size. Your hemoglobin level is measured as well. The CBC also provides a count of your white blood cells and platelets.

Red blood cells (RBC) and hemoglobin

Red blood cells, also called erythrocytes, are very small. There are typically 4.5 to 6 million of them in just 1 cubic milliliter of blood. Their main purpose is to transport oxygen to your body's tissues and carry carbon dioxide to the lungs. In active cases of ulcerative colitis or Crohn's of the colon, the number of red blood cells is often low, because blood is frequently lost through intestinal bleeding. In addition, chemicals produced by the inflammation from either type of IBD tend to reduce the production of new erythrocytes.

Red blood cells contain hemoglobin, a substance composed of iron and protein. Hemoglobin is what enables red blood cells to carry oxygen. Its iron component attracts oxygen from the air you breathe. Thus, your level of hemoglobin reflects your blood's ability to transport oxygen to all the cells of your body.

Normal levels of hemoglobin for men range from approximately 13.5 to 18 grams per deciliter. A normal value for women is typically from 12 to 16. In otherwise healthy adults with no heart or lung problems, most doctors order blood transfusions for people when their hemoglobin drops to 8 or below. Although your hemoglobin can be low for a number of other reasons, a low level in combination with other signs and symptoms may suggest IBD.

White blood cells (WBC)

White blood cells are another major component of your blood. They are larger than red blood cells and are responsible for defending your body from infection. During flares of IBD, white blood cell counts are often elevated, reflecting the immune system's increased activity. Normally, your blood has 5,000 to 10,000 white blood cells per cubic millimeter. Some medications for IBD may raise your WBC, whereas other drugs that suppress your immune system may lower your count.

Your body produces several different types of white blood cells. If your doctor wants a count of the different types of white cells, a test called a differential is sometimes performed along with your CBC.

Platelets

Platelets are the components in the blood that are necessary for clotting. If a blood vessel is damaged somewhere in your body, your platelets clump together and adhere to the injured area to stop the bleeding. They are smaller than red blood cells, and typically 350,000 to 500,000 of them are found in a cubic milliliter of blood. Platelet levels are often elevated in people with Crohn's or ulcerative colitis who have frequent bleeding in their bowel.

Erythrocyte sedimentation rate (ESR or sed rate)

The sed rate (erythrocyte sedimentation rate, or ESR) is a test that measures the amount of inflammation in the body. When present, inflammation can cause red blood cells to clump together and become heavier than normal. As a result, the clumped erythrocytes fall at a faster rate (compared to normal, nonclumped erythrocytes) when they are put in a special type of test tube. The rate at which they fall—measured in millimeters per hour—is called the sedimentation rate. Sed rates are frequently high in people who have significant inflammation, because they tend to have more clumping of their red blood cells.

One technique for measuring the sedimentation rate is called the Westergren method. Using this procedure, normal rates for men are 0 to 15 millimeters per hour, and 0 to 20 for women. Someone with an active case of IBD can have a sed rate of 50, 75, or more. A high rate, however, is not specific to Crohn's or ulcerative colitis; any inflammatory illness can increase the sed rate. As with other blood tests, your doctor uses the sedimentation rate in conjunction with other criteria when trying to make a diagnosis.

C-reactive protein (CRP)

Many doctors are now using the C-reactive protein (CRP) test in addition to or in place of sed rates. Like the sedimentation rate, CRP measures the level of inflammation in the body and is not specific to IBD. However, some doctors prefer it to a sed rate, because C-reactive protein provides a more direct measure of inflammation in the body. Normal values typically range from 0 to 1 milligram per deciliter.

Serum albumin

Serum albumin is a type of protein in the blood that is generally a good indicator of the body's protein stores. Someone with a severe case of IBD is often malnourished; thus she will probably have a low albumin level. The normal range for adults is about 3.5 to 5 grams per deciliter. Anything less usually indicates that a person is receiving inadequate nutrition or that he is losing protein through his inflamed intestine.

Managing results

Some people with IBD like to keep track of their test results. There are many ways to do this, such as entering data into a computer spreadsheet or by keeping a notebook. Managing results this way gives some people a sense of control over their illness, because they can monitor results over a period of time and spot trends. However, although some people may feel more comfortable knowing all their results, others prefer not to bother with these details. For them, tracking numbers only escalates anxiety.

It's important to tell your doctor how much you want to know. If you are newly diagnosed, it's possible you may not have a good sense of how much you want to hear.

This is completely normal. Over time, you'll have a much better idea of how you want to manage this kind of information.

Craig, who has had Crohn's for almost twenty years, explains:

> As a young adult, I had multiple flare-ups of my disease. I am a take-charge kind of person when it comes to my health so I always want to know the results of blood tests. There were periods where I would get lab work done weekly, and then even more often if I was in the hospital. For whatever reason, I seemed to latch on to my sed rate since it tended to correlate with my symptoms—most of the time. But sometimes it didn't. I can remember many times when I knew I was feeling better, but my sed rate hadn't gone down, or just hadn't gone down as much as I thought it should. I would then worry about it and end up feeling worse. It got to the point where I would always stress myself out every week just before hearing what the new value was.
>
> I finally decided enough was enough. I told my doctor to feel free to keep monitoring it, but I no longer wanted to know the result. It was difficult at first not knowing, but it turned out to be a wise decision. Over time, I learned not to care about it, and now I no longer lose energy to worrying about my sed rate. I love the freedom of not letting a number dictate how I am going to feel. I let my doctor worry about the numbers, and I just focus on getting and staying well.

Stool tests

Stool tests are used to check for blood, parasites, and harmful bacteria. This section describes some of the basic tests your physician may order and then gives tips on how to provide a stool sample.

Occult blood

The word "occult" means hidden. Your stool may appear normal and brown, but many people with IBD who have inflamed colons have at least a small amount of blood hidden in their stool.

The occult blood test—sometimes called a stool guaiac test—is done very easily. It usually involves putting a small sample of stool on a thin, cardboard test card. Then all you have to do is return the card to your doctor or to the laboratory. Or you can just mail it to either of them. The lab technician adds a few drops of a special solution on the other side of the card. If the area on the card turns a certain color, then you have tested positive for blood in your stool.

Stool guaiac tests are also sold over the counter. They are very similar to the ones your doctor uses, except you add the drops to the card yourself and observe any color change. If you use the over-the-counter product and test positive, be sure to inform your doctor of your results.

Parasites

Parasites are small, primitive organisms that live off other life forms, usually to their host's detriment. Even if you haven't been roughing it in the woods and drinking water straight from rivers or creeks, your doctor will probably order a parasite test, because some of these small life forms can cause symptoms similar to IBD. You'll generally have to collect samples of your stool for three consecutive days. Your doctor (or the lab) will provide you with test tubes filled with a preservative solution. You simply place your stool samples in these test tubes each day, and return them to your doctor or lab after your third day of collection.

Your doctor can order a number of parasite tests. She'll probably suggest one that specifically looks for a chemical produced by *Giardia lamblia,* one of the most common parasites that people have. Another test can check for amebic dysentery, which can cause symptoms very similar to ulcerative colitis. A third test involves smearing a sample of stool on a slide and then examining it under the microscope. The lab technicians specifically look for cysts, which look like small capsules. They are a stage in the life cycle of some parasites. If you test positive for giardia, amebic dysentery, or cysts, it's unlikely that Crohn's or ulcerative colitis is the source of your bowel problems.

Harmful bacteria

Your lower digestive tract is full of bacteria. They are a natural part of your system and necessary for proper digestion and bowel function. But if the wrong kinds of bacteria get into your system, they can produce a colitis that resembles IBD. An infectious colitis is produced by various types of bacteria, including *Salmonella, Shigella, Campylobacter, Clostridium,* and *Yersinia.* Your doctor will test for these to rule out any chance of a bowel infection.

Candida

Candida is a type of fungus. *Candida albicans* infection is often a controversial subject in medical circles. Some healthcare practitioners think candida overgrowth in the intestines can contribute to many different problems such as chronic fatigue syndrome, irritable bowel syndrome, or even IBD. Most gastroenterologists, however, do not believe candida in the bowel causes Crohn's disease or ulcerative colitis.

Tips on stool tests

Stool tests aren't invasive, but they are also not exactly the kind of thing people look forward to doing. Although most people would probably prefer not to have contact with their feces in this way, consider that elimination is a natural process in which every living creature participates. Here are a few tips to help you with stool collection:

- **Don't go in the toilet.** It's probably best to avoid eliminating directly into your toilet and then trying to get samples. Even if you've just cleaned the toilet bowl, it's possible other bacteria or parasites are present there that might interfere with the results of your test. Instead, try to go in a clean, relatively large plastic container. It's also much easier to gather a sample this way.

- **Have everything ready ahead of time.** The call to go to the bathroom can happen any time; so it's probably wise to have everything you need in your bathroom ahead of time. Items to have in place include your stool test kit, your plastic container to catch the stool, a clean plastic spoon, and a large plastic bag. Use the plastic spoon to transfer samples to the various slides or containers that you need to fill for the different tests. When you're through, empty the remaining stool contents into the toilet, put the plastic container into the plastic bag, seal it, and then dispose of it.

- **Have a sense of humor.** A sense of humor can really help in situations like these. You may feel a little uneasiness when collecting your stool, but if you can, consider taking a lighter attitude toward the process.

Craig, who's done many stool tests over the years, shares how humor has helped him accept what he needs to do:

> *Stool tests used to bother me but not anymore. Since it's something that just comes with the territory when you have IBD, I figured I might as well use a humorous approach to deal with it.*

When you think about, it's kind of funny what you are doing. Someone is essentially telling you that your stool is so important that not only do they want you to collect it, but they have given you a postage paid box in which to put it so that it can be shipped to them by first class mail. How many people get to experience that? Yes, if you're using a local lab you may have to bring it in yourself, but if not, it's possible a private carrier will literally come right to your door to pick it up.

One time as I was getting ready to mail a sample, I noticed the address label said it was being shipped to North Carolina. I've never even been to North Carolina! Who would have thought my stool would make it there before me?

Imaging procedures

X-rays are a form of energy discovered in 1895 by a German physicist named Wilhelm Roentgen. They are able to penetrate deeply into various forms of matter, including the human body. As a result, they are often very useful in medical settings, particularly in the area of diagnostic imaging. Imaging tests frequently use x-rays to take pictures of the organs inside your body.

X-ray pictures, also called radiographs, are produced when x-ray beams are passed through someone and onto film that is placed on the other side of the person. The shadow of dense structures, such as bones, generally appears quite clearly on x-ray film because they absorb more of the rays. The bowel, however, which is not particularly dense, absorbs few rays and generally casts no shadow onto the film. Thus, x-rays alone can't provide much information on the condition of your intestines.

Physicians therefore have to rely on special x-ray tests when trying to identify various diseases, including IBD. The following are the most common imaging exams used to help diagnose ulcerative colitis or Crohn's.

Barium contrast studies

A contrast medium is a material that absorbs x-rays. Your intestines are not dense enough to cast much of a shadow onto regular x-ray film, so a contrast medium is necessary in order to view the bowel.

Barium sulfate, a white, chalky substance, is an excellent contrast medium for x-raying the digestive tract. It is dense and also cannot be absorbed by the human body. When x-ray beams are passed through a barium-filled intestine, the barium casts a well-delineated shadow onto the x-ray film. Your doctor can then see the outline of your bowel with great detail. For example, if ulcers are present in the inner lining of the bowel, barium will fill into the sores and show up on the x-ray. Barium contrast studies also show any narrowing of the intestine or thickening of the bowel wall.

Barium is administered through either end of your body, depending on what part of your GI tract your doctor needs to see. The major barium studies that are commonly performed to diagnose IBD are an upper GI series, a small-bowel enema, and a barium enema.

Upper GI series with small bowel follow-through

An upper GI series is an x-ray examination of the esophagus, stomach, and duodenum (the first part of the small intestine). The procedure is easily performed on an out-patient basis. Preparation usually involves fasting for at least four to eight hours before the exam. When you arrive, a radiological technician positions you next to a fluoroscope. A fluoroscope is an x-ray machine that displays your insides onto a screen for the radiologist to view during the test. You are then asked to drink several cups of barium sulfate. As you swallow, the radiologist can view your esophagus, stomach, and duodenum as the barium flows down. Still photographs are also taken so your doctor has pictures for your records and to view at a later time.

A small bowel follow-through is often performed as a continuation of the upper GI series. The barium you drank continues to flow through your small intestine. This provides an excellent opportunity to view the lower areas of your small bowel. Because it may take some time for the barium to make its way through, pictures are taken at set intervals, such as every fifteen to twenty minutes. You may have to go in and out of the x-ray room for several hours, depending on how quickly it takes the barium to reach the end of your small intestine.

Small-bowel enema

A small-bowel enema is another way to view the small intestine. A tube is inserted up a person's nose, threaded down the esophagus and stomach, and placed in the duodenum. Barium is then injected through the tube so it empties right into the small bowel. The x-rays generally come out better this way, because a concentrated amount of barium is deposited right into the duodenum.

Sometimes, if a person has trouble drinking enough barium the pictures are not always the highest quality. Also, even if a person can drink a sufficient amount of barium, digestive juices may dilute it by the time it reaches the lower part of the small intestine, and this can affect the quality of the photographs, too. The small-bowel enema helps prevent these problems and consistently delivers the best images.

The downside of a small-bowel enema is that placing the tube is often very uncomfortable. Drinking the barium is sometimes unpleasant as well. Even with added flavoring, most people find the taste unpalatable.

Stacy has had extensive medical testing during the 25 years she's had Crohn's:

> I've probably had about ten upper GIs with a small bowel follow-through. With each one, I've always found the barium very difficult to consume. They want you to drink it relatively quickly, but if I drink it too fast, it makes me gag. Somehow, I always manage to drink it all. I think it has something to do with the alternative. If you can't drink it, they have to insert a nasogastric tube and then infuse it. When I think of it this way, drinking the barium doesn't seem so bad.

Craig has also had to drink barium many times and shares his feeling on the subject:

> I've probably done about five barium drinks since I was first diagnosed with Crohn's. They try to make it seem like a milkshake, but after about the second sip, you definitely know it's not. It's very thick, and tastes more like liquid chalk with an extra bitter flavor added to it. I know this sounds so cliché, but if we could put a man on the moon over 30 years ago, why can't we make the drinks for medical tests taste better?

Barium enemas

Barium enemas are used to examine the colon. This procedure requires an extensive preparation to clean out the entire large intestine (see the section later in this chapter called "Preparing for barium enemas and colonoscopies"). After you lie down on the x-ray table next to the fluoroscope machine, a plastic tube is inserted into your rectum. A combination of both barium sulfate and air is then pumped into you. You may feel some discomfort, almost as if they were blowing your colon up like a balloon. You'll also have the urge to pass gas, but will be unable to do so with the tube in your rectum. If the discomfort becomes too great, let the doctor or x-ray technician know. They can control the release of the air from your colon.

During the procedure, they move you and the table in different directions so the barium can coat the inner lining of your entire colon. They may also ask you move into various positions while you are on the table. At appropriate times, they take x-ray pictures so that these films are available later for the doctor to examine. Once the procedure is over, they send you to a bathroom where you have an almost pure white bowel movement. Because you were cleaned out before the test, the barium is just about the only thing in your colon to eliminate.

Stacy, who has had Crohn's throughout her lower GI tract, shares some of her frustrations and tips regarding barium enemas:

> The barium enema was one of the more difficult tests for me to handle. I've probably had close to ten of them over the years. The problem is that they expect you to move around and get into what seems like—at the time at least—different yoga positions. They'd ask me to roll over one way, then the other, and then move my hip a certain way. All the while, the tube was still in my bottom, I was blown up with barium and air, and was quite uncomfortable. Many times I couldn't move myself the way they requested. Fortunately, they were always able to see what was necessary, but it was often a physically and emotionally draining experience.
>
> When it was over, I'd usually have cramps for a while, since the test would irritate my colon. I also learned I needed to drink a lot of water afterward to wash the barium out. And after the first time, I always brought baby wipes with me. The barium is very sticky and can be a problem when you are trying to wipe your bottom.

Computerized tomography (CT) scans

CT scans—sometimes called CAT scans, for computerized axial tomography—provide detailed views of the structures inside your body. CT scans use a special x-ray machine in combination with high-powered computers to produce sharp, high-quality images. CT scans are most often used to identify complications of Crohn's disease, such as abscesses (areas of infection) and fistulas (abnormal connections from the intestines to other organs).

The preparation for this test usually involves the ingestion of a contrast agent, a substance that absorbs x-rays. The contrast agent makes the images of your intestines more visible, just as it does when using a regular x-ray machine (see section earlier in this chapter, "Barium contrast studies"). Typically, you'll have to drink a few cups of a mildly sweet clear liquid that most people find unpleasant but relatively tolerable. If you are allergic to iodine, let your doctor know ahead of time.

The CT scanner is a large machine with a circular opening in its center. The technician places you on a table that slides into this hole, with your feet pointing toward the scanner. Because your abdominal region is of most interest, you probably won't have to go all the way into the machine. Instead, the technician will slide the table until your upper abdomen is just inside the hole. A rotating frame at the opening spins, thus allowing the x-ray tube mounted in it to emit x-rays 360 degrees around you. The table will then move a very small distance—perhaps 0.5 to 1 centimeter each time—so that the next section of your abdomen is imaged. During the procedure, the technician tells you when to breathe and not breathe, or a light near you may signal when you need to hold your breath.

Computerized tomography takes multiple pictures of your body, one "slice" at a time, and then pieces them together to create an accurate, detailed image that can help your doctor identify potential complications of your disease. The test usually takes from 15 to 30 minutes.

Jamie, who has had multiple complications with her Crohn's, shares her experience with CT scans:

> I've probably had more than a dozen CT scans during the last ten years. Compared to other tests, it's not so bad. I'd take one any day over a barium study. Also, my doctor and I have generally found them to be very useful. I've had a propensity to develop fistulas and also abscesses that form in my abdominal cavity. The CT scans have been very helpful in locating the areas of infection. We've even used them to help place tubes to drain the abscesses.

Radiation exposure

Some people with IBD have concerns about radiation exposure. Those who have frequent barium procedures or CAT scans may particularly fear the cumulative effects of these tests.

Jamie has had many x-ray procedures and shares her thoughts on the subject:

> I've had many CAT scans, upper GIs, small bowel follow-throughs, and barium enemas since the time I was first diagnosed. I admit that when I think about it, I do have concerns about all the radiation exposure. But what can I do? I feel that almost every test I've had has

*been necessary. X-ray procedures have often provided valuable
information that has helped me and my doctor determine the
appropriate treatment for my illness. At times, the tests lead to even
more questions about what's happening in my body, but overall,
they've been quite useful. So I just have to trust that we're making
the best decisions given the circumstances.*

It sometimes helps to put things in perspective. The American Nuclear Society (ANS) states that the average American is exposed to approximately 360 millirems of radiation each year.[1] (A millirem is one type of unit measuring radiation exposure that takes into account the relative harmfulness of different types of radiation). The average barium enema gives you a dose of 405 mrems, and the average upper GI gives you 245 mrems. However, national standards allow people who work with radioactive material to receive as much as 5,000 mrems per year.[2] Thus, people undergoing a few diagnostic procedures in one year are still receiving an amount of radiation well below this national standard.

A conscientious doctor carefully weighs the benefits of a particular test against its risks. Discuss any concerns you have with your doctor. Here are a few suggestions on ways to reduce your exposure to radiation:

- Ask your doctor if the results of the test will significantly affect what treatment he will recommend. If not, perhaps you really don't need the test at this time.

- Ask for a lead shield to cover parts of your body that don't need exposure. Your genital area is especially important to protect.

- Ask the technician or radiologist to do what she can to minimize your radiation exposure. One study found that a radiologist's technique can affect the amount of radiation you receive during a barium enema.[3]

- Request minimal use of the fluoroscope. One researcher found that when radiologists knew radiation exposure was being measured, less time was spent using the fluoroscope, and the person receiving the test was exposed to less radiation.[4] Perhaps having your request and concern fresh in the radiologist's mind might have a similar effect. It certainly couldn't hurt.

- Make sure to mention if you are pregnant or if you think you may be. Special precautions are then taken during the procedure, or your doctor may suggest avoiding the test altogether.

Endoscopic procedures

Endoscopy uses a thin, flexible instrument that transmits images from inside a person's body to either an eyepiece or a monitor screen. Previously, endoscopes were primarily fiber-optic instruments. This technology uses tiny, flexible glass fibers that transmit light end to end, regardless of how many twists and turns they undergo. With multiple fibers bundled together, equipment manufacturers made a thin, flexible scope that allowed gastroenterologists to see the GI tract through an eyepiece. Today, most endoscopes make use of charge-coupled device (CCD) chips, which are special image-sensing devices. They produce high-quality images that are then projected on to a video monitor.

Endoscopy is very useful when diagnosing IBD. It's also helpful for monitoring IBD because your doctor can directly view the lining of your GI tract. You can watch your own endoscopy on the video monitor if you are awake or care to watch. It's even possible to take home a videotape or some photos from the procedure. Endoscopes also have other parts that allow for suctioning, blowing air, tissue sampling, and cauterization (a burning procedure used to stop bleeding)—all of which may be needed during the examination.

Several different endoscopic procedures are used for people with IBD.

Esophagogastroduodenoscopy (EGD)

An EGD is a test that uses a flexible scope to view the esophagus, stomach, and duodenum (upper portion of the small intestine). This exam is frequently used when people have recurring upper GI symptoms, such as nausea, vomiting, difficulty swallowing, or a burning sensation in their esophagus or stomach. Although those with IBD usually have problems with their lower digestive tract, Crohn's disease of the upper GI tract can occur. If someone with IBD has upper GI symptoms, an EGD is useful in identifying whether the problem is Crohn's or another disorder, such as gastroesophageal reflux disease (GERD) or stomach ulcers.

The only preparation needed is to fast for four to eight hours before the exam. When you arrive, you lie on an examining table on your side. A nurse starts an IV (intravenous line) and a short-acting tranquilizer such as Versed is often given to make you drowsy. The doctor sprays your throat with a numbing agent that helps reduce gagging. He'll then gently insert the endoscope into your mouth and throat and ask you to swallow while he continues to thread the tube down into your esophagus.

Because it's normal to want to bite down on the scope, a mouthpiece is used so you won't damage the equipment. The doctor maneuvers the scope into your stomach and duodenum to see if there are any abnormalities.

A friend or family member should take you to your EGD appointment, because most doctors require that you have someone to drive you home after the test.

Stacy, who has had IBD for almost 25 years, shares her experience with this procedure:

> *Before the test I can remember thinking, "How am I going to breathe? Am I going to choke? What if I gag?" The whole idea of putting a tube down my throat frightened me. But as soon as I got in and they started the IV, I went out completely. I honestly don't recall anything during the exam. So I guess it was really more the anticipation of the test—not the actual procedure—that was difficult for me.*

Sigmoidoscopy

Sigmoidoscopy is a common procedure used to diagnose and monitor some forms of IBD. As the name implies, the area examined is the sigmoid colon, the S-shaped part of the lower large intestine. The anal/rectal area is also seen, because the scope must pass through this region to reach the sigmoid colon. Although preparation procedures vary from doctor to doctor, you'll probably be instructed to consume only clear liquids the day of the exam. You're also frequently asked to take a Fleet enema a couple hours before the test so your lower colon is clean for the examination.

During a sigmoidoscopy, you'll lie on your left side with your knees up toward your chest. Sedation is rarely used. But if you feel you'll need sedation, discuss it with your doctor when you make the appointment for the procedure. Once you're in position, the scope is inserted into your anus. The procedure is somewhat uncomfortable but is not usually painful. With a flexible sigmoidoscope, your doctor can view the entire left side of your large intestine—well past the sigmoid colon—if necessary.

The sigmoidoscopy is a valuable test, providing your doctor with a clear, direct view of your bowel mucosa. Tissue samples can be taken, and if inflammation is present, a sigmoidoscopy can provide good information about the extent and pattern of disease. The procedure only takes ten to twenty minutes. Sedation generally isn't required, so you can usually resume normal activity following the exam.

Carla, who has had ulcerative colitis for 33 years, shares how sigmoidoscopies have changed since the late 1960s:

> Sigmoidoscopies have improved quite a bit since I was diagnosed well over 30 years ago. I have painful memories of them putting this cold, metal tube up my rear. It was extremely painful, and it was very difficult for a teenage girl to have to go through. It really was just horrible.
>
> Sigmoidoscopies today, in comparison, are a breeze. The flexible tube that they use now makes the examination so much more comfortable. Not that it's something that I look forward to, but I really don't mind having the procedure now. The difference between 30 years ago and now is literally like night and day.

Colonoscopy

A colonoscopy is similar to a sigmoidoscopy, except that it is used to examine the whole colon. In many cases, your doctor can view the end of the small intestine as well. Unfortunately, it's necessary to completely clean out your large bowel before the examination. (See section later in this chapter, "Preparing for barium enemas and colonoscopies.") And because the procedure is often quite uncomfortable—even painful—sedation is recommended. Typically, people are given a combination of Versed (a short-acting sedative) and Demerol (a pain medication).

The test begins with your doctor positioning you on your left side with your knees toward your chest. He then inserts the long colonoscope into your anus. The procedure is generally more painful than a sigmoidoscopy, because the scope, as flexible as it is, must go around many turns in your large intestine. During the exam, your doctor can view the entire inner lining of your large intestine. He may also inject air to inflate the colon so he can see details in the mucosa more clearly. He can also pass a special instrument through the scope to take tissue samples or remove any small growths. The test usually takes 30 to 60 minutes. You'll probably have to spend at least another hour in a recovery room for observation. Most doctors and hospitals require that you have a ride home, because your body may take many more hours to eliminate the drugs.

Trish, who's had several colonoscopies to monitor her ulcerative colitis, shares her feelings on this procedure:

> Now that I've had a few colonoscopies, I really don't worry about having them anymore. With the drugs they give you for the procedure, it's

not that bad. In fact, two years ago I really wanted to watch it on the TV monitor while they were doing it, but the medications put me to sleep.

I've also found colonoscopies to be very informative. The test tells you exactly where your inflammation is. One time, we learned that my inflammation was only in my rectal area and that there was nothing further up. We therefore started using enema medication to treat the disease. I was then able to taper off my oral medication, which had a lot more side effects. So colonoscopies have been very useful in helping us know how to treat my disease.

Endoscopy in a pill

Researchers have developed a pill that has a tiny camera built into it. You swallow the endoscopic capsule, and for the next five hours it takes pictures of your GI tract. This pill transmits images via a signal that's picked up by a recorder worn around your waist. The data are later downloaded to a special computer that can convert the recording into a video. You and your doctor can then watch the video of your GI tract.

This pill won't eliminate the need for cleansing preparations or traditional endoscopic procedures. It can't take tissue samples, and it can only image the small intestine. Sometimes the capsule can reach the first part of the colon, but then the battery soon runs out. Thus, the endoscopy pill is currently not useful for people with ulcerative colitis or Crohn's disease of the colon. However, it can be a helpful diagnostic tool for those who have Crohn's in their small bowel. As of early 2003, endoscopy capsules are available in the United States, Japan, and western Europe. However, they are still relatively new and not yet routinely used. For more information on this new technology, visit *http://www.ccfa.org/news/wireless_endoscopy.html.*

Risks of endoscopic procedures

Endoscopic procedures are relatively safe, but they do involve some risk. EGDs and sigmoidoscopies cause the fewest problems, because they both involve shorter distances and have fewer curves to maneuver. Colonoscopies, because they examine a lengthy area of the GI tract and require a number of turns in the colon, are more risky. The most serious risk for any of these tests is perforation, or tearing, of the GI tract. Other effects may include local bleeding or exacerbation of disease—either from the procedure itself or the preparation needed for it.

Denise, who has ulcerative colitis, describes how colonoscopies have affected her:

> *I have found that having a colonoscopy can aggravate my condition.*
> *I suppose it could be a part of the disease just running its natural*
> *course, but I have noticed a worsening of symptoms after it.*
> *Specifically, I've found that after the examination I have more pain,*
> *more bleeding, and more diarrhea.*

It's wise to ask questions about any procedure that can possibly harm your body. Although most doctors would never jeopardize the health and safety of those under their care, the following suggestions can help you determine if a proposed procedure is necessary:

- Ask your doctor if the benefits of the examination outweigh the risks. If your doctor can't give you an answer that satisfies you, consider seeking a second opinion.

- Ask if the results of the test will affect decisions regarding treatment. For example, if an upper GI has already shown inflammation in the small intestine, and a sigmoidoscopy has already found inflammation in the rectum, do you really need a colonoscopy just to see if there is inflammation higher in the colon? Unless you've had IBD in your colon for more than eight to ten years and thus require a colonoscopy to check for cancer, you probably wouldn't need one.

- Ask your doctor how many colonoscopies he has performed over his entire career and within the last year. If the numbers seem too few, you might consider finding someone else who has more experience.

- Keep in mind that the risk of perforation generally increases when the bowel is more inflamed and diseased, because of its fragile condition. If your doctor has suggested a test and you suspect your colon is in a delicate state, ask if you can postpone the exam to a later time.

Preparing for barium enemas and colonoscopies

Preparing for a colonoscopy or barium enema generally requires a complete cleanout of the lower digestive tract. It's very important that your colon be free of all stool, or it will be difficult for your doctor to properly perform either procedure. Unfortunately, many people with IBD find this necessary process quite unpleasant. In fact, many say the worst part of these diagnostic procedures is not the actual tests but instead the preparation for them. Although there are many different methods to cleanse your colon, the three used most frequently today are sodium phosphate drinks, magnesium citrate, and electrolyte lavage solutions, such as GoLytely, CoLyte, or NuLytely.

Sodium phosphate

Sodium phosphate is a type of salt, sold over the counter, that is used as a laxative. When using a sodium phosphate solution, doctors generally recommend you go on a clear liquid diet for the two days before your test date. The evening before your exam, you take three tablespoons of sodium phosphate mixed in water. It tastes rather salty, but you only need to drink one glass. It's then a good idea to follow it with more water throughout the night, while remaining close to the toilet. Early the next morning, you take three more tablespoons in water and can continue drinking water up till four hours before your examination.

Sodium phosphate is harsh on some people's system. If you have significant inflammation in your colon, it's probably better to go with another option. It's also not recommended for people with illnesses such as congestive heart failure or kidney disease. If you have any other health problems or concerns, definitely check with your doctor before taking sodium phosphate solutions, as they can cause serious side effects in some people.

A new type of sodium phosphate preparation became available in 2001 by prescription. Visicol, sodium phosphate in tablet form, is only recommended for adults. The standard dose is 40 pills taken in two separate doses. The first dose of 20 tablets is usually taken the afternoon or evening before the examination. You then take the second round of pills about twelve hours later, making sure it's at least six hours before your procedure. It's recommended that you take each dose of 20 pills over a 90-minute period. During this hour and a half, it's suggested you take 3 tablets every 15 minutes with an 8-ounce glass of water. This means you have to drink at least seven cups of water during each 90-minute dosing period.

The same precautions for the standard sodium phosphate solution mentioned earlier also apply to Visicol. Thus, if you're having a significant flare-up or have other health problems or concerns, discuss with your doctor whether Visicol is appropriate for you.

Magnesium citrate

Magnesium citrate somewhat resembles a carbonated lemon/lime drink, except that it feels more heavily carbonated and it has a stronger, more sour taste. One advantage of magnesium citrate is that you don't have to drink so much—usually 10 ounces the night before your exam. Within a few hours, you'll have diarrhea that may last all night. The following morning, your doctor will probably ask you do an enema to ensure the colon is clean. Sometimes it's also suggested to eat lightly or go on clear liquid diet the two days before the test.

Magnesium citrate's effect on people varies. Some find it harsh and capable of aggravating their disease, whereas others do well with it and prefer it over electrolyte lavage solutions.

Stacy, who recently had a colectomy, had to clean out her colon many times before she had her surgery:

> I definitely preferred magnesium citrate over drinking a gallon of the lavage solution. Even though my doctor said I didn't have to drink all of it and could stop it after my stools were clear, it was still too much to consume. What worked best for me was to go on a two-day liquid diet, and then take the magnesium citrate the night before. It was much easier for me this way.

Electrolyte lavage solutions

Most doctors currently recommend electrolyte lavage solutions, such as Go-Lytely, Colyte, or NuLytely. These solutions are usually gentler on your system and are a better choice if you have concerns about dehydration or exacerbating your disease. The major disadvantage is that you have to drink three or four liters in a relatively short period of time. An 8-ounce glass every ten to twenty minutes is recommended. This means it will take you three to six hours to drink all the solution. This is often not easy, because it has a salty, plastic-like flavor.

Gina, who has Crohn's disease, has had difficulties with electrolyte drinks:

> I'm supposed to have colonoscopies on a regular basis but I find myself stalling on them since I dread the preparation. I need to get another one soon but it's hard for me to make the appointment since drinking a gallon of that salt water is so traumatic for me! It's especially bad when you are already feeling so sick. I have these horrible memories of sitting on the toilet with diarrhea while crying and sipping on my next glass of the drink. My husband has tried to be supportive and drink a little of it with me, but still, it's so difficult.

Here are some tips to help you consume all your electrolyte drink in a timely fashion:

- **Chill it.** Prepare the solution a few hours ahead of time and place it in the refrigerator. Many people say it is at least slightly more palatable when chilled.

- **Add some flavoring.** Nonnutritive flavorings, such as Crystal Light drink mix, may help a little. Check with your doctor to see if it's okay to do this, and then follow her directions. She may want you to avoid any red-colored flavoring. Some lavage solutions already come in different flavors, such as lemon-lime, pineapple, or cherry.

- **Change the taste in your mouth.** Another idea is to suck on an orange slice before drinking each glass. The flavor of the orange can help mask the taste of the solution. So can rinsing your mouth out with a pleasant-tasting beverage.

- **Eat lightly beforehand.** Consider eating lightly for the few days before your test. Even if directions say you can eat normally up till a certain time, start eating less a little earlier. If you can, try taking in less solid foods and consuming more liquids. This will make the cleansing process easier.

- **Pinch your nose and drink quickly.** Sometimes blocking the smell makes the flavor less intense. Also, try drinking each glass as quickly as you can. Drinking too slowly only prolongs the time you are exposed to the taste.

- **Have support on hand.** Have a friend or family member around for moral support. Also, consider calling a variety of people on the phone to keep occupied. If you know others who have been through the same thing, it might be a good idea to call them.

Craig shares his experiences using electrolyte drinks:

> *At support group, we always laugh at the name GoLytely, since it makes you go quite heavily! And there's little doubt that for most people, the preparation for the colonoscopy is worse than the actual test. The first time I needed to have one I had to cancel the exam because I could not drink the gallon of solution. It tasted as if someone had boiled salt water and melted a few plastic bags in with it. Anyway, I was quite sick, and by the time I got a third of the way through, I was in tears. I just couldn't drink another sip.*
>
> *Another time, I already had a feeding tube up my nose so we took advantage of it. We infused all the solution right through the tube and I didn't have to taste a drop! It's almost worth getting a tube up your*

nose just to get down the electrolyte drink—but that's probably an exaggeration.

Before the surgery to remove my colon, I also had to cleanse my colon. Although, I knew it would be my last time I'd ever have drink the stuff, I did everything I could to ensure I would be able to drink enough of it. What made the biggest difference was having a support system in place. I kept myself distracted the whole time by having my family around and talking to others on the phone. All afternoon and evening I spent time talking with people who love and support me. Much of the time was spent talking to my IBD buddies who have all been through this as well. I obviously had to bring the cordless phone into the bathroom with me and spent much of the time there. But before I knew it, my bowel movements were clear and I had drunk all I needed. I am so glad I'll never have to drink one of those solutions again, but it's nice to know that with good support I can do it.

CHAPTER 4

Complications

IBD CAN CAUSE many problems in and beyond the bowel. Fortunately, people with mild Crohn's or ulcerative colitis experience few—if any—complications with their disease. Those with moderate to severe IBD have a greater chance of additional difficulties occurring sometime during the course of their illness.

This chapter begins by looking at what else can occur within the bowel of those with IBD, beyond the basic problems presented in Chapter 2, *Signs and Symptoms*. It then examines how Crohn's and ulcerative colitis can affect other organs of the body. Throughout the chapter, people with IBD share how these complications have affected their lives.

Complications in the intestine

A variety of bowel complications can occur in people with IBD, most of which are quite serious. A few are even life threatening. Some of the more common occurrences include strictures, bowel obstructions, abscesses, and fistulas. Some less common problems are toxic megacolon and short bowel syndrome. Lastly, colorectal cancer is a real possibility, especially if you have had IBD in your colon for many years.

Craig, who had many IBD flare-ups with various complications for over fifteen years, comments:

> The basic symptoms of Crohn's and ulcerative colitis are already
> a lot for most people to deal with. But as if diarrhea, bleeding, pain,
> nausea, fever, and weight loss weren't enough, IBD has other
> complications in store for those with severe disease. I have suffered
> from abscesses, fistulas, and a complete bowel obstruction. It's a lot
> of problems for one person to go through.

The following sections discuss each of these complications, and how they affect those with IBD.

Abscesses and fistulas

Inflammation from IBD can slowly wear away the lining of your bowel. Small holes can gradually develop, allowing intestinal contents to dribble out bit by bit. When this happens, your body can usually contain the resulting infection by forming an abscess (a localized collection of pus, mostly made up of bacteria and white blood cells). Abscesses are more common in Crohn's, because the inflammation penetrates through all the layers of the intestine.

Inflammation sometimes burrows deeply through the bowel wall. Occasionally an abnormal channel forms between it and a nearby organ. These unusual tracts are called fistulas, and they can cause different problems based on the organs to which they attach. Connections made to the bladder are often troublesome, because fecal matter empties there and can cause infection. In women, a fistula connecting to the vagina is particularly distressing, because sexual relations can be affected. When fistulas connect to the skin, the result is very annoying because the drainage patterns are so unpredictable.

Richard, who has had a fistula for almost ten years, describes his experience:

> I have a fistula in my rectum that drains out to my skin on the inner cheek of my bottom. Since I never know when it's going to drain, I always have to wear pads in my underwear. I've had some good laughs about it over the years with friends and family. It's always interesting as well to observe reactions in the check-out line when I'm buying them at the store. Thankfully, the thin kind suffices so no one can tell I'm wearing them.
>
> Overall, I've adapted to having to wear the pads. I hardly think about it anymore. But really it's a nuisance, and I look forward to the day I no longer need them. Once when I was putting a pad in my underwear and pulling off the paper to reveal its sticky backing, I noticed on the paper it said repeatedly, "Kotex understands, Kotex understands . . ." Somehow, I don't think they really do!

Gina recounts her experience with a fistula going to her bladder:

> I kept getting urinary tract infections. As soon as I'd finish a course of antibiotics, the infection would return. I also started noticing that I might be passing air after I urinated. My doctor told me to sit in a

bathtub while voiding, to check for air bubbles. Sure enough, I had them. He explained that the inflammation in my intestine was so severe that it created a hole and formed a tract to my bladder. So intestinal contents were actually leaking into my bladder. We had hoped the fistula would close by itself, but ultimately I needed to have surgery to remove the tract and repair my bladder.

Fistulas can also link to other segments of the bowel. In some situations, you may not experience any symptoms.

Fistulas are generally treated by surgery or antibiotics. Medications that suppress your immune system, such as azathioprine or 6-MP, are also sometimes used. Infliximab, a drug that blocks the production of tumor necrosis factor (an inflammatory chemical made naturally by your body) can also help close fistulas. These treatments are discussed in Chapter 5, *Medications,* and Chapter 6, *Surgical Treatments.*

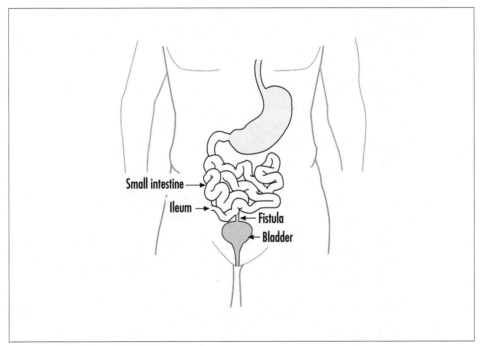

Figure 4-1. Fistula to the bladder

Cancer

One of the most feared complications of IBD is cancer. Much research has been conducted on this topic, yielding variable information. People with both ulcerative colitis and Crohn's disease of the colon appear to have increased risk for developing a malignancy in the large intestine. Previously, researchers thought that people with Crohn's colitis were at less risk than those with ulcerative colitis. Although some debate still goes on, recent research suggests that if the extent and duration of colonic inflammation is similar, people with either illness have about the same chance of getting colorectal cancer.[1] Overall, it's estimated that less than 5 percent of all people with ulcerative colitis will develop a malignancy in the large bowel.[2] The risk for those with Crohn's is lower, because not everyone with this disease has inflammation in their colon.

Heather developed colon cancer at a young age:

> *I was about 15 when I started having bloody stools and was soon diagnosed with colitis. A few years later, I was diagnosed with Crohn's disease. During a colonoscopy I had fourteen years later, my doctor said she saw cancer. I was only 29 years old. I was suddenly faced with surgery, and the possibility that I might have to wear a bag the rest of my life. I was scared and devastated. It helped to talk to people who had undergone the colectomy procedure, but it was still difficult since all of this came up so suddenly. When I went in for surgery, we still didn't know whether I would come out with a bag or not. But it turned out they didn't need to remove my whole colon. They were able to cut the cancer out and resect my colon. So fortunately for me, I can still eliminate the normal way after having colon cancer.*

People with Crohn's have a higher risk of small-bowel cancer than those who don't have Crohn's. Overall, though, malignancies in the small intestine are extremely rare, even if you have Crohn's disease.

The risk of colorectal cancer in people with IBD depends on many different factors. Following is a list of items that are thought to affect risk.

Diagnosis at a young age

Some studies suggest that people who develop IBD in their colon at a young age are at a higher risk for colorectal cancer than are those diagnosed later in life. For example, one group of researchers found the risk was higher for people with both types of IBD if their colon inflammation began before age 25.[3] This risk is independent of the length of time since diagnosis.

Extent of colon involvement

The more pervasive the inflammation in the colon, the greater the chance of developing colorectal cancer. One study of people with ulcerative colitis found that those with pancolitis (inflammation throughout the whole colon) had a higher risk of developing cancer than those who had left-sided colitis. People with proctitis—but no other colonic involvement—had a smaller risk of getting cancer.[4]

Length of time since diagnosis

A long duration of IBD is a major risk factor for the development of colorectal cancer. Most experts agree that for the first eight to ten years with either illness, there is little increased risk of cancer. Starting around eight to ten years after diagnosis, however, the risk of developing colorectal cancer gradually increases.[5] For this reason, regular colon examinations are recommended annually for those who have had IBD in the colon for more than eight to ten years.

Presence of dysplasia

Dysplasia means "malformation." In IBD, it refers to benign but abnormal tissue growth in the cells lining the intestine. As tissue in the bowel progresses from a normal state to cancer, dysplasia is the intermediate phase between these two stages. This is why it's sometimes thought of as a precancerous condition. Dysplasia itself also has different stages, including low and high grade, with the latter being more serious, because the tissue is often on the verge of becoming cancerous. However, not all dysplasia necessarily turns into cancer. And even if it does, the time it takes to progress from low grade to high grade to cancer varies widely among people.

Dysplastic tissue itself is not malignant, but it's often a predictor of an undetected, early-stage cancer elsewhere in the colon. High-grade dysplasia is thought to be the most predictive of a malignancy already present, but large-bowel cancer can exist in people with low-grade dysplasia as well. Another problem is that experienced pathologists' opinions vary widely when classifying dysplasia. In other words, if one pathologist identifies a sample as low grade, there's a good chance another may classify it as high. For these reasons, many doctors recommend immediate colectomy if either low- or high-grade dysplasia is diagnosed.[6]

Another possible diagnosis is indefinite dysplasia. This means you may have dysplasia, but the pathologist couldn't make a definite determination. If your pathology report comes back as indefinite, your doctor will probably recommend frequent colonoscopies with multiple biopsies (tissue samples) to closely monitor the status of your colon. However, with this diagnosis some physicians may recommend removal of the large intestine.

Krystal was diagnosed with dysplasia after several years of ulcerative colitis:

> One time after a colonoscopy, it was discovered that I had a polyp with dysplasia. I don't know whether it was high grade or low grade. Although that polyp was removed, my doctor said that it was very possible that dysplasia could be lurking elsewhere in my large intestine. We could do regular colonoscopies and take tissue samples, but he said that trying to find dysplasia or even a very early stage of cancer in a colon with severe ulcerative colitis is often like trying to find a particular blade of grass in a baseball field. You can look and take a lot of samples, but if you miss that one blade of grass, you're in trouble. It wasn't worth risking my life to save my colon.

Knowing the risk factors is important, but knowing what you can do to help prevent colorectal cancer is even more important. Although no one knows the optimal strategy for preventing colon cancer in people with Crohn's disease and ulcerative colitis, the following sections offer several suggestions for decreasing your chances.

Colectomy

Having your colon removed is probably the only sure way to prevent colon cancer. Of course, this would never be recommended for the average person. However, for some people with long-term colitis, having the large intestine removed may be a reasonable option. If you and your doctor determine that a colectomy is appropriate for you, know that you can lead a normal, healthy life after the surgery. For more information on this topic, please see Chapter 11, *Life with an Ostomy*.

5-ASA drugs

Drugs used to treat IBD such as sulfasalazine and mesalamine that contain a 5-aminosalicylic acid (5-ASA) component (an aspirinlike substance) have been found to reduce the chances of colorectal cancer in individuals with IBD. In one recent study, researchers found that regular 5-ASA therapy reduced cancer risk by 75 percent in people with ulcerative colitis.[7] Some experts believe that the protective effects of these drugs is similar to aspirin's ability to help prevent colon cancer in the general population.[8]

Folic acid

Research indicates that supplementation with folic acid (a B-vitamin, also known as folate) may help prevent dysplasia and cancer in people with ulcerative colitis. One group of researchers found that in people with ulcerative colitis, supplementation with folic acid was associated with a lower rate of colon cancer, compared to a group not receiving the supplement.[9]

Healthy diet

A diet low in fruits and vegetables is considered a risk factor for colorectal cancer in the general population. Although no study has specifically examined whether people with IBD can reduce their chances of colorectal cancer with a diet high in fruits and vegetables, there's little reason to doubt that what's true for people in general wouldn't also be true for those with IBD. Of course, some people with Crohn's and ulcerative colitis have trouble digesting fruits, vegetables, or other high-fiber foods. If this is the case, you might consider pureeing fruits and vegetables in a high-power blender. Juicing is also another way to derive the benefits of nutritious foods that you might not otherwise consume.

Surveillance

Surveillance itself can't prevent colorectal cancer from developing. However, frequent colonoscopies with multiple biopsies throughout the large bowel help keep you and your doctor aware of changes in your colon. Many physicians recommend yearly colonoscopies beginning eight to ten years after a diagnosis of ulcerative colitis. It's a good idea for people with Crohn's who've had colonic involvement for the same amount of time to follow the recommendations given for ulcerative colitis. Please note that being in remission—whether you have Crohn's or ulcerative colitis—is not a reason to forgo your annual exam, because you are still at risk. Frequent surveillance can help detect dysplasia or cancer at an early stage, when it's easier to treat successfully.

Short bowel syndrome

The average length of small bowel in adults is approximately 20 feet, although it can range from 9 to 27 feet, depending on your size. Short bowel syndrome is caused by extensive resectioning (cutting out pieces and re-attaching the remaining ends) of the small intestine. Because ulcerative colitis doesn't affect this part of the gut, this complication occurs in those with Crohn's disease who have had multiple surgeries. Fortunately, trends in Crohn's management now emphasize medical over surgical treatment, so short bowel syndrome is rare today.

There's no clear definition of what constitutes short bowel syndrome. Some define it as having more than 50 percent of your small bowel removed, whereas others point out that the functionality of remaining bowel is the key determinant. Most people can digest and absorb their nutrients appropriately, even if half or more of their small intestine is gone. This is especially true if a good portion of the ileum remains intact. As more bowel is removed, though, your chances of malnutrition and dehydration increase. In some situations, people may need intravenous (IV) supplementation to compensate. However, one group of researchers reports that if people have at least 60 to 100 cm of small bowel (24 to 45 in inches), long-term IV feeding is usually not necessary.[10] These researchers also report that glutamine (an amino acid) and growth hormone may help increase nutrient absorption and improve prognosis. Although they also mention intestinal transplant as a possible therapy, the prognosis for people undergoing this procedure is currently not good. As medicine advances, however, newer drugs that prevent organ rejection may eventually make this procedure a better option for people with this syndrome.

Melanie, who has had multiple surgeries, describes how she manages with a short bowel:

> In addition to having my colon and most of my small intestine out over 28 years ago, I've also had five resections to the remaining part of my small intestine. I have about four and a half feet of small bowel left. I'm fortunate that I am able to eat most things and absorb nutrients, except for vitamin B_{12}. In addition to supplementing my diet with a good powdered multi-vitamin and mineral formula, I give myself monthly vitamin B_{12} injections.
>
> I must be constantly aware of dehydration because I do not absorb liquids very well. When it is hot or when I overexert and sweat, I lose electrolytes very quickly. I try to avoid carbonated beverages because

they run through me rapidly and wash out my electrolytes. I keep water and Gatorade with me wherever I go. When my electrolytes depletion is severe, I use Pedialyte to restore balance.

Because I don't have a colon and can't absorb salt easily, I need to snack on salty foods to increase my salt intake.

I have been frightened by my health problems more times than I care to think about. I've been ill for many years. Through the years I've come to the realization that I can't live in continual fear. I'm very healthy physically and emotionally and I lead a full and active life. The quality of my life is excellent. I have peace of mind and happiness. I've had more than one doctor tell me to not change anything that I'm doing. When I had my ileostomy done the doctors told me that I would not live past 40 years of age because of the severity of my disease. I'm now 58 years old and healthier than most people I know.

Strictures and bowel obstruction

A stricture is an abnormal narrowing of a tubular structure. In IBD, the tubular structure is usually the small intestine, although the inside of the colon can narrow as well. Because Crohn's is the form of IBD that affects all layers of the bowel and causes a great deal of thickening and swelling, strictures are more common with this disorder than in ulcerative colitis.

If the narrowing is minor, you may not even have symptoms. But as the intestine becomes more blocked, you may experience more and more cramping. Peristalsis of the gut continually moves bowel contents along. If there is a narrowed section, pressure will build up behind the area and cause pain and bloating. Nausea and vomiting are common, too, especially if the stricture is higher up in the small intestine. If the intestine becomes completely blocked (obstructed), nothing—not even gas or liquid—can pass by. This situation is very dangerous and extremely painful. Hospitalization is necessary and treatment depends on the type of blockage.

Strictures and obstructions can result from inflammation. When the lining of the intestine swells, the interior of the bowel narrows. If you become obstructed for this reason, you'll likely need IV anti-inflammatory drugs as well as a tube put down your nose and into your stomach to draw out air and fluids. Usually this treatment will suffice, and soon you can resume liquids and then solid food again.

Scar tissue that builds up after years of disease can also cause strictures and obstructions. In addition, scar tissue from a previous surgical procedure might generate adhesions (fibrous bands that may attach to the intestine) that can create partial or complete obstruction. If there is a total blockage, surgery is usually necessary to resolve the situation.

Melanie, who has had many surgeries for her Crohn's, explains how she manages when she develops a stricture:

> I have a severe case of Crohn's. I lost my colon many years ago and have an ileostomy. I currently have a narrowing in one of my small intestines that is caused by scar tissue. This area of my bowel blocks occasionally. When I suffer from bowel obstruction, my pain is very intense. If I'm lucky, the obstruction resolves on its own. If it does not resolve, I am admitted to the hospital. There, they take off the appliance and flush the small intestine to try to clear the blockage. They also give me medication to stimulate peristalsis to try to get the bowel to pass the obstructed material through. Fortunately, the majority of the obstructions cleared as a result of these treatments. The ones that didn't, required major surgery.

Toxic megacolon

Toxic megacolon is a serious complication of severe colitis. The term "megacolon" refers to the dilation (stretching beyond the normal range of expansion) of the colon. When inflammation in the colon becomes widespread and severe, the large bowel can lose its muscular tone and can become paralyzed. Gas produced by bacteria is unable to pass out of the body, and the colon begins to inflate. This condition is dangerous because it can easily lead to perforation, which means the colon tears open, spilling its bacteria-filled contents into the abdominal cavity. Perforation can then lead to peritonitis, a potentially fatal condition in which the lining of the abdominal cavity is both inflamed and infected.

Toxic megacolon is uncommon but life threatening. It occurs in approximately 6 percent of people hospitalized with IBD, more of whom have ulcerative colitis than have Crohn's of the colon. Approximately 15 percent of the people who develop toxic megacolon die, and the death rate is highest in people who are older and who develop a perforation in their colon.[11] Because the condition is so dangerous, if the problem does not resolve within 48 hours most people have to undergo emergency surgery to remove the colon.

Conservative measures, such as IV steroids, IV fluids, IV antiobiotics, and decompression (releasing the trapped gas with a rectal tube) are sometimes used to treat toxic megacolon.[12,13] Even if these conservative measures prevent the immediate need for a colectomy, many people who've had one episode of toxic megacolon eventually need to have surgery. After developing this complication, therefore, frequent follow-ups with a gastroenterologist are necessary.

Complications outside the intestine

IBD is not just a bowel disease. Crohn's and ulcerative colitis can cause problems well beyond the gut. When signs and symptoms occur in other parts of the body, they are called extra intestinal manifestations. This means the disease is manifesting, or showing, itself in areas outside the GI tract. Researchers estimate that about 25 percent of people with IBD develop some type of extra-intestinal complication.[14]

The following sections review the major problems outside the GI tract that are sometimes associated with IBD.

Eye problems

Eye problems occur in about 13 percent of people with IBD.[15] The most common complication is episcleritis, a disorder that involves inflammation in the white part of the eye. It's generally not serious and is characterized by mild burning and redness. Another eye problem associated with IBD is uveitis, which involves inflammation in the colored part of the eye. It's sometimes called iritis, because the iris is part of the uvea. Uveitis is potentially more serious than episcleritis. It causes pain in the eyes, blurred vision, increased sensitivity to light, and sometimes headaches. Other eye problems include conjunctivitis, an inflammation in the lining of your eyelid that covers the eyeball, and cataracts, a clouding of your eye's lens that's often caused by long-term corticosteroid medication. For further information on how corticosteroids can affect the eyes, see Chapter 12, *Coping with Prednisone.*

Eye complications sometimes correlate with bowel disease activity, especially if it is in the colon. Although general treatment for IBD usually helps relieve eye problems, doctors often recommend treating with medicated eye drops. Even if you're unaware of any eye problems, you should have regular eye checkups from an ophthalmologist.

Joint problems

Peripheral arthritis, which causes painful, swollen, and/or stiff joints in the arms and legs, develops in about 20 percent of people with IBD.[16] Overall, this type of joint problem occurs more frequently with ulcerative colitis. But when it strikes in Crohn's, it generally affects people who have the disease in their colons. Peripheral arthritis tends to correlate directly with disease activity in the intestine. Thus, when bowel symptoms are brought under control, joint symptoms often disappear as well. Fortunately, the peripheral arthritis that develops in IBD, even if it is particularly painful and debilitating, generally leaves no lasting damage to the joints.

Approximately 5 to 10 percent of people with IBD develop ankylosing spondylitis, a type of arthritis that affects the spine.[17] Back pain and stiffness are common with this complication because the vertebrae are inflamed. Sacroiliitis, which causes inflammation in the joint connecting the sacrum (the base of the spine) and the ilium (the upper part of the hip bone), can occur in conjunction with ankylosing spondylitis. Sacroiliitis can also develop independently. Ankylosing spondylitis and sacroiliitis both tend to occur more frequently in those with IBD in the colon. They progress slowly and are not related to bowel activity.

Jamie, who has had a variety of complications over the years with her Crohn's, explains how joint problems have affected her during flare-ups:

> During flare-ups, I've had joint problems in my knees, hips, elbows, and shoulders. It can be very debilitating. Just getting out of a chair or walking around was sometimes a struggle. I can recall times at work when walking to the printer was a painful task. I had to really plan ahead before I got up to do anything. I'd also try to enlist others to help me do things so I'd avoid having to get up and move. It's very draining when you're so immobile. Moving around is hard enough, but when you have to make so much effort in just planning to move, that's almost even worse.

People with IBD are generally advised by their doctors not to take nonsteroidal anti-inflammatory drugs (NSAIDs), such as aspirin, ibuprofen, or naproxen. NSAIDs are associated with GI bleeding and inflammation in the colon, even in people who do not have Crohn's or colitis. In addition, taking NSAIDs has also been found to provoke flare-ups of IBD.[18] If your arthritis is causing significant discomfort, discuss with your doctor what other options are available to treat your pain. One small study suggests the relatively newer COX-2 inhibitor drugs—celecoxib (Celebrex) and rofecoxib (Vioxx)—may be safe for people with ulcerative colitis and Crohn's disease.[19] However, larger studies are needed. Consult your GI doctor if you have questions about the latest safety data on these drugs for people with IBD.

Liver problems

Liver disorders occur in approximately 5 to 10 percent of people with inflammatory bowel disease.[20] Liver conditions that can develop in IBD include fatty liver, gallstones, and primary sclerosing cholangitis (PSC).

Fatty liver

Fatty liver, a condition commonly associated with alcohol abuse, sometimes occurs in IBD. No one knows exactly why fat accumulates in the liver, but one theory is that the disorder is associated with malnourishment. Another is that inflammation itself may contribute to fat accumulation in the liver. In most cases, people aren't aware they have it, because it generally doesn't cause symptoms. It tends to disappear when one's health improves.

Gallstones

Gallstones sometimes form when there is an excess of cholesterol in bile, a digestive juice made in the liver. Cholesterol is normally a soft, waxy substance produced by the liver for use around the body. But if there is too much in the bile, not all of it can dissolve. The undissolved cholesterol can then form a stone in the gallbladder, where bile is stored.

People with IBD—particularly those with Crohn's near the end of the small bowel—are sometimes more prone to developing gallstones. If the end of the small intestine is inflamed, it may not be able to absorb enough bile salts (a major component of bile) to return to the liver. Because bile salts help dissolve cholesterol in bile, having less bile salts increases the chances of gallstones forming.

You can have gallstones for years and never know it. Other times the gallstones cause nausea or discomfort in the right side of the upper abdomen. The most serious complications occur when a stone leaves the gallbladder and lodges in the common bile duct, which connects the liver to the small intestine.

Jamie, who has Crohn's in her ileum, describes her experience with a gallstone that became stuck in her bile duct.

> I had many episodes of severe pain. I had some discomfort in my upper abdomen, but what was much worse was this unusual pressure and pain in my midspine that radiated to my rib cage. My doctors ruled out any heart problems. It was then suspected I might have gallstones since my Crohn's was in my ileum. My doctor said that if gallstones occur in IBD, it's generally with this type of Crohn's. So I decided to have surgery to remove my gallbladder. Unfortunately, this did not solve my problem.
>
> I continued having these painful episodes. Finally, after another year, it was suggested that I might have a gallstone stuck in my common bile duct. The only way to find out was through a procedure called ERCP, where a scope is maneuvered through your mouth, throat, stomach, and intestine. Then they insert a catheter through the scope and into the bile duct. It was a difficult procedure to go through, but they found the gallstone and removed it. Sure enough, that was the problem, and I've never had that type of pain again.

Primary sclerosing cholangitis (PSC)

The most serious liver complication that can occur in Crohn's and colitis is primary sclerosing cholangitis (PSC). The disorder involves inflammation and scarring of the bile ducts, the channels that carry digestive juices from the liver to the small intestine. It may progress to cirrhosis, a term used to describe a heavily scarred liver. PSC occurs in about 5 percent of people with IBD, most of whom having ulcerative colitis. However, over half of individuals with PSC have IBD. PSC is very difficult to treat and can cause liver failure. When PSC is advanced, the main treatment option is a liver transplant.[21] A more conservative therapy that shows promise is high-dose ursodeoxycholic acid (UDCA), but larger studies are needed.[22]

Kidney stones

Kidney stones occur more frequently in people with IBD than in the general population. The most common stones are made of calcium oxalate—a type of mineral salt. They tend to develop in people with Crohn's who have trouble digesting fats. Undigested fats in the intestine compete with oxalate to bind with calcium. As a result, excess oxalate remains unbound in the bowel. It gets absorbed into the bloodstream and ends up in the kidney, where it can bind with calcium to form stones.

It's sometimes possible to prevent kidney stones, or at least reduce the number of them that form. Here are a few suggestions that have worked for some people:

- **Increase fluid intake.** The simplest way to help reduce kidney stones is to drink more water. Researchers have found that a low urinary output is a major risk factor for kidney stones in people with IBD.[23]

- **Increase citrates.** Citrates are derived from citric acid, a substance that's produced by your body and found naturally in citrus fruits, such as lemons and limes. Citrates bind to minerals such as potassium or magnesium. Research suggests that taking citrate supplements may reduce your chance of developing kidney stones.[24] Another group of experts says that drinking lemonade might also raise citrate levels enough to help reduce stone formation.[25]

- **Increase magnesium.** Magnesium is an essential mineral found in many foods, such as green vegetables, whole grains, almonds, and seafood. Researchers have found supplemental magnesium can decrease one's risk of getting kidney stones. In one study (not specifically of individuals with IBD), only 15 percent of people taking extra magnesium formed new stones compared to 59 percent of those not taking it.[26] If you are considering taking this mineral, it's a good idea to discuss the topic with your gastroenterologist. Supplemental magnesium can cause diarrhea in some people.

- **Reduce oxalate intake.** Avoiding foods rich in oxalates may also help prevent kidney stones. Foods that may increase your chances of developing calcium oxalate stones include beets, rhubarb, spinach, chocolate, and nuts.[27]

Kidney stones are sometimes described as causing one of the worst pains known to human beings. Melanie, who's had a severe case of Crohn's with a number of intestinal resections, describes her experience with kidney stones:

> *The pain of kidney stones is very intense. It feels as if someone is taking a sharp knife, stabbing it in your back where your kidney is, and dragging it down to your bladder. All of the kidney stones I've had were so big that they would not pass on their own. I have had to undergone outpatient procedure called a lithotripsy. In this procedure, shock waves are used to break up the stones into smaller pieces so that the stones will eliminate naturally. I've had this procedure twice in the last three years to break up my stones.*

Skin problems

One of the most troublesome complications of IBD involving the skin is erythema nodosum. This disorder is characterized by painful red nodules that develop on your shins, although they can also occur on other areas of your body. Erythema nodosum occurs in ulcerative colitis about twice as frequently as in Crohn's, and is more common in women than men.[28] This painful disorder tends to occur with increased bowel disease activity; thus it often goes away once the IBD is under control. When these nodules develop, they are usually quite debilitating.

Richard, who had an active case of IBD during his teen years, explains:

> After a couple of years of remission in high school, I developed these mysterious red bumps on the front of my lower legs. It felt as though someone had just kicked me in the shins. It got to the point where it was so painful I could barely walk. The bumps throbbed excruciatingly even when I stood in the shower. There wasn't much I could do other than to put my legs up, which at least helped to relieve some of the throbbing. Fortunately, the bumps disappeared once we got the IBD under control. With repeated flares over the years, they never returned after that one episode.

The other major nonintestinal skin disorder associated with IBD is pyoderma gangrenosum. It occurs in about 5 percent of people with ulcerative colitis and 1 percent of those with Crohn's.[29] Ulcers can occur anywhere on the skin, although they typically develop on the lower body. Although they usually don't become infected, the ulcerations can spread rapidly and grow quite large. The condition is frequently disfiguring and can destroy tissue. Unlike erythema nodosum, it doesn't necessarily occur with active bowel disease. Steroid and other drugs that suppress the immune system are used to treat it, but it's usually a difficult condition to manage.

Heather, a young woman with Crohn's, shares her experience with pyoderma gangrenosum:

> Many years ago I was dealing with some arthritic symptoms, and I also developed these lesions on the back of my legs. They looked like some type of flesh-eating wound. They were really disgusting, and grew quite big. I had to get many rounds of cortisone shots to treat them. I also had to use these special bandages that are similar to ones used by burn victims. Overall, I was a pretty good trooper dealing with this complication on an emotional level. They were difficult to

treat, but they finally went away after about a year and have never returned.

Melanie sums up her philosophy about complications of her Crohn's disease:

> It has been rough over the years with the severity of my Crohn's disease and all its complications. At times I've gone through many periods where I've been extremely frightened. As my struggle with my health evolved, I realized that I couldn't live with fear my entire life. I found out that there is no quality of life when you live in a constant state of terror. For about the last twenty years my attitude has been that when I am well I am going to get the best quality out of my life that is possible. When I'm ill I rest so that I can recover and continue enjoying my life. I listen to my body so that it tells me what I need. I have worked extensively with many psychotherapists so that I understand myself enough to cut down on my stress level. I exercise avidly by walking and participating in a body pump class two mornings a week. I'm also hooked on golf and I love to travel to Europe. My attitude has given me a wonderful quality of life. I have a zest for life that I don't see in many people.

CHAPTER 5

Medications

MOST PEOPLE WITH IBD require medication at some point during the course of their disease. Some briefly require small amounts of a single medication, whereas others may need to take high doses of several drugs for an extended period. Unfortunately, no medication currently available can cure Crohn's disease or ulcerative colitis. Instead, the goal of drug therapy is either to reduce inflammation and other symptoms or to help maintain remission.

Drug therapy has come a long way during the last century. Before World War II, no medications existed to treat IBD. By the 1950s, there were two. In the 1980s, doctors began using a few more medications successfully. The 1990s brought even more advances. Today, people with IBD have more options than ever, with many more on the way.

This chapter reviews the major drugs used to treat IBD. It discusses how they work and what side effects they cause. It then covers experimental therapies under evaluation.

5-aminosalicylic acid (5-ASA) drugs

5-ASA drugs are a group of aspirin-like substances that have an anti-inflammatory effect on the bowel. Sulfasalazine, the oldest drug in this class, was the first drug used to treat IBD. It was initially developed for people with arthritis, but physicians found it worked very well in controlling colitis. Newer 5-ASA medications are now more commonly prescribed than sulfasalazine.

Sulfasalazine

Sulfasalazine is made from two components: a sulfa portion (a derivative of sulfur) and a 5-aminosalicylic acid part (the aspirin-like part). At first, doctors weren't sure which component was responsible for helping colitis. Some thought it was the sulfa portion, because sulfa has antibacterial properties. However, they now generally agree the active ingredient is 5-ASA. Although the exact mechanism of action is not fully understood, 5-ASA inhibits the production of chemicals associated with bowel inflammation.

Dosage and benefits

The major advantage of sulfasalazine over the newer 5-ASA drugs is that it is both inexpensive and has a long history of treating IBD. Moreover, none of the newer 5-ASA drugs are proven more effective than sulfasalazine. If you have active disease, a normal adult dose of sulfasalazine is 2 to 4 grams a day (four to eight pills). A common remission-sustaining dose is 2 grams per day.

Sulfasalazine is used for mild to moderate ulcerative colitis. It's also used to treat Crohn's of the colon. In addition, doctors have found it works very well for maintaining remission once colitis is brought under control.

Carla describes her experience on sulfasalazine:

> As someone who's had ulcerative colitis for well over 30 years, I clearly remember the years when prednisone and sulfasalazine were the only choices. Fortunately, sulfasalazine worked well for me for a long time. When I'd flare, I'd take it and have things under control within a week. I had no side effects other than the drug left a bad taste in my mouth. After several months, I'd stop it and be fine until the next flare. I kept with this pattern for many years until one time the sulfasalazine didn't work. I was sick for nine months straight. Fortunately, we finally got the colitis under control, but it was scary. Today, I feel fortunate now that I'm able to stay well with 6-MP, Asacol, and occasional short courses of prednisone.

Side effects

The most common side effects of sulfasalazine are nausea and headaches. Taking the drug with food sometimes helps prevent nausea. Men can have a reduced sperm count while on the drug, but normal counts usually return within a few months of discontinuing it. People can also have allergic reactions that may cause a rash or hives. Notify your doctor immediately if this happens. She'll probably want you to stop taking the drug. However, she might re-start you later on a much lower dose and try to gradually desensitize you.

The most serious side effects—although rare—involve the blood. Sulfasalazine can cause your body to destroy your own red blood cells. It can also depress the production of all types of blood cells. To watch for these side effects, your doctor will monitor your blood work closely while you're on the drug.

Gina had difficulty with sulfasalazine's side effects:

> *I had the worst headaches and nausea on sulfasalazine. It was frustrating back in the early days because it was my only other choice besides prednisone. It helped my symptoms, but sometimes the headaches and nausea were so bad that I'd rather just deal with my Crohn's symptoms instead. For years I went on and off it, and I always developed the same nausea and headaches. I tried taking other medications for the side effects, but they didn't help. What a relief it was when 5-ASA became available without the sulfa! I finally could take a medication that helped without giving me other problems.*

Newer 5-ASA drugs

New 5-ASA drugs were developed in the 1980s. The difference between these medications and sulfasalazine is that the newer ones do not contain sulfa. The first one to hit the US market was olsalazine (Dipentum) in 1990. It was followed by mesalamine (Asacol and Pentasa), which were also approved by the Food and Drug Administration (FDA) in the early 1990s. Balsalazide (Colazal) came out in 2000.

Each of these drugs delivers 5-ASA to the lower GI tract, but through different means. Because Asacol doesn't dissolve in an acidic environment, its 5-ASA is not released until it reaches the end of the small bowel or the colon, both of which are more alkaline. Pentasa relies on a time-release formula, and Dipentum and Colazal require colonic bacteria to release the 5-ASA.

Dosage and benefits

All the 5-ASA drugs have demonstrated effectiveness in treating mild to moderate ulcerative colitis. They are also helpful for Crohn's disease of the colon. Like sulfasalazine, 5-ASA medications can help maintain remission. They are not typically used for small-bowel Crohn's, though, because the 5-ASA is not generally released till it reaches the end of the small intestine or the colon. However, Asacol and Pentasa can dissolve in the lower end of the small bowel. Thus, they are worth a try if you have inflammation in your ileum.

Dosages can vary, but if your disease is active, your doctor will probably prescribe between 2 and 5 grams of 5-ASA per day. Depending on which drug you are taking, this can add up to a lot of pills. For example, Pentasa comes in 250-mg capsules. So some people have to take sixteen pills (four of them four times a day).

Gina comments on Pentasa:

> When I first heard that I'd have to take sixteen pills a day, I
> freaked. Four pills four times a day was quite a hassle. It seemed like
> too much medicine, and the regimen dominated my daily life. Plus it
> made me feel so dependent on a medication. However, since it worked
> and gave me no side effects, I quickly learned to get used to it. It was
> nice when after a year I was able to taper the dose—first to twelve,
> then nine. Today I only take four—two twice a day. That little bit
> makes a difference. If I'm not good about taking it, I'll start noticing
> some loose stool.

Some people like Gina can maintain remission on less than the standard dose of
5-ASA. However, many people require the full dose to stay well. Because 5-ASA
medications generally have few side effects, your doctor might recommend against
tapering so that you don't risk flare-ups. Maintenance therapy is important because it
can help prevent recurrences and future complications.

You can also take 5-ASA by suppository or enema. If you have proctitis, Canasa
suppositories are often helpful. For those with colitis limited to the left side of the
colon, Rowasa enemas can provide relief. Some people find a combination of both
oral and rectal 5-ASA works best for controlling their symptoms.

Side effects

The major advantage of these newer 5-ASA drugs is that they have far fewer side
effects than sulfasalazine. Allergic reactions are uncommon. There is a small risk of
kidney damage on higher doses, but this is also rare. However, 5-ASA drugs can
cause diarrhea. In rare instances, they can also aggravate colitis. If you think this is
happening, call your gastroenterologist and let her know.

Corticosteroids

Corticosteroids are powerful anti-inflammatory drugs used to treat moderate to
severe IBD. Because they work so reliably despite significant short- and long-term
side effects, many—but not all—doctors prescribe them frequently. Even with the
introduction of newer IBD medications, including budesonide (a corticosteroid with
fewer side effects), traditional corticosteroids such as prednisone continue to play a
significant role in IBD management, albeit less so than in the recent past.

Prednisone

Prednisone is a highly effective drug for treating IBD. Although it can work like a miracle, many people experience side effects. Chapter 12, *Coping with Prednisone,* contains detailed information on prednisone.

Budesonide

Budesonide (Entocort EC) is a rapidly metabolized corticosteroid that received FDA approval in October 2001. This medication is a major advance, because it is effective for certain people and has fewer side effects than prednisone. However, it's still uncertain if budesonide is safer in the long term than prednisone.

Dosage and benefits

Budesonide is used to treat mild to moderate Crohn's disease of the ileum and ascending colon. Some researchers report that budesonide is as effective as conventional corticosteroids, and others have concluded it is less beneficial. One recent study summarized previous research and found that budesonide induces remission in 51 to 69 percent of people with Crohn's.[1] The standard dose is 9 mg (three capsules) once daily. It's generally agreed budesonide is not useful in maintaining remission.

Many people who are dependent on prednisone wonder if they can switch to budesonide. Research shows that if Crohn's is relatively inactive, most people can make the switch without relapse.[2]

Cathy has had success with budesonide:

> I was on prednisone for thirteen years and thought I'd never get off. I was excited when budesonide became available because it was my chance to finally eliminate prednisone from my life. At the time I was making the switch, I had my usual level of symptoms, but I was stable. Fortunately, everything went smoothly. My symptoms stayed the same. Although they say it doesn't necessarily work well long-term, so far it's worked as well as prednisone. I was hoping I'd lose some weight, but that hasn't happened. But at least the puffiness in my face has gone down.

Side effects

Budesonide is a nonsystemic corticosteroid, meaning it has minimal effects on your body as a whole. Instead, it works locally in the intestine. Very little of the medication ends up in your bloodstream, so it has fewer side effects than prednisone or other traditional corticosteroids. The most common side effects are headaches, nausea, and respiratory infection.

Immunosuppressive drugs

Drugs that suppress the immune system are playing an increasingly important role in IBD management. Because an overactive immune system is thought to contribute to IBD inflammation, it makes sense that these medications might help. Their primary value is in helping people reduce or eliminate the need for corticosteroids. In addition, they can help maintain remission. The most common immunosuppressive drugs used to treat IBD are discussed next.

Azathioprine and 6-MP

Azathioprine (Imuran) and 6-MP (Purinethol) are chemically similar drugs. If you take azathioprine, your liver converts it into 6-MP. Both drugs appear to work equally well when treating IBD.

Researchers have studied the drugs' effect on IBD since the 1960s. However, because of concerns about potential side effects, most gastroenterologists didn't prescribe them regularly until the 1980s.

Dosage and benefits

Doctors usually prescribe these medications to those who do not respond favorably to 5-ASA or prednisone. In addition, your doctor may want you try them if you require a high prednisone dosage to remain symptom free. Most people start on 50 mg of 6-MP or 100 mg azathioprine once a day. Assuming you have no unusual reactions and your blood work looks good, your doctor may decide to gradually increase your dosage. To calculate your maximum dose of 6-MP in mg, you multiply 1.5 times your weight in kilograms. For azathioprine, you multiply by 2.5. These dosages are significantly lower than those given to people with other medical conditions, such as certain forms of cancer.

The research on these medications shows they are helpful for both Crohn's disease and ulcerative colitis. Not only can they effectively treat active disease, but they also help people stay in remission. They also allow many prednisone-dependent people to significantly reduce their prednisone dosage, or even come off of it altogether. Others have found their fistulas heal and close up when taking either drug.

Carla describes her success with 6-MP:

> Before I was on 6-MP, my flares would escalate rapidly. I'd have to take high amounts of prednisone to treat them. Since I've been on 6-MP, I'll still get occasional flares, but they don't spin out of control. I also stay well for longer between episodes. And if I do need prednisone, the highest I need is 40 mg. and I can usually taper off fairly quickly.

Gina has done well with 6-MP, too:

> In addition to Pentasa, 6-MP is an integral part of my treatment. Eight years ago, I was stuck on prednisone and couldn't get off without re-flaring. My doctor and I agreed I'd try 6-MP to see if it could help me get off the steroid drug. Within a few months, I slowly began to taper the prednisone. I got all the way to zero without any problems. I have never had to take prednisone since.
>
> I continue to take a very small amount of 6-MP every day. I toy with the idea of coming off. But I'm doing so well. I've never had any side effects and my blood work has always been good. Maybe some day I'll try and come all the way off, but for now, I'm keeping with it and enjoying my good health.

One major disadvantage of these drugs is that they take a long time to start working. Most people need to take them for at least three to six months before they can begin to see benefit. So if you are acutely ill, your doctor will have to prescribe another form of treatment first.

Side effects

Side effects of 6-MP and azathioprine are generally minimal—especially compared to corticosteroids. However, about 10 to 15 percent of people can't take these drugs because they produce specific reactions, such as a rash, severe headaches, nausea, or inflammation of the pancreas or liver. Moreover, some peoples' levels of white blood cells drop too low, thus compromising their immunity. Once the medication is stopped, all these effects are reversible. Your doctor will monitor you and your blood work very closely the first few months to check for side effects.

Cathy had to stop taking 6-MP:

> I had been on prednisone a long time and needed to get off or at least reduce my dosage. My doctor thought it would be a good idea to try 6-MP since it has helped a lot of other people. I agreed and started on the standard dose. Within only a few weeks, however, my liver enzymes shot

up very high. My doctor was not comfortable with this so he
recommended that I stop the drug. It's a good thing I was getting blood
tests to check my liver or else we wouldn't have caught the problem early.
I was disappointed it didn't work, but that's just the way it went.
Fortunately, I eventually was able to try budesonide, and this drug
allowed me to get off the prednisone.

Perhaps the most feared side effect of 6-MP and azathioprine is cancer. Although people with organ transplants on higher doses of the drugs have an increased risk of various cancers—especially non-Hodgkin's lymphoma—the data on people with IBD are less clear. However, there may still be a small risk.[3]

The use of 6-MP and azathioprine during pregnancy is somewhat controversial. Although a recent study found the doses used to treat IBD appear to be safe during pregnancy,[4] some doctors are still cautious about the drugs' use in expectant mothers. Despite some remaining uncertainties, though, many IBD experts currently feel 6-MP and azathioprine can be taken during pregnancy if needed to manage very active IBD. Your gastroenterologist can help you make an educated decision about taking the drug based on the current data. For more information on this topic, see Chapter 14, *Fertility and Pregnancy.*

Methotrexate

Methotrexate was developed in the 1940s as a treatment for cancer. Today, it's still used to treat certain malignancies. However, in the 1980s, new uses were discovered for diseases such as psoriasis, rheumatoid arthritis, and IBD.

Dosage and benefits

The doses of methotrexate used to treat IBD are much lower than those used to treat cancer. Although the drug is available in pill form, most doctors prescribe a weekly injection, because it is more effective this way. A typical dose is 15 to 25 mg per week. Methotrexate is either injected into a large muscle or subcutaneously (just under the skin). Most people can learn to give themselves shots.

Methotrexate is somewhat effective for treating active Crohn's disease. Like 6-MP and azathioprine, it also can help people lower their prednisone dose while maintaining remission. Its benefit for ulcerative colitis is less clear. Although researchers generally consider methotrexate not that helpful for ulcerative colitis, a recent study of 70 people with IBD suggests it may work as well for individuals with ulcerative colitis as it does for those with Crohn's.[5]

Methotrexate has greatly helped Terri's daughter:

> *Methotrexate has been the magic bullet for Kristy. She's had Crohn's since her pre-school years and nothing else has worked to control her illness so well. She's no longer on prednisone or any other medications and her health is great. We are very thankful that we found something that works.*

Side effects

In the United States, methotrexate is generally reserved for those who do not respond well to azathioprine or 6-MP. Although it tends to work more quickly—usually within two months—doctors have concerns about its side effects. In the short-term, the drug can cause nausea, vomiting, headaches, and diarrhea. It can also elevate your liver enzymes and lower your white blood cell count. Hair loss or thinning is a possibility as well. Inflammation in the lungs is a rare side effect.

Methotrexate gave Cathy diarrhea:

> *I hoped that methotrexate might work for me, but it didn't. I developed diarrhea on it, which is a known side effect. Obviously, that's not something you want when you already have Crohn's!*

Methotrexate sometimes causes liver damage over time. In addition to monitoring your liver enzymes, your doctor may suggest a liver biopsy to make sure you are not developing liver disease.

Methotrexate should never be taken if you are pregnant, because it can cause severe birth defects or miscarriage. After discontinuing methotrexate, men should wait at least three months before trying to father a child.

Cyclosporine

Cyclosporine (brand names Sandimmune and Neoral) is an immunosuppressive drug that has revolutionized organ transplantation. Many more people survive kidney, liver, heart, and other transplants, because cyclosporine prevents the body from rejecting transplanted organs. Like methotrexate, cyclosporine can help control symptoms in diseases such as rheumatoid arthritis, psoriasis, and IBD.

Dosage and benefits

A typical cyclosporine dose for people with IBD is approximately 5 mg for every kilogram you weigh. Your dose may vary, however, depending on whether you are receiving the drug orally or intravenously. You need less intravenously to achieve the same therapeutic blood level, which is usually between 150 to 400 nanograms (a nanogram is a billionth of a gram) per milliliter. Over time, your doctor will adjust your dose accordingly, so your blood level of the drug stays in this range.

Cyclosporine's main advantage is that it can rapidly produce results in very sick people. One review study reports IV cyclosporine induces remission within two weeks in 50 to 80 percent of people with severe ulcerative colitis who were unresponsive to IV corticosteroids.[6] The data are not as clear for Crohn's disease, although some evidence suggests it works quickly for these people, too, when IV corticosteroids don't.[7]

Cyclosporine's role in preserving remission is unclear. However, it's currently not used as a remission-sustaining drug. Doctors usually prescribe it to get severe symptoms under control so they can prevent an unwanted surgery. They then introduce another therapy concurrently, such as azathioprine or 6-MP, in the hope one of these drugs will maintain remission once cyclosporine is stopped. Hence some doctors refer to cyclosporine as a "bridge therapy" to other drugs. Sometimes this formula is successful, but other times surgery is still needed.

Side effects

Cyclosporine can cause numerous side effects, some of which are quite serious. Because it is a potent immunosuppressive drug, people who take it have a higher risk of infection. It may also increase the chance of developing certain types of cancer.[8] Kidney and liver damage is also possible. Other side effects include tremors, high blood pressure, headaches, nausea, and vomiting. Because of these potential problems, your doctor will monitor you very closely when taking this drug.

Antibiotics

Antibiotics are sometimes useful for treating IBD. Although no specific bacteria are known to cause Crohn's or ulcerative colitis, your doctor may suggest you try an antibiotic, particularly if you have Crohn's. The most commonly prescribed ones are metronidazole, ciprofloxacin, and antituberculosis drugs.

Metronidazole

Metronidazole (Flagyl) is the most frequently used antibiotic to treat Crohn's. It's effective against anaerobic intestinal bacteria—ones that don't require oxygen to survive. Doctors generally don't prescribe it for ulcerative colitis because it usually doesn't help this form of IBD.

Dosage and benefits

A typical dose of metronidazole is 1 to 2 grams per day, taken in three or four doses. Most people are used to taking antibiotics for ten days or two weeks to treat infections. In contrast, metronidazole is usually taken daily for several months to treat IBD.

Metronidazole is most effective for treating fistulas (abnormal connections between the bowel and other organs) in people with Crohn's disease. Research also suggests that taking it for several months after having a small-bowel resection may help prevent recurrence.[9] Its value for treating active Crohn's is unclear.

Cathy found metronidazole useful:

> I had a fistula on my bottom on and off for many years. Flagyl would make it go away, but then it would come back when I stopped it. It was hard for me to tell, but I also thought at times that it was helping the Crohn's in general, too.
>
> Fortunately, I was able to tolerate the drug, since I sometimes was on it for months or years. It left a funny, metallic taste in my mouth, but that was about it. I was also careful to avoid all alcohol while on it since I heard having even a little can make you really sick.
>
> Finally, after the last time I discontinued the medication, the fistula has not returned. I hope it's gone forever.

Metronidazole is generally not useful for people with ulcerative colitis. However, for those who've had a colectomy with the ileal pouch-anal anastomosis (see Chapter 6, *Surgical Treatments*), metronidazole is helpful for controlling pouchitis.[10]

Side effects

Side effects are common with metronidazole. The most frequent problems are headache, nausea, loss of appetite, and a metallic taste in your mouth. You also may notice a furry substance growing on your tongue. This is due to changes in the balance of microbes in your mouth.

Gina had lots of side effects when taking metronidazole:

> Flagyl made me extremely nauseated. It was so bad I couldn't eat. With my Crohn's, I was often nauseated already. This drug made it so much worse. I had to stop it after three days. Fortunately, other medications such as Pentasa and 6-MP have worked much better for me.

The more serious side effects are neurologic. These include numbness and tingling in the hands and feet, and difficulties with balance and motor coordination. These neurologic problems are generally reversible once people stop taking the drug, but it may take months before they fully resolve.

You must avoid alcohol while on the drug. Mixing alcohol and metronidazole usually causes vomiting and makes most people feel extremely ill.

Ciprofloxacin

Ciprofloxacin (Cipro) is an antibiotic used to treat many different kinds of infections throughout the body. Doctors have also found it helps some people with IBD.

Dosage and benefits

A common dose of ciprofloxacin is 500 mg twice daily. As with metronidazole, your doctor will probably prescribe it for an extended period (at least several months) to see if it helps. Indeed, research has shown a six-month course of ciprofloxacin may improve symptoms in people with ulcerative colitis and Crohn's disease when added to their treatment regimen.[11,12] A recent study also supports its use over metronidazole for pouchitis, because ciprofloxacin has fewer side effects.[13]

Nathan has been on ciprofloxacin for a long time:

> Pouchitis has been a problem for me since a year or two after my surgery. My doctor would prescribe either Flagyl or Cipro. However, the pouchitis would always return within a year. When it became chronic, my doctor suggested I just stay on a maintenance dose of Cipro all the time. It's been almost seven years and the pouchitis has not returned.

Side effects

People usually tolerate ciprofloxacin fairly well. Side such as nausea, diarrhea, vomiting, and headache can occur, but they typically don't prevent people from continuing the medication.

Antituberculosis drugs

Antituberculosis drugs, such as clarithromycin (Biaxin), have recently gained attention because a type of bacterium, *Mycobacterium paratuberculosis,* has been found in the GI tract of some people with Crohn's. However, as mentioned in Chapter 1, *Introduction to*

IBD, most gastroenterologists aren't convinced this bacterium is responsible for causing Crohn's.

Dosage and benefits

Clarithromycin acts against many types of bacteria. Thus, the fact that it helps you doesn't mean *Mycobacterium paratuberculosis* is responsible for your illness. If clarithromycin is prescribed, gastroenterologists typically recommend 250 or 500 mg twice daily. Research on its effectiveness so far is mixed. Although some researchers have found it helpful for Crohn's,[14] a recent, well-designed study of clarithromycin and ethambutol (another antituberculosis drug) found no benefit.[15] Further research is needed to clarify what role clarithromycin and other antituberculosis medications can play in treating Crohn's.

Clarithromycin has worked well for Rhonda:

> *I was diagnosed with Crohn's nine years ago, but have probably had it about sixteen. One drug that has consistently helped me is the antibiotic Biaxin. Not only does this medication agree with me, but it effectively controls my symptoms, and has done so for the last four years. I was on prednisone for three years previously and am glad I don't have to take that anymore. Budesonide worked at first but its effect wore off after about two years. 6-MP isn't an option since I had a bad reaction to it (elevated liver enzymes). I'm very thankful that I found a medication that works for me.*

Side effects

Clarithromycin's side effects include nausea, vomiting, and stomach cramps. It can cause colonic inflammation in some people.

Biologic therapies

Biologic therapies are made from proteins and other products of living organisms. They are a major advance in medicine because they are designed to specifically block particular chemicals in the body associated with disease.

Infliximab (Remicade) is currently the only biologic therapy approved for Crohn's disease. Released in 1998, it's a special type of antibody made from both human and mouse proteins. It blocks the body's synthesis of tumor necrosis factor alpha (TNFα), a chemical associated with Crohn's inflammation.

Dosage and benefits

Infliximab is administered by a two- to three-hour-long infusion through an IV. You'll need to visit your doctor or local infusion clinic to receive it. The standard dose is 5 mg per kilogram of weight. Initially, your physician will probably give you three doses within a six-week period. If you require repeated infusions, your doctor will usually space them in eight-week intervals.

Infliximab offers people with moderate to severe Crohn's another option if they don't respond well to other drugs. One large, recent study found that 58 percent of people improved markedly within two weeks of their first infusion. With follow-up infusions every eight weeks, significantly more of those taking infliximab maintained remission than those receiving a placebo.[16]

Michael has found infliximab very helpful:

> *I've had Crohn's since 1996. I've never thought of my condition as that severe, but my other medications—prednisone, 6-MP, and Pentasa—weren't enough to keep me symptom-free. My doctor kept suggesting Remicade, so I finally decided to give it a try. I had some concerns, but I figured it was worth a shot.*
>
> *I've had excellent results. Since my first infusion, all my pain has gone away. I've also gotten off prednisone and there's been no sign of a flare. For now, the plan is to keep taking it every eight weeks.*

Infliximab helps heal fistulas. One major study found the standard dose closed all fistulas in 55 percent of those taking it. This compares to 13 percent of people receiving a placebo.[17] Infliximab is currently undergoing testing on those with ulcerative colitis. A small, recent study reports that taking infliximab is beneficial for these people, too.[18]

Side effects

Infliximab can cause a variety of side effects. Common ones include headache, nausea, vomiting, and respiratory infection. Reactions such as itching, fever, chills, rash, chest pain, or breathing difficulties can also occur following an infusion. Most doctors recommend getting a chest x-ray and tuberculosis skin test before receiving the first dose, because infliximab may activate a latent tuberculosis infection.[19]

Mary's son had a reaction to infliximab:

> My son was diagnosed with Crohn's 13 years ago as a young
> teenager. He's also had arthritis along with his GI symptoms. Not too
> long ago, he had his first infusion of Remicade and it worked
> wonderfully. However, he didn't have a second infusion till six months
> later. Within the first minute of this second infusion, he developed
> shortness of breath, a fast heart rate, and his face turned bright red.
> The Remicade was immediately stopped and the nurse gave him
> intravenous Benadryl, an antihistamine. This brought the reaction
> under control. Within a half-hour, he was able to resume the
> Remicade infusion at a much slower rate. The doctor recommended
> that from now on he receive Remicade every eight weeks to prevent
> this kind of allergic reaction.
>
> Having the regular infusions has been a good thing for him. He still
> takes a Benadryl with each infusion, but he doesn't have any reaction
> anymore. Even better, the Remicade works like a miracle for him. It's
> very effective for controlling both his Crohn's and arthritis. It's given
> him a new lease on life.

Antidiarrheal drugs

Many people with IBD highly value antidiarrheal drugs such as loperamide
(Imodium) and diphenoxylate with atropine (Lomotil) because they minimize one of
IBD's most dreaded symptoms. Loperamide is especially popular because it is avail-
able over the counter.

Antidiarrheal drugs slow down the mechanical motion of the bowel; they don't eliminate IBD inflammation.

Dosage and benefits

Before taking any over-the-counter medication, talk with your doctor about the drug
and the proper dosage. Most people take an initial 4-mg dose (two capsules) of
loperamide. You can then take another 2 mg (one capsule) after every loose stool, as
long as you don't exceed 16 mg in one day. A typical starting dose of diphenoxylate
with atropine is two tablets four times a day (20 mg per day).

Once diarrhea has improved—usually within two days if not sooner—most people take lower doses on an as-needed basis. Others start with lower amounts, or only take an antidiarrheal drug when they need to get through an important event without having to run back and forth to the bathroom. Some people take their antidiarrheal drugs before bedtime, to ensure a good night's sleep.

Side effects

Side effects of antidiarrheal drugs include constipation, abdominal pain, and nausea. They can also cause drowsiness or dizziness, but this is uncommon. Doctors generally recommend people not take these medications during severe flare-ups because they can—although very rarely—cause toxic megacolon. Even though these antidiarrheal drugs don't cause dependence, most gastroenterologists prefer to use other therapies to treat IBD inflammation, rather than just treat the symptoms. When inflammation subsides, loose stools improve or go away without your needing to take an extra antidiarrheal drug.

Jamie uses antidiarrheal drugs cautiously:

> I've occasionally taken Imodium when my diarrhea is bad.
> However, most of the time, I don't. I dislike taking so many drugs, and
> I certainly don't want to mask what's really going on with my disease.
> I reserve it for times when I need to be out doing things and I don't
> want to have an accident.

Pain medication

Pain medications can play an important role in managing one of IBD's most unpleasant symptoms. Some people with Crohn's and ulcerative colitis use oral pain medications such as hydrocodone with acetaminophen (Vicodin) or acetaminophen with codeine (Tylenol with codeine) to get through difficult periods until other IBD medications bring their disease under control. Drugs such as IV morphine are commonly prescribed following surgery. Used properly, these medications are not habit forming. It's best to work closely with your doctor to determine the right drug, dose, and duration of time you should take such drugs. Common side effects of prescription pain medications are dizziness, disorientation, nausea, constipation, and sweating. Some gastroenterologists prefer not to prescribe pain medications because they can cause bowel spasms or a rebound of more pain as they wear off.

Jamie uses pain medication sparingly:

> *I really don't like taking pain medication. My first choice is always just plain Tylenol, but that doesn't really work for serious Crohn's pain. So when it gets bad, I'll take a Vicodin. It makes me feel strange. It's hard to describe, but I feel rather disassociated from my body. I suppose that's actually a good thing when you're in severe pain, but I honestly don't like that doped-up feeling. However, it does help with the pain. But like Imodium, I reserve it for times when I really need it.*

Antispasmodic drugs

Antispasmodic drugs such as dicyclomine (Bentyl) or propantheline (Pro-Banthine) are occasionally used to control cramping. Like antidiarrheals, they do nothing to treat IBD inflammation. They inhibit a particular chemical in the body that slows down the GI tract and its secretions.

Dosage and benefits

A common starting dose for dicyclomine is 20 mg four times per day, taken on an empty stomach. If this isn't effective, most adults can take as much as 160 mg per day. Doctors typically prescribe 7.5 to 15 mg of propantheline three times per day. These medications are best used to provide temporary relief from cramping until other IBD therapies bring the disease under control.

Side effects

Dicyclomine and propantheline have similar side effects. In addition to constipation, they can cause dry mouth, dry skin, decreased sweating, and sensitivity to bright light.

Experimental therapies

Many other therapies for Crohn's disease and ulcerative colitis are undergoing testing. Some agents are commercially available, because they are already approved for different uses. However, this doesn't necessarily mean they are safe for people with IBD. Newer compounds are unavailable for commercial use, because they are unapproved by government agencies. Researchers are still testing them for safety and effectiveness.

The following sections review some of the more promising therapies that are either already available or will perhaps arrive on the market soon.

Natalizumab (Antegren)

Natalizumab (Antegren) is one of a new group of medications called selective adhesion molecule (SAM) inhibitors. Like infliximab, it is also a biological agent. Natalizumab binds to a specific molecule—known as alpha-4 integren—which is present on the surface of certain types of immune cells. By attaching in this manner, it prevents these immune cells from traveling to inflamed intestinal tissue where they can cause more damage. A recent study of 248 people with moderate to severe Crohn's found that 71 percent of people who had two infusions of natalizumab (at a dose of 3 mg per kg body weight) experienced a significant improvement in their symptoms.[20] Larger studies with it over a longer period of time are currently underway. Natalizumab may be the next drug approved by the Food and Drug Administration (FDA) to treat Crohn's disease.

Onercept

Onercept is a protein that binds to tumor necrosis factor alpha ($TNF\alpha$). As mentioned in the infliximab section earlier in this chapter, $TNF\alpha$ is a chemical associated with IBD inflammation. By binding to $TNF\alpha$, onercept may effectively neutralize the effect of this inflammatory chemical. One small study demonstrated onercept was helpful for the majority of people with Crohn's.[21] However, larger and more controlled studies are needed to determine its safety and effectiveness.

Thalidomide

Thalidomide is a sedative originally introduced in the early 1960s. It was quickly pulled off the market because it was found to cause severe birth defects. The FDA approved the drug in 1998 to treat a skin disorder associated with leprosy, but doctors who prescribe it must register with a special thalidomide prescription safety program.

Thalidomide is currently undergoing study for people with Crohn's disease. It's unknown exactly how it works, but it's thought to inhibit tumor necrosis factor alpha. Doses of 50 to 300 mg per day seem to help reduce Crohn's symptoms and may help close fistulas.[22] However, more studies are needed. Very strict protocols are used when taking thalidomide, because it can cause severe birth defects.

Newer immunosuppressive drugs

Tacrolimus (Prograf) and mycophenolate mofetil (Cellcept) are two newer immuno-suppressive drugs that are approved to prevent rejection of transplanted organs. Because doctors have had some success using cyclosporine to treat IBD, it was only natural to hope these drugs might have something to offer people with Crohn's and colitis as well. Initial reports on tacrolimus indicate it may work better than cyclosporine. One small study found it induced remission quickly in the majority of people taking it.[23] It also seems to maintain remission, and may help heal fistulas. More studies are needed.

Mycophenolate mofetil has been used as a substitute for azathioprine or 6-MP. So far, it appears less effective overall and is associated with more side effects.[24] Like other experimental therapies, researchers need to design well-controlled studies to properly assess the drug.

Nicotine

The relationship between smoking and IBD is interesting. As mentioned in Chapter 1, *Introduction to IBD,* smoking seems to reduce ulcerative colitis symptoms. Some have therefore proposed that nicotine therapy might prove effective for treating this form of IBD. One study found that nicotine patches were beneficial for 39 percent of people with mild to moderate ulcerative colitis who were also taking other medications. Only 9 percent in the group using placebo patches experienced improvement.[25] Nicotine patches, however, may not be useful for maintaining remission. A well-designed study found them no more beneficial than a placebo.[26]

Nicotine patches have many side effects. Thus, researchers have developed a nicotine enema that works topically and has fewer negative effects. A preliminary study found it reduces inflammation and helps with symptoms,[27] but more research is needed to demonstrate its true effectiveness.

Because the hazards of smoking are so numerous, do not start or resume the habit to help your IBD. The terrible cost of smoking is not worth the theoretical benefit it might offer those with ulcerative colitis.

Helminths

Helminths are parasitic worms. Researchers at the University of Iowa are currently studying whether ingesting helminth eggs can help people with IBD. In 1999, when five of the first six people to receive this experimental treatment went into remission, major newspapers throughout the United States reported this interesting story. The doctors involved with the study suspect IBD may result from living in an environment that is too "clean." This theory helps explain why IBD is generally present only in Western, industrialized societies that have high sanitation standards. The researchers believe parasitic worms and their eggs somehow reduce the production of chemicals that cause inflammation.[28] Thus, they feel that failing to acquire parasites in the GI tract may somehow predispose people to IBD. Controlled studies are needed to see if this theory is correct.

Treatments for IBD have come a long way over the last 60 years. Although still far from ideal, people with IBD have many more treatment options than in the recent past. With continued research, many more will be coming soon.

Gina, who's had Crohn's for over twenty years, sums up her feelings on taking medication for her disease:

> *I've taken a lot of medication over the years. I have to say that for a long time, I was quite resentful that I had to do so. It's especially frustrating when you're doing everything right, and taking your medications like you're supposed to, and yet you still remain sick. It's not fair, but I guess that's just the way it sometimes is.*
>
> *In recent years, I've become more at peace with taking medication. Of course, it's been much easier now that I've been well for so many years and don't have to take as much as I used to. However, I can accept the fact that these drugs have helped improve the quality of my life. In fact, I may have not been able to get so healthy without them. So I'm very thankful that I have these options available.*
>
> *I'm one of the lucky ones. Not everyone can find a combination of medications that works without experiencing side effects. For this, I am extremely grateful.*

For a list of reference books on the medications used to treat IBD and other illnesses, see the "Drugs" section in the *Resources* appendix.

CHAPTER 6

Surgical Treatments

PEOPLE WITH IBD generally respond favorably to medications. However, some individuals with severe Crohn's disease or ulcerative colitis develop excessive inflammation or complications that require surgical intervention.

Having an operation is a major undertaking. Risks are involved and complications are possible. People with IBD facing complete removal of their colon may have concerns about living with a bag attached to their abdomen for the rest of their life. Yet for many people with Crohn's and ulcerative colitis, surgery is sometimes the passport to a life free of disease. The renewed health made possible by surgery can last for many years or a lifetime.

This chapter begins with a discussion of how people with IBD determine whether surgery is a good choice. It then reviews the many different surgical procedures currently available for treating ulcerative colitis and Crohn's. Next, it covers how to prepare for your surgery, including what to expect before, during, and after your operation.

Reasons for surgery

Surgery is usually performed for one of two reasons: It's an urgent or emergency situation in which without the operation either you might die or suffer serious consequences, or you've decided on an elective procedure to try to improve the quality of your life. The following sections discuss these two situations.

Emergencies or urgent situations

Surgery is sometimes unavoidable. At other times, your life may not be in immediate danger, but you still need surgery as soon as possible, to have the best chance of preventing long-term problems. Following are some examples of emergencies or urgent situations that warrant surgery.

- **Abscess.** An abscess is a collection of pus, consisting of mostly white blood cells and bacteria. Abscesses often form when intestinal contents leak out of the bowel into the abdominal cavity. If not drained from the body, infection can spread throughout the abdomen and eventually lead to septicemia (infection in the bloodstream).

Jamie's Crohn's disease was diagnosed when she needed emergency surgery to drain an abscess:

> *I was feeling so sick that I felt I needed to go to the emergency room.*
> *I had a high fever, I was vomiting, and I was in horrible pain. It turned*
> *out I had a grapefruit-sized abscess in my abdomen. While cleaning it out*
> *during surgery, they also discovered I had Crohn's disease, something I'd*
> *never heard of before. It was good thing I went to the ER when I did. If the*
> *infection had spread, I might not have survived.*

- **Cancer or dysplasia.** Cancer and dysplasia (precancerous changes in the lining of the bowel that often predict the presence of cancer elsewhere in the intestine) usually don't require emergency surgery. However, there is a sense of urgency when they are discovered. Because cancer is life threatening, it's best to remove it as soon as possible.

Heather felt unprepared to face her diagnosis:

> *It was difficult to accept that I had colon cancer. It seemed so unreal.*
> *I didn't want to have surgery since I knew there was a chance I'd have*
> *to wear a bag the rest of my life. But if I wanted to have a rest of my life,*
> *I knew I had to have the surgery. My surgeon was able to remove the*
> *cancerous section of my colon and reconnect the two healthy ends—*
> *so I can still eliminate normally. Fortunately, throughout all of this I*
> *'ve had very supportive parents.*

- **Fistulas.** Fistulas, which are abnormal channels between the bowel and other organs, generally don't require emergency surgery. But they can create urgent situations, especially if the intestinal contents are emptying into the bladder.

Gina describes her experience:

> *After having Crohn's for many years, I began to notice a strange*
> *sensation when urinating. It felt as if I were passing some air just as I*
> *finished voiding. During this time I also had a urinary tract infection.*
> *I was given antibiotics and they helped. But the infection returned soon*
> *after I finished the course of medication. My doctor was concerned and*

*suspected a fistula to my bladder. However, he really wanted to
make sure this was the problem. He told me to sit in a bathtub while
urinating to see if any air bubbles came also came up. Unfortunately,
some did. TPN and bowel rest were discussed as an option, but my
doctor and I decided to go with the surgery right away. Since the
Crohn's wasn't getting better either, I had to have an intestinal
resection during the same surgery as the fistula removal and bladder
repair. Everything is fine now and the fistula has never returned.*

- **Obstruction.** Obstructions—especially complete blockages in the intestine—are very dangerous. Often surgery is immediately performed to remove the obstructed portion of intestine.

- **Perforation.** Perforations—or holes in the intestine—that develop slowly generally lead to abscesses or fistulas. If a tear develops suddenly, however, intestinal contents quickly escape from the bowel. This usually results in peritonitis, a potentially fatal condition involving infection and inflammation of the abdominal cavity.

Stacy describes a sudden perforation:

> *During a flare several years after my diagnosis, I suddenly felt a
> very intense pain. I knew something really bad had just happened, but
> I didn't know what. My husband tried to drive me to my doctor's
> hospital some distance away, but we had to stop at one closer. From
> there, they sent me in an ambulance to my doctor's hospital. My
> memory at this point isn't too clear, but I recall they did some tests
> and determined I had a perforated bowel. I had emergency surgery,
> but I already had peritonitis. When I came out, they told my husband
> that they didn't know if I would make it. I was in ICU for three days,
> and then stayed in the hospital for a month. I made it, but it was a
> close call.*

- **Severe bleeding.** Some people with severe inflammation can lose a lot of blood quickly. Surgery is often necessary to remove the severely inflamed intestine.

Nathan explains:

> *After having bouts of ulcerative colitis for about a year and a half,
> I was hospitalized. I was on complete bowel rest, receiving TPN, and
> on high doses of intravenous corticosteroids. Despite these measures,
> I was still having a lot of rectal bleeding and required several blood*

transfusions. But the bleeding wouldn't stop. I essentially had no choice but to have a colectomy since the bowel rest and IV medication weren't working.

- **Toxic megacolon.** Toxic megacolon is a complication of severe colitis in which the colon loses its muscular tone and becomes paralyzed. Perforation can result if the colon is not removed in time. For more information, see Chapter 4, *Complications*.

Elective surgeries

Deciding whether to have surgery is difficult, especially if your life is not immediately at stake. People usually choose to have an operation once they and their physician determine that the benefits outweigh any risks. However, making this decision is not always easy. What one person is willing to put up with is often quite different from what another will tolerate. It all depends on how you view the quality of your life.

Here are some situations that may indicate IBD is significantly affecting your quality of living:

- **You are unable to work or go to school.** Although it's common to miss a few days of work or school due to an IBD flare, some people with Crohn's or ulcerative colitis may have to take weeks or months off when they get sick. Some become so chronically ill that they are unable to hold a job or keep up with their studies.

- **You have developed other problems from long-term use of medications.** Long-term use of certain drugs, such as prednisone, can cause serious side effects. Unfortunately, some people with IBD have difficulty tapering off medications without having a major flare-up. However, if they remain on high doses of drugs to keep IBD under control, they may develop problems such as cataracts, depression, or osteoporosis.

- **You've missed out on too many things for too long.** Some people with IBD are frustrated they are unable to participate in activities that make them happy. Those with severe cases of Crohn's or ulcerative colitis may have difficulty just getting out of the house, because of low energy or frequent diarrhea. Others may have to avoid or limit pleasurable activities such as travel, sports, and other hobbies or recreation if their IBD symptoms interfere.

- **You are not growing or developing normally.** Some children or teenagers with Crohn's or ulcerative colitis are physically small for their age. IBD can cause loss of appetite or inability to digest foods appropriately, so malnutrition may result. Lack of nutrients is especially harmful for children, because it almost always affects their growth and development.

Some people with IBD have difficulty making a decision whether to have surgery, even if they fall into one of the categories just described. This is normal. For elective procedures, there's generally no need to make a quick decision. It's okay to take the time you need to make a decision with which you feel comfortable.

Clarissa tells how she came to her decision:

> Ten years ago, my Crohn's became very severe. I had a lot of diarrhea and was so fatigued that I had difficulty taking care of my family. I have four kids. At the time they ranged from one to ten years. On most days when my husband went to work, I'd have friends and neighbors take my children to their houses since I could barely tend to my basic needs, much less theirs. It was very frustrating to be unable to care for my children. I was also on a lot of medication, and my body was not responding to it. It became clear to me that I needed to have surgery.
>
> The only problem was that I was under pressure from certain friends and family members not to have it. They thought I shouldn't take the risk. I took their arguments into consideration, but concluded that I didn't agree with them. I decided to have the surgery, and I have no regrets. I've still had plenty of problems with Crohn's since the operation, but at least I've been well enough to raise my children.

Cathy chose not to have surgery:

> I have a major case of Crohn's, but so far have decided not to have surgery. I have extensive inflammation throughout my bowel. They could do surgery to remove the worst part, but my doctor was not optimistic about this providing me much relief for very long. He said it might help for six months. Maybe up to two years if I was lucky. Those odds don't sound good to me. It wouldn't be worth going through surgery.
>
> To be honest, I'm not happy with the quality of my life. However, I am able to maintain my weight. I'm coping with my situation and making the best of it. I'm not saying I wouldn't ever have surgery, but right now it doesn't seem like the best option.

Surgeries for ulcerative colitis

About one third of people with ulcerative colitis have surgery to remove their large intestine. Because ulcerative colitis doesn't affect the small bowel, removing the entire colon prevents the disease from recurring. Having a complete colectomy is considered a cure for ulcerative colitis.

People with ulcerative colitis usually have several surgical options. The two most commonly used today are the Brooke ileostomy and the J-pouch.

Brooke ileostomy

An ileostomy is a surgical creation of an opening in the abdomen that allows for the elimination of intestinal contents from the ileum (end of the small intestine). It is usually performed in conjunction with the removal of the colon. This procedure was perfected by a British surgeon named Bryan Brooke in the early 1950s. Although there are now other options, it is still a commonly performed surgery for those whose ulcerative colitis does not respond to medications.

Julie had ileostomy surgery in the late 1950s:

> I've had an ileostomy for well over 40 years. I was very sick with ulcerative colitis in the years before my surgery, and missed a lot of school. My growth was severely delayed, and I even dropped to 50 pounds at one point. When I finally had my surgery at the age of 16, I quickly regained my health. For a while, I gained a pound a day, and eventually caught up with my peers. I have never had a recurrence of my disease.
>
> I know there are other options now. But it's interesting how they are still doing the same surgery over 40 years later. One thing that has changed, however, is the choices we have for appliances. Back then, there were few options—and none of them were particularly good, at least by today's standards. But now, they have bags to suit almost anyone's needs. There are so many choices that it is almost overwhelming.

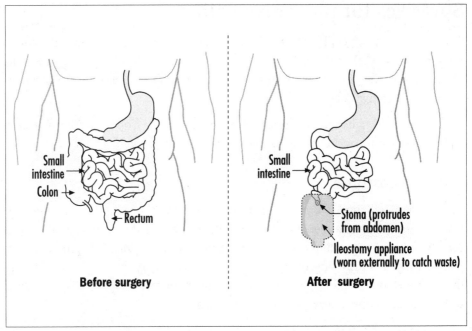

Figure 6-1. Colectomy with Brooke ileostomy

The procedure

A Brooke ileostomy is performed in one operation. First, the colon is surgically removed. Depending on the person's condition and whether there is a chance he can eliminate through his anus in the future, the rectum is sometimes left in place. The surgeon then takes the end of the ileum, pulls it through the abdominal surface, and then folds it back on itself, much like you'd fold the end of your shirtsleeve if it were too long. He then attaches the end of the ileum to the abdomen. This end segment of intestine, which protrudes about ½ to 1 inch, is called the stoma. The stoma is bright red, because it is made from the inner lining of the small bowel. Intestinal contents drain from the stoma into a bag—sometimes called an appliance—that the person wears on his abdomen. The consistency of ostomy output varies. Typically, it ranges from semiliquid to a thick, pasty consistency.

What to expect after surgery

Recovery time after ileostomy surgery can vary, but many people can return to school or work in six to eight weeks. If you were very sick before your surgery, you may need more time to regain your strength.

People who have ileostomy surgery generally have fewer long-term problems than those who undergo other procedures for ulcerative colitis. However, complications such as postoperative infection or small-bowel obstruction can occur. For more information on this topic, see "Complications" in the "After surgery" section later in this chapter.

It's important to learn as much as you can about living with an ostomy—or at least as much as you feel comfortable learning—before your surgery. This way, there will be few surprises after your operation. To assist you in this effort, your surgeon will refer you to an enterostomal therapy (ET) nurse. ET nurses specialize in ostomy care and are a valuable resource for people undergoing this type of surgery Of course, in an emergency situation there is little time to prepare.

Adjusting to an ostomy is difficult for some people. It's only normal that you will require some time to adapt to your new way of eliminating. For more information on living with an ostomy, please see Chapter 11, *Life with an Ostomy*.

J-pouch

The J-pouch, also known as the ileal pouch-anal anastomosis (IPAA) or ileoanal pull-through, is the number one choice today for people with ulcerative colitis facing surgery. Developed in the late 1970s, this surgery involves removing the colon and then creating an internal pouch attached to the anus. Most people prefer it because it lets them eliminate feces the normal way. There's no need to wear a bag to catch waste.

Nathan explains why he chose the J-pouch:

> *I had three choices: the standard ileostomy, the Kock pouch, or the J-pouch. I decided against the Kock pouch, as I had heard of people having valve slippage problems. I knew I could handle a standard ileostomy, but I figured I'd try the J-pouch first. If that didn't work, they could always convert it to a standard ileostomy. I wasn't too concerned with body image. But since I had a choice between having an external appliance or not, I chose the J-pouch. I have large dogs, and when we play, it's probably better not to have a stoma on my abdomen. I've had the J-pouch now for fourteen years and all is well.*

The J-pouch procedure

J-pouch surgery is performed in either one or two operations. If done in two steps, the first surgery involves removal of the colon and rectum. However, the upper anal canal and anal sphincter muscles are left in place. A J-shaped pouch is then made from approximately the last 30 cm of ileum (end of the small intestine). The surgeon then brings the pouch down and attaches it to the anus. To let this newly connected area heal properly, the surgeon creates an opening in a section of the ileum above the pouch. She then brings this opened loop of bowel through the abdominal wall. As a result, intestinal contents are diverted away from the internal pouch and empty through this new, temporary opening, called a loop ostomy. An external pouch is worn on the abdomen to catch the waste. However, this external appliance is only needed for a short time.

After about three months of healing and regaining strength, the person has the second surgery, in which the temporary loop ostomy is removed. Intestinal contents can now empty into the internal pouch and are eliminated through the anus.

Some people can have J-pouch surgery with only one operation. After the colectomy and construction of the pouch, no temporary ostomy is created. Intestinal contents are not diverted and instead flow directly into the pouch as soon as the person resumes eating.

The best candidates for having one surgery are those who are in good physical condition and are not too sick at the time of the operation. The major advantages of having it done all at once are that you only undergo one surgery and you don't need the temporary ostomy. The major disadvantage is that it is sometimes difficult recovering from a colectomy while dealing with the multiple bowel movements that are common during the first months after the surgery. In addition, there is a greater chance of having a serious infection after a one-stage procedure.

When to avoid J-pouch surgery

Not everyone with IBD is an ideal candidate for the J-pouch. This procedure is not recommended for people with Crohn's disease. If Crohn's were to recur in the pouch—and it could, because it is made from the small intestine—excessive diarrhea, bleeding, abscesses, and fistulas might result. The risk to quality of life is too great. Also, someone who has excess fat in the abdominal area is not a good candidate. In these cases, it sometimes isn't possible to stretch the end of the ileum to the anus. Abdominal fat also makes surgery more difficult and slows healing.

People with ulcerative colitis whose anal sphincter muscles are damaged should not have the procedure, because the risk of incontinence is too high. Also, anyone who has had cancer in the rectum cannot have a J-pouch. It's necessary to remove all of

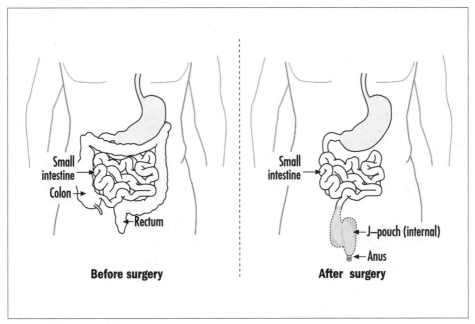

Figure 6-2. Colectomy with J-pouch

the rectum and anus to eliminate the malignancy; therefore, there would be no way to eliminate normally.

What to expect after surgery

Recovery time from J-pouch surgery varies. If you're having the two-step procedure, the first surgery is the major one. You'll probably need at least six to eight weeks to recover. Between your first and second operation, you'll also have to wear a bag on your abdomen at all times to collect your waste products. Some people have difficulty adjusting to an ostomy, even when they know they'll only have it for a short time. For information on coping with an ostomy, see Chapter 11.

The second operation is less complex. However, it can sometimes take just as much time to get back to your normal routine as it did after the first surgery. It depends on how long it takes your stools to normalize. It's not uncommon to have ten to fifteen watery stools per day in the weeks following your surgery. Soiling your underpants during this period is a possibility as you learn to figure out whether you have to pass gas, go to the bathroom, or can hold it. In time, however, your bowel movements will thicken and have a pasty consistency. Once fully recovered, most people have somewhere between four and nine bowel movements per 24-hour period. Some people may have to get up and eliminate overnight, whereas others don't.

Many people with the J-pouch have burning or discomfort around their anal area. Because your stool—fresh from your small intestine—contains many digestive enzymes, it can irritate your perianal skin. Your doctor or other member of your health care team can recommend specific creams or ointments that easily solve this problem.

Krystal recalls what it was like after her second surgery:

> Initially, I had a lot of bowel movements—well over ten a day. They were very watery. I always had what I call burning butt syndrome. It was just awful. Sitz baths helped, and so did using a special over-the-counter cream. It took about four or five months till I achieved what I now call normal. I go about seven or eight times a day. My stools aren't runny, but they are soft. I also take Lomotil, a drug that slows down my digestive tract. Additionally, I eat Metamucil wafers since they help to bulk up my stool.

Complications are a possibility after J-pouch surgery. One problem specific to this procedure is pouchitis, an inflammation of the ileal-anal pouch. Symptoms can include diarrhea, bleeding, fatigue, and fever. Approximately a third of people who've had J-pouch surgery develop pouchitis at least one time. And unfortunately, about half of these people have pouchitis chronically. No one knows exactly why this inflammation occurs, but most doctors agree it is not a recurrence of ulcerative colitis. Instead, many physicians believe an overgrowth of bacteria in the pouch is a major factor, because antibiotics such as Flagyl and Cipro are often effective remedies. Doctors have also recently discovered that probiotics—bacteria beneficial to the digestive tract—can help prevent flare-ups of chronic pouchitis.[1]

Nathan describes his problems with pouchitis:

> After a year and a half with my J-pouch, I developed my first episode of pouchitis. It almost felt like I had colitis again. I went from my normal five times a day to at least ten or twenty urgent bowel movement per 24-hour period. I had cramps, gas, a slight fever, and a yellowish discharge in my stools. My doctor gave me a ten-day course of antibiotics, and it went away. However, it came back about once every year for the next several years. Each time, I took either Flagyl or Cipro for ten days. However, after a while, the pouchitis came back as soon as I stopped the medication. I consulted with my surgeon, and

> *he recommended that I stay on a maintenance dose of Cipro all the time. I've been on this now for almost seven years, and the pouchitis has not returned.*

Other serious complications can result after having J-pouch surgery, such as abdominal infection and small bowel obstruction. For information on these problems, see "Complications" in the "After surgery" section later in this chapter.

People who have a J-pouch are generally very happy with their quality of life. In one study comparing people who had colectomies, people who opted for the J-pouch reported the highest quality of life.[2] Furthermore, despite the risk of complications, the pouches have held up well over time. One study found that after ten years 91 percent of people who had had this procedure still had a functioning pouch.[3]

Kock pouch

A third but less common option for people with ulcerative colitis facing surgery is the Kock pouch. It's commonly called a continent ileostomy because a person can control the release of his waste products, unlike what is possible with the standard Brooke ileostomy. Developed by a Swedish surgeon in the late 1960s, the Kock pouch procedure involves removing the colon and creating an internal pouch that empties via a valve on the abdominal surface.

Laura decided the Kock pouch was her best option:

> *The Kock pouch was the best choice for me. I had years of unrelenting diarrhea with my ulcerative colitis. When I heard that people with the J-pouch still go the bathroom seven or eight times a day, I knew I wouldn't be able to handle that. Although I could live with a bag, I preferred not to have one. So the Kock pouch was the logical choice. I have continence, and only need to empty it about three or four times a day. I'm fairly quick with emptying it; I only take about three minutes. I spend a lot less time in the bathroom than most people with healthy colons!*

The procedure

A Kock pouch procedure generally involves only one operation. First, a colectomy is performed. Then the surgeon takes 45 cm of the ileum to construct a pouch that connects to the abdominal surface. The end of the ileum is then used to make a stoma that is flush with the abdomen. This stoma also acts as a one-way valve that

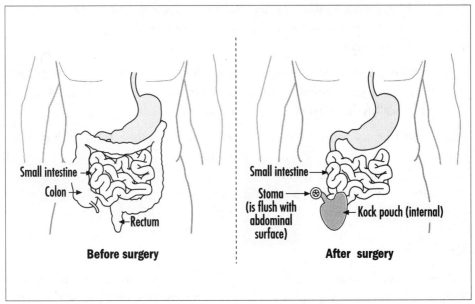

Figure 6-3. Colectomy with Kock pouch

keeps intestinal contents from draining out. The person uses a special catheter to empty the pouch when full. He must carry the catheter with him at all times.

Reasons to have the procedure

Kock pouches are an appropriate alternative for people with ulcerative colitis who have poor or no anal sphincter function. Those who already have ileostomies can also convert to one if they no longer wish to wear an external appliance. The Kock pouch is not recommended for anyone with Crohn's disease. Because the pouch is made from small-bowel tissue, the risk of inflammation developing in the pouch is high.

What to expect after surgery

The Kock pouch procedure requires the usual six- to eight-week recovery period that's typical after major surgery. For the first couple of weeks after the operation, a catheter is placed through the stoma so the pouch is free to drain. After this period, it's a good idea to empty the pouch every couple of hours. Because the ileostomy is continent, there's no need for an external appliance. However, most people put some sort of covering over the stoma—such as gauze—as it discharges mucus from time to time.

The pouch's capacity is limited at first. However, after a few months, it generally can hold about a half a liter (two cups) of stool. In time, you'll probably only have to intubate (place the catheter in to drain) four or five times per 24-hour period. It generally takes most people approximately five minutes to empty the reservoir, and then wash the catheter.

Complications

Postoperative infection and small-bowel obstruction are possible, as they are after other major abdominal operations. However, certain complications are specific to continent ileostomies.

One of the most common problems is valve slippage. When this happens, not only does it become difficult to drain the pouch, but gas and stool can leak out between intubations. Slippage can occur for various reasons. Excessive pressure in the abdominal region—from certain types of exercise, heavy coughing, or sneezing—can promote valve slippage, especially in the months after surgery. So can waiting too long between intubations. If you notice signs of slippage, contact your surgeon immediately. Surgery to revise the valve is sometimes necessary. In one large study, 22 percent of people with Kock pouches required surgery to fix their valves within one year of their surgery.[4] This operation generally requires a short hospital stay, and recovery is much quicker compared to the original surgery.

Laura feels fortunate she's never required a valve revision:

> I've been lucky that my valve still functions perfectly after fourteen years. However, I'm sure a lot of it has to do with the fact I had a very skilled surgeon. Also, I treat my Kock pouch with great care. I always rub a generous amount of K-Y jelly lubricant on the end of my catheter before inserting it. I never press on the pouch while emptying it, and never do regular sit-ups. Hopefully, it will continue to do well for a long time to come.

Another common problem is pouchitis. Like people with a J-pouch, those with a Kock pouch can also develop inflammation in their internal reservoir. Symptoms include diarrhea, bleeding, fatigue, and fever. Pouchitis occurs with approximately the same frequency as it does in people with the J-pouch. No one knows what causes it, but overgrowth of bacteria and waiting too long to empty the pouch are correlated with its development. Pouchitis usually responds well to antibiotic treatment. Irrigation—the injection of water into the pouch and then draining it—helps as well. Emptying your pouch more frequently also helps reduce levels of bacteria. Lastly, probiotics are likely to be as useful for preventing recurrences of pouchitis in people with Kock pouches as they are for those with J-pouches.

Thick stool is sometimes a problem for people who have a Kock pouch. If intestinal output is too thick, it can become difficult to drain your reservoir. Or it simply may take too long. To prevent this problem, it's a good idea to keep well hydrated. You may also find certain foods and drinks make your stool more watery. Lastly, if altering your input is not helping, you can always irrigate your pouch. Diluting its contents will make your reservoir much easier to drain.

Laura describes how she handles this problem:

> Thick stools sometimes pose a difficulty. However, there are ways to treat the problem. Everyone is different, but I've found that coffee, seafood, and prune juice help to thin my output. Grape juice used to work for me, but not anymore. I also carry a syringe with me everywhere I go. Most of the time, I inject 60 cc of water to dilute my stool. It then flows out very easily.

Sometimes fistulas can occur in either the pouch or the valve. Depending on where the fistula connects, surgery is often required to fix the problem.

The long-term durability of the Kock pouch is a major concern among people who have chosen or who are considering this surgical option. One follow-up study found that 60 percent of people who underwent this procedure still had their continent ileostomies.[5] The average length of time since their surgery was 15 years, with one person having it almost 22 years. Thirty-six percent had to undergo conversion to a standard ileostomy after an average of 5 years. The rest died of causes unrelated to their surgery.

Kock pouch procedures are not performed very frequently anymore. Since the early 1980s, the J-pouch has become the treatment of choice. With the J-pouch, you not only avoid wearing a bag, but you can eliminate the normal way. Plus, you don't have to worry about carrying a catheter around with you wherever you go. But for certain people with ulcerative colitis, a Kock pouch can be a good choice. If you are considering a Kock pouch, however, make sure to discuss the pros and cons with your surgeon, including how long he expects it will last.

Surgeries for Crohn's disease

People with Crohn's disease require surgery more frequently than those with ulcerative colitis. Over two-thirds of individuals with Crohn's need to have an operation at some point in their life. And up to half undergo a second surgery. Furthermore, surgery does not cure Crohn's disease as it does ulcerative colitis. Because multiple surgeries over a lifetime can result in significant loss of intestine, doctors are cautious about recommending an operation unless there's a good chance it will improve quality of life.

Surgeons perform several different procedures to treat Crohn's. This disease can strike more than just the colon, so the type of operation depends on what part of the GI tract is affected. The following sections describe the most common operations people with Crohn's undergo.

Colectomy with ileostomy

Some people with Crohn's have a very ulcerative colitis-like disease. However, if you have severe Crohn's in your colon, you don't have the same surgical options as those with ulcerative colitis. Instead, you usually have one choice: colectomy with a permanent ileostomy. People with Crohn's colitis are strongly advised to avoid the J-pouch or a continent ileostomy. Because Crohn's can recur anywhere in the GI tract, the internal pouches for these alternative procedures have a high risk of failing, as they are made from small-bowel tissue.

If only part of your colon is diseased, you can elect to have the inflamed section removed. The healthy ends are then sewn or stapled together, and you'll eliminate normally. The problem with this choice is that Crohn's frequently recurs in the remaining parts of the large intestine. If it does, you'll once again face more medical treatment and possibly another surgery. Some people, however, prefer this option, especially if they want to avoid an ostomy for as long as possible.

The worst of Stacy's inflammation was in her rectum:

> I lost a lot of weight and was extremely malnourished. The inflammation was the most severe in my rectum, and the rest of the colon was not great either. My doctor explained that if my rectum had to go, it only made sense to take out my whole large intestine. There'd be no point having an ostomy and still keeping some of my colon. I'd probably still be just as sick and eventually need another surgery. So we decided on a total colectomy with ileostomy. It's been four years now and I'm doing great.

For information on the colectomy with ileostomy procedure, please see the section on Brooke ileostomy earlier in this chapter. If you wish to learn more about living with your ostomy, see Chapter 11.

Operations for abscesses and fistulas

Abscesses and fistulas are caused by perforations (tears) in the GI tract. Unfortunately, people with Crohn's are prone to developing perforations in their intestine, because inflammation commonly penetrates all layers of the bowel.

Abscesses

An abscess is a localized collection of pus, which is made up of mostly bacteria and white blood cells. If you have an abscess in your abdomen, drainage of the resulting infection is necessary.

Hollie had this done in the operating room through an abdominal incision.

> *Twenty years ago I was extremely sick and in the worst pain of my life. My parents rushed me to the hospital, where they determined I had an abscess. Unfortunately, it burst before they had a chance to do anything. I was rushed to the operating room, where they had to open me up to clean out the infection. It was a very dangerous situation, and I almost didn't survive. I'm fortunate to be alive and well today.*

A surgeon can also drain an abscess by inserting a long, thin needle through the abdomen and into the abscess. This method will temporarily relieve the infection, but it sometimes doesn't solve the problem. Because the source of the infection is usually a hole in the bowel, the abscess is likely to recur. Thus, it is often necessary to remove the segment of intestine containing the perforation. The remaining, healthy ends are then sewn or stapled together.

Fistulas

A fistula is a tract between the bowel and another organ, such as the bladder, vagina, skin, or another section of intestine. Not all fistulas require surgery. Some, such as those between two segments of bowel, are often not even noticed. Others are treated successfully with medications such as Flagyl, 6-MP, or Remicade. Also, although it's sometimes a nuisance, some people live with fistulas draining to their skin for many years without much impact on their day-to-day life.

Cathy was fortunate her fistulas responded to medical treatment:

> *I've had a recurring rectal fistula for many years. It came out to my skin, not far from my anus. I'm fortunate that it has always responded*

to Flagyl. I've stayed on the drug for months—and even years—at a time. When I've come off, the fistula has sometimes returned. However, when I go back on the medication, it goes away again. Currently, I've been off Flagyl for many years. Fortunately, there's been no sign of it coming back again.

Surgery is necessary to remove some types of fistulas, such as those connecting to the bladder. The bladder is not designed to hold fecal matter. If intestinal contents empty there, chronic bladder infections—among other problems—result. Your surgeon will remove the perforated segment of intestine, as well as repair the wall of your bladder where the fistula was attached.

Fistulas to the vagina (called rectovaginal fistulas) are often difficult to treat. Occasionally the medications mentioned earlier resolve the problem. But most of the time, surgery is required to eliminate the problem. If the rectal tissue is in otherwise good condition, a flap of rectum can be used as a patch to cover the perforated section, preventing drainage into the vagina. This type of surgery is performed transanally (through the anus). However, if this operation isn't possible, removal of the colon and rectum with an ileostomy is another option.

Stacy never got rid of her rectovaginal fistula until she had surgery:

I had a rectovaginal fistula for ten years. Medication didn't do anything to help it. I didn't specifically have the surgery just to remove the fistula. My Crohn's reached a point where I had little choice other than to have a total colectomy with ileostomy. Since this included the rectum, we got rid of the fistula at the same time.

Resection and anastomosis

A resection and anastomosis is the most common surgical procedure performed on people with Crohn's. It involves removing the diseased segment of bowel and rejoining of the two remaining ends of intestine. The most frequently resected area of the GI tract is between the end of the small bowel and beginning of the large intestine, called the ileocecal region. The length of bowel removed depends on the extent of the inflammation. Your surgeon should operate conservatively, usually cutting no more than 5 cm of healthy intestine on either side of the inflamed section. This ensures that the rejoined ends will have the best chance of healing properly, with minimal loss of healthy bowel.

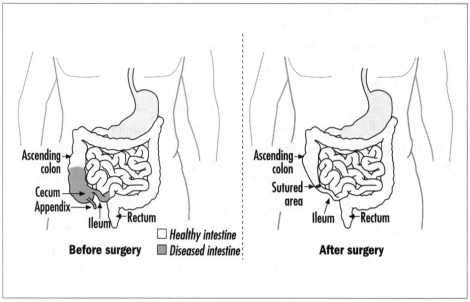

Figure 6-4. Resection and anastomosis

Clarissa describes her experience:

> I've had two small-bowel resections. Each time, they had to take out quite a bit of intestine since the inflammation was so widespread and unresponsive to medication. Normally, they don't like to take out so much, but in my case there wasn't an alternative. Although I've had recurrences and still require medication, the surgeries greatly improved my condition. Without them, I could have never raised my children, much less have been healthy enough to have them in the first place. I know I made the right decision both times.

A resection is a major surgical procedure. For details on what to expect when having a major abdominal operation, see the section called "What to expect" later in this chapter.

Strictureplasty

Strictureplasty is a procedure for widening strictures (narrowed segments of small intestine). Its main advantage over a resection is that it does not involve removal of any bowel. Thus, you don't need to sacrifice precious small intestine to eliminate areas that are partially obstructed.

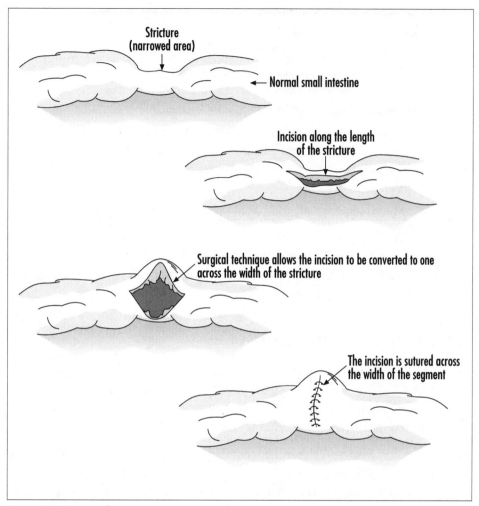

Stricture
(narrowed area)

← Normal small intestine

Incision along the length
of the stricture

Surgical technique allows the incision to be converted to one
across the width of the stricture

The incision is sutured across
the width of the segment

Figure 6-5. Strictureplasty

The procedure is performed by cutting the intestine along the length of the narrowed section. However, the incision is then closed transversely, or across the width of the segment. This widens the previously constricted region (see Figure 6-5). If you have multiple strictures, your surgeon will perform all the strictureplasties in a single operation.

Chuck had this procedure two and a half years ago:

> *I suffered with narrowed areas in my small intestine for seven years. My symptoms included pain and bloating after meals. I was*

fortunate not to have a total obstruction anywhere, but the strictures gradually worsened. I could tell from my symptoms, and my doctor could tell from my barium x-rays.

We decided on strictureplasty since it preserves bowel. I also knew there was a chance that they might have to do a resection if the narrowed areas were too long or too close together.

It turned out I had about a half a dozen strictures. A few of them were close together, so my doctor decided to resect that region. The others were in short segments where he was able to perform stricureplasties.

My recovery went smoothly, and none of the strictures have returned.

Strictureplasty is a major operation, because it involves opening the abdomen. For information on what to expect when having abdominal surgery, see the "What to expect" section later in this chapter.

Recurrence after surgery

People with ulcerative colitis don't have to worry about their disease coming back after surgery (assuming the entire colon is removed). Those with Crohn's who have had any type of surgery, however, frequently have concerns about their disease returning. And the threat of recurrence is very real.

Many researchers have studied recurrence rates of Crohn's following surgery. One large study of almost 2,000 people with Crohn's found that 33 percent had a recurrence of their disease within five years of their resection surgery.[6] The recurrence rate was 44 percent at ten years. Another study reported a rate of 60 percent after fifteen years.[7] The numbers are somewhat better for those people having colectomies with ileostomies. Their recurrence rate is approximately 15 percent, with most of their relapses happening in the first ten years after their operation.[8]

Jamie had a resection five years ago:

I had a rather classic Crohn's flare involving my ileocecal region. I became quite ill and was running out of options. My surgeon described my choices as all "short straws." I didn't want to spend months on TPN, so I opted for a resection. They took out about a foot of intestine from the end of my ileum to the beginning of my colon. I was only in the hospital for five days, which seemed rather short to me. Although I've had some other medical problems following my operation, I didn't have another flare till approximately a year and a half later. We've been able to treat the Crohn's with medications, and I have not needed another operation for my IBD.

Hollie has never had a recurrence after her colectomy and ileostomy:

I had my original ileostomy surgery over twenty years ago, but I didn't have the total colectomy until eight years ago. Since then I have had no recurrence. My doctor said that since the only evidence of Crohn's was in my colon, there's a good chance that it will never come back. I'd say eight years with no problems is a pretty good sign!

Researchers have tried to isolate what factors increase a person's chance of having a relapse after an operation. Variables such as age, sex, duration of disease before surgery, previous surgeries, and extraintestinal complications have been studied. Yet none of them consistently correlate with having a recurrence. One factor that does, however, is smoking. The risk of relapse increases with the number of cigarettes smoked and the number of years a person has smoked.[9,10]

What to expect

It's completely normal to have fears about surgery. No matter how convinced you are that you need it, and no matter how much confidence you have in your surgeon, you may still find yourself worrying about your upcoming operation. However, you can take steps to allay at least some of your concerns. One way is to educate yourself on your particular procedure. When you know what to expect at each stage of the process, your anxiety will probably lessen.

The following sections take a general look at what people with IBD can typically expect before, during, and after most major abdominal surgeries.

Before surgery

Preparation for your surgery frequently begins well before you're admitted to the hospital. With the exception of emergency operations, most of what you need to do is typically done at home or at clinic visits.

Educating yourself

It's a good idea to begin educating yourself about your particular operation as soon as possible. Many resources are available to you:

- **Your healthcare team.** Your primary care physician, gastroenterologist, surgeon, nurse, dietitian, and other healthcare personnel are all wonderful resources. To make the best use of your time with them, take a few moments to prepare your questions before appointments. If you think of more questions later, you can always call and arrange for another appointment. Or perhaps your concerns can be addressed over the phone.

- **Other people with IBD.** Others with Crohn's or ulcerative colitis are great to have around during this time. It's very comforting to know someone who has already been through what you are about to experience. If you don't know anyone who's already undergone your surgery, call your local Crohn's and Colitis Foundation of America (CCFA) office and ask the staff to connect you to a volunteer. The CCFA web site also has links to web sites where people can post messages and receive answers from other people with IBD. Go to *http://www.ccfa.org/* and click on "links."

- **Published resources.** Information on your surgery is available from a variety of sources. Your hospital library is a good starting point for books, brochures, and videotapes. You can also search the Internet. The CCFA web site contains excellent information and has links to many other reputable sites.

Stacy took advantage of all the resources just mentioned:

> *I read as much as I could, and I spoke to as many people as I could. I met a number of people through a CCFA support group who were a great help. In addition to my doctor and enterostomal therapy (ET) nurse, I also asked my doctor if he knew of other patients of his who'd be willing to talk to me. He got their permission, and then I was able to speak to others who had already been through the same surgery. I can't imagine going through such a major thing without all these resources.*
>
> *It's nice now to be on the other side. I tell my doctor to put others in touch with me if they need someone to talk to.*

Preoperative evaluations

Your surgeon will ask about your medical history and will give you a thorough physical examination. The purpose is to identify any other health problems that might affect your surgery. For example, if you have diabetes, heart disease, or lung problems, your surgeon may need to take special precautions during your operation. If you smoke, your doctor will encourage you to quit as soon as possible. If you can't completely stop, reducing the amount you smoke can at least reduce your chances of a postoperative respiratory infection.

It's also very important for your medical team to know of any allergies you have to specific drugs, such as antibiotics or anesthetic medications. Most hospitals also require that you have a separate preoperative appointment with an anesthesiologist.

You may also need to consult with other healthcare professionals before your operation. If you are having ostomy surgery, for example, you'll see an enterostomal therapy (ET) nurse, who specializes in ostomy care. Also, if your doctor suspects you are nutritionally depleted, he may suggest a consultation with a dietitian. Because recovery often takes place more slowly in a malnourished state, a dietitian may suggest taking an oral supplement to supply extra calories and nutrients. If you are unable to eat, intravenous feeding, such as total parental nutrition (TPN), may be recommended.

Tests

It's necessary to undergo various tests before your surgery. Most of this testing involves blood work, but you may also need to have other tests. For instance, your doctor may request an electrocardiogram to evaluate your heart's rhythm and/or a chest x-ray.

Your doctor will order many different blood tests, including a complete blood count (CBC) and a blood-typing test. Even if you have plenty of red blood cells and hemoglobin, blood typing is essential because during major abdominal surgery, transfusion is always a possibility. You'll also need one last blood draw within 48 hours of your surgery. This blood is used for cross-matching. Cross-matching involves mixing your blood with potential donor blood to make sure there are no negative reactions. If you are worried about the safety of donor blood, keep in mind that blood banks in Western, industrialized countries test blood very thoroughly for things such as HIV and hepatitis. However, if you still have concerns, there are sometimes other options. For example, in some areas, you can have trusted friends or family members as designated donors. Because this is not available everywhere, check with your doctor to see if you have this option. It's unusual for people with IBD to donate their own blood a few weeks before surgery because they are often too sick or anemic to do so.

Stacy has used both designated donors and the blood bank:

> I had one transfusion in 1983 at a hospital in San Francisco. This was a couple of years before they tested blood for HIV. Needless to say, I was concerned for many years after it. However, I was tested for HIV several times, and the results always came back negative. Since then, I've had many more transfusions using both the blood bank and blood from family members. I got blood from both my dad and father-in-law. My husband also has the same blood type, but they don't let spouses donate to each other.

Final preparation

The final 24 hours before major abdominal surgery is sometimes difficult. Besides the general stress associated with the anticipation of your operation, you also need to clean out your GI tract. This usually means drinking unpleasant-tasting laxative products, and then spending the next several hours running back and forth to the bathroom. (For information on various alternatives for cleansing your bowels, see Chapter 3, *Diagnostic Procedures*). Your doctor will also prescribe antibiotics. Previously, oral antibiotics used to be given beginning the day before surgery. Now, usually only IV ones are started after you arrive at the hospital. The antibiotics, along with a well-cleaned bowel, help reduce the chances of developing a postoperative infection.

Clarissa recalls having to cleanse her bowel:

> Cleaning out your intestines is never easy. We often think of it only for diagnostic procedures, but you have to do it before surgery, too. I recall I had to drink a gallon of this horrible tasting solution. It had sort of this burnt, oily taste. I'm not sure how I managed to drink it all. But I knew I had to do it—so it was probably sheer determination.

Your doctor will let you know what time to come to the hospital. Once you arrive, a nurse will start an IV so you are well hydrated by the time you enter the operating room. The IV antibiotics are then administered as well. A drug to reduce secretion of stomach acid is usually given, too. If you are currently on corticosteroid drugs such as prednisone—or have been on high doses within the last six months—your doctor may prescribe additional amounts of the medication. Corticosteroids impair your adrenal glands' abilities to produce their own stress hormones. The extra boost of medication may be necessary, because surgery is a major stress on the body. For more information on corticosteroids and how they affect your adrenal glands, see Chapter 12, *Coping with Prednisone*.

The only thing left to do is to wait. And delays are not uncommon. Emergencies can happen any time, and they take precedence over surgeries that aren't. If you find yourself in this situation, try to use the extra time in as positive a way as possible. Instead of worrying or getting stressed out, consider focusing on all the wonderful and fun things you'll be able to do after you recover from your operation. You have a whole new life ahead of you.

Craig waited for a long time before his surgery:

> I was told to come to the hospital around 7:00 A.M., and arrived even earlier. They connected me to all the IVs and I was soon ready to go. However, there were a number of emergencies that day. I waited for hours and hours. By afternoon, I was concerned that my surgery might be canceled. It was frustrating, especially since I drank all that Go-Lytely the day before! I certainly didn't want to go through that again. I tried to relax and focus on my healthy life after my surgery. It wasn't easy. I just wanted the surgery to be over with. However, there really wasn't much I could do to control the timing of the surgery. Finally, around 6:00 P.M., they took me to the operating room. Everything worked out fine, but eleven hours was a long time to wait.

During surgery

There's obviously not much you can do once they wheel you into the operating room. Once you're on the operating table, the anesthesiologist begins giving you medication to put you to sleep. She may use IV medication, inhaled drugs, or a combination of both. The anesthesiologist then carefully monitors you throughout the surgery and continues giving you just the right amounts of medication to maintain your unconsciousness.

Before your operation can begin, a few more tubes are inserted. A catheter is placed in your bladder, because urination isn't possible during or immediately after surgery. A plastic tube is inserted through your mouth and placed in your trachea (your wind pipe, leading to your lungs). This tube is then attached to a machine, called a ventilator or respirator, which breathes for you during surgery. A nasogastric tube (NG tube) is also inserted through your nose, threaded down your esophagus, and placed in your stomach. A suction machine is attached to this tube to remove stomach juices. Lastly, if you require any other IVs, your surgeon or operating room (OR) nurse will place these as well. Aside from the tubes, the only other remaining tasks are to shave your abdomen and then clean it with an antiseptic solution.

Your surgeon can now perform your operation. Typically, most abdominal surgeries for IBD take from two to five hours. You might consider the following:

- **Request music or tapes.** Some people believe that having soothing music or positive affirmation tapes playing in the background can help facilitate a successful surgery. Some audio programs are specifically geared toward people undergoing an operation. Of course, check with your surgeon first to make sure it won't distract him while he's operating.

- **Ask for positive affirmations.** You might consider asking your surgeon or other surgical team members to repeat positive affirmations directly to you during your operation. Some suggestions might include "You have tremendous healing capacity" or "You'll live a long, healthy life."

- **Know who will be performing the surgery.** Your surgeon is always the one in charge of your surgery. However, other doctors, including those who are learning how to perform abdominal procedures, sometimes do a significant portion of the surgery under the head surgeon's supervision. If you're not comfortable with this, talk to your surgeon ahead of time to discuss the pros and cons. Although your surgeon will likely perform the critical portions of the operation, many surgeons prefer to work with one of their colleagues or residents. If after careful consideration you still only want your surgeon performing all of the operation, or prefer that the second surgeon be a colleague rather than a resident, make sure to specify this on the consent form you sign.

Jamie wasn't happy to learn a resident had performed a significant portion of her surgery:

> *I wasn't aware that other surgeons might do some of my operation. I recall while recovering that one resident kept checking in on me. I wasn't sure why. Later, after I was out of the hospital, I read my medical records regarding my operation. I then figured out why that resident kept checking in on me. From what I could tell, she did quite a bit of my surgery. Of course, my surgeon was there the whole time, and he was the one still in charge. But I would have liked to know*

*ahead of time if someone else was going to be operating on me—
especially if it was a resident. I would not have been comfortable
with that. Of course, my operation went fine and there were no
complications. But if I ever have surgery again, I'm going to make
it clear who I want operating on me.*

A gastrointestinal surgeon shares his view:

*Surgery is a bit like riding a tandem bicycle. One person can do it,
but you should consider that it is designed for two if you require the
best performance. I am very prescriptive with our chief residents and
feel that it is both helpful and a good idea to have them assist with
surgery. We do tell patients if a resident will be involved so that they
are aware of who will be performing their operation.*

After surgery

When the surgeon is finished, the anesthesia drugs wear off, thus allowing your
normal bodily functions to resume. Once you are breathing on your own, the anesthesiologist will unhook the respirator and remove the plastic tube from your
trachea. However, the NG tube is usually kept in place, because it may take a few
days for your GI tract to begin working again. The catheter to your bladder will also
remain, because it's often difficult to get up and go to the bathroom for several days
after major abdominal surgery.

Before you wake up, a feeding tube, narrower than the NG tube, may also be placed
up your other nostril, threaded down your esophagus, passed through your stomach,
and set in your duodenum (the first part of your small intestine). Some doctors like
to begin tube feeding—at a very low rate, such as 10 ml per hour—almost immediately after surgery. It sometimes helps the GI tract to return to normal function more
quickly. The NG tube going up your other nostril and down to your stomach is still
necessary, though, to suction gastric juices and any other GI contents that get pushed
back to the stomach. It's not easy having two tubes up your nose, but try to keep in
mind it's only temporary.

You will wake up in a special recovery room. The nurses caring for you will provide
you with medications to keep pain to a minimum. They will also carefully monitor
you for any signs of postoperative complications. During this time, you'll probably
drift in and out of sleep. If your pain becomes too uncomfortable, let one of the
nurses know; they can usually give you more pain medication. Assuming no major
complications, they'll transfer you to a regular hospital room within a few hours.

Richard describes his immediate postoperative experiences:

> *I've had two major surgeries. The first one was a planned colectomy. Everything went fine during the surgery. When I awoke, it felt as if no time had passed. It was a very strange sensation. I couldn't believe that they had time to do anything.*
>
> *My second surgery was an emergency one due to a complete obstruction. There were a number of complications during the surgery, and I was fortunate to survive. Awakening from this one though was a different experience. Perhaps due to the complications arising during the operation, my brain woke up before the paralyzing drugs wore off. It was the weirdest thing. The only thing I could do was hear. I couldn't move, I couldn't open my eyes, and the scariest thing was that I couldn't breathe. I seriously wondered if I was dead. However, I could continue to hear people talking. Since I didn't feel as though I was suffocating, it occurred to me that maybe I was still on the respirator. Although I have no idea how long I was like this, I recall trying to focus on opening my eyes, and soon I was able to do this. I then recall people around me saying, "Oh . . . he's coming around." Indeed, I was in the recovery room, and I was still hooked up to the respirator. My first thought was "Weren't you suppose to take this out before I woke up?" My surgeon was right there and must have read my mind. He said it had been a very difficult surgery and he had to leave the breathing tube in since I was having difficulty breathing.*
>
> *I eventually made a complete recovery from this operation. But it shows how sometimes not everyone has the same experience upon awakening from surgery.*

Recovering in the hospital

Most people having major abdominal surgery for their IBD spend approximately five to ten days in the hospital. The time you spend in the hospital may vary depending on your circumstances. If you were very ill or on corticosteroid medication before surgery, you might have to stay a little longer.

Controlling postoperative pain is instrumental to your recovery. When you have your pain under control, you'll sleep better, feel more relaxed, and have the ability to move around more easily. Today, most people coming out of surgery have the advantage of patient-controlled analgesia (PCA). PCA allows you to control how much pain medication you receive. All you need to do is push a button, and a small amount of medicine is automatically infused intravenously. The PCA is set up so you cannot overdose. Pain medications—even ones such as morphine—are not addictive when used in this manner. Most people only require them for a short period and then taper off gradually.

Clarissa has had two surgeries. She had PCA with the second one:

> I had my first resection in the early 80s. I didn't have PCA with that one. As far as I know, they didn't have it back then. I recall the nurse had to come in and give me some IV pain medicine whenever I needed it.
>
> My second surgery was ten years later. By this time, they had PCA. I must say it was very nice having it. I could control exactly how much I received. I didn't have to worry about getting too much, too little, or having to wait till the nurse had time to bring it to me. PCA is definitely a great advance for giving people some control during their recovery.

Many hospitals also use continuous epidural anesthesia. It's often started in the operating room and maintained postsurgically. A needle is inserted into your back between your vertebrae and placed in an area called the epidural space. A thin catheter (tube) is then threaded through the needle until its tip is also in the epidural space. The needle is removed, but the tube is kept in place and then taped so it doesn't slip out. Anesthetic medication is now infused through the catheter to numb the nerves in your abdominal area. This comes in handy postsurgically, as it greatly reduces the need for IV pain medication. People can be comfortable, yet not have to deal as much with the side effects of intravenous medications.

Major abdominal surgery can cause the normal peristaltic contractions of your GI tract to temporarily cease. Interestingly, having the epidural anesthesia often prevents this from happening. Your nurse will place her stethoscope on your abdomen several times a day to listen for bowel sounds. As soon as she begins to hear normal sounds—which can occur as soon as the first day following surgery but may take longer—you'll start you on a clear liquid diet, consisting of things, such as juice, gelatin, and broth. Assuming all goes well, you can progress to a full liquid diet (puddings, cream of rice, supplement drinks) and then a diet consisting of solid, but soft foods. Once you can eat sufficiently without problems, your nurse can remove both your NG and your feeding tube.

Your medical team will encourage you to get up and move around as soon as possible. Although you may have difficulty imagining yourself standing up and walking the day after your surgery, this is the goal. The more you are sitting up, standing, and walking, the quicker you will recover. You will also lessen the chance of developing a respiratory infection. Even while lying in bed, it's a good idea to move your muscles as much as possible. You can also practice deep breathing exercises with the aid of a small device, called a spirometer, that measures the volume of your breaths. Once you are moving around more easily, your nurse can remove your urinary catheter. At first, you might have some mild burning when eliminating, but it should go away soon. If the burning persists, inform your nurse or doctor. This symptom can indicate a urinary tract infection. You may also experience some cramping in your bladder when urinating, which also is temporary.

It's common to have a fever after surgery. Your body temperature should gradually come back to normal within a week or so. If a fever persists longer or starts going up, it could indicate an infection.

Complications

Complications are always possible after any major surgery. One of the most common of these problems is a postoperative infection, which typically occurs in the surgical wound or inside the abdominal cavity. One study of people with Crohn's found approximately 10 percent had a postoperative infection after surgery.[11] For people with ulcerative colitis undergoing J-pouch surgery, the rate can range from 3 to 7 percent.[12]

Jamie shares what happened to her after her operation:

> Although my surgery involved draining an abscess, others were
> discovered post-surgically. Most likely they were already there before,
> but I would think they would have found them when they were doing
> the original surgery. Anyway, I didn't need to have another major
> surgery. Instead, the surgeon placed a drainage tube into my
> abdomen, using a CAT scan and fluoroscope to guide it into the right
> place. The drainage tube was left in three weeks, allowing any
> drainage to flow into a little bag attached to it. I had to flush the tube
> twice a day with sterile water to help clear out the infection. During
> this time, I was also taking antibiotics. It was uncomfortable have the
> tube in me, but at least it resolved the infection.

One major factor that increases your chance of early complications, such as a post-operative infection, is long-term corticosteroid therapy prior to surgery. Corticosteroids suppress your immune system and can impair your body's ability to heal.

The other major complication of having an abdominal operation is small-bowel obstruction. Bands of scar tissue—called adhesions—can form after intestinal surgery. And unfortunately, the small intestine can sometimes become entangled in these adhesions. When this happens, partial or complete obstruction can occur. Sometimes the obstructions resolve by themselves, and other times further surgery is necessary. One study of people who had Crohn's resections found 14 percent had small-bowel obstruction within fifteen years of their surgery.[13] Another study on people with ulcerative colitis who had J-pouch surgery revealed about 31 percent had problems with obstruction during their first ten years following their operation. Almost 8 percent had to have another surgery to remove the blockage.[14]

Craig was someone who had to undergo a second surgery for his adhesions:

> *I thought after my colectomy and ileostomy that I wouldn't have any more problems. Well, I didn't have any more directly from IBD, but I did have a very dangerous situation happen with adhesions.*
>
> *Eleven months after my surgery I was doing great. There was no sign of IBD and I was once again in good shape. One afternoon, out of the blue, I developed the worst abdominal pain I'd ever had. This says a lot, after all the years I was sick with Crohn's. I knew it wasn't the normal IBD pain—it was something much worse. Within a couple of hours, I had no choice but to go to the emergency room. As soon as I arrived, I began throwing up. I was admitted right away. They put in a nasogastric tube, which helped at first with the pain. The next day they ran some tests, and it was determined I had some sort of blockage. The pain continued to get worse. No pain medication would help. When they noticed that my abdomen was starting to get hard, I was rushed to surgery. It turned out my small intestine had become entangled in some adhesions that developed after my first surgery. Two and a half feet of my intestine had turned gangrenous. I could have easily died. Fortunately, I survived and made a complete recovery. It was amazing how quickly I went from being perfectly fine to almost dead. It was scary.*

The decision to have my first surgery was still a good one, and I'd make it all over again. But I hadn't realized the very real risk of intestinal obstruction following abdominal surgery. What happened to me was extreme, and fortunately it doesn't happen too often.

Recovering at home

Once you are eating and eliminating without complications, your physician will discharge you from the hospital. If you were on IV antibiotics, you can generally switch to oral ones when you go home. If you have special needs that require a home health nurse, your doctor will make these arrangements as well. On discharge, you'll also receive a list of instructions that have many good suggestions for helping you recover as quickly as possible. Here is a list of tips, many of which are probably included in your recommendations:

- Eat a soft diet for six weeks. Then gradually add foods to your diet one by one, making sure they each agree with you.

- Consider eating six or seven small meals throughout the day until you can eat larger amounts of food.

- Drink plenty of fluids. Include drinks with sodium and potassium—such as sports drinks or vegetable cocktail juices—especially if you've had your colon removed.

- Avoid heavy lifting (usually no more than 5 to 10 pounds) for six to eight weeks.

- Avoid exercises that put pressure on abdominal muscles, such as crunches, for at least several months. Regular sit-ups should be permanently avoided. Check with your surgeon to clarify what abdominal exercises are safe for you, given your particular operation.

- Don't drive until you are off all pain medication and feel strong enough to do so.

Most doctors say you should be able to return to your normal activities within six to eight weeks. However, some people with IBD, such as Jamie, take longer:

My surgeon told me I should be back to normal within six weeks. However, I did not feel strong enough to go back to work until after eight weeks. Even then, I could only work half time during the first six weeks I was back. So it took quite a bit longer than they told me. It may have had to do with the fact I was very sick and was on prednisone for a while before the surgery. Anyway, my advice is that each person should listen to his own body, and to try not to worry if they're not at 100 percent by six weeks.

Gina had a similar experience:

> *I really didn't feel I recovered till about four months after my surgery. I've also found talking to others that they have needed longer than what their doctor said, too. I think it is unrealistic to expect that you can just jump back into things so soon. I now always tell people facing surgery that the healing process can take a while. But although it can be a slow process, you do get better. Patience comes in handy.*

Chuck recovered right on schedule:

> *I had a resection and a few strictureplasties to fix the narrowed areas in my small bowel. I was lucky that I had no complications following my surgery. I stayed in the hospital for a week, and recovered at home for the next five. I was fortunate that I was able to return to work as planned.*

Most people with IBD who undergo an operation are glad they did. Although it's a difficult process, surgery has allowed many people with both Crohn's and ulcerative colitis to return to a normal, productive life.

Nathan comments:

> *Surgery was a very positive experience for me. I had severe ulcerative colitis that required a colectomy. I know this might sound unusual to some, but when I woke up in the recovery room, I felt great. I knew that I was going to be well and that the disease was gone. Of course, my recovery took a while, but it was worth it. The surgery is not a perfect solution, but it is so much better than colitis.*

Clarissa expresses her gratitude:

> *I've had two surgeries for my Crohn's. Both of them greatly improved my quality of life. I am so thankful. I'd do them both again in a heartbeat.*

CHAPTER 7

Diet and Complementary Therapies

WESTERN MEDICINE currently has no cure for IBD, with the exception of complete colectomy for those with ulcerative colitis. Although drug and surgical treatments are often helpful, they are usually not completely effective. In addition, they are sometimes risky or cause serious side effects. It's therefore understandable why many people with Crohn's disease and ulcerative colitis use various diets, supplements, and other therapies in an effort to help manage their condition.

This chapter covers how diet and nutritional supplements can help treat IBD. It then reviews the increasing role that complementary therapies are playing in the management of Crohn's disease and ulcerative colitis.

Dietary changes

Many people with IBD change their diet to try to control their symptoms. Although it would be nice if just one diet worked for everyone, this isn't the case. What works wonderfully for your friend at the support group may not necessarily work for you. Moreover, an individual person can have inconsistent reactions to the same foods at different times. However, if you are open to trying different things and can be disciplined about your eating, dietary therapy might help.

The only way to determine whether a specific diet or dietary change is helpful is to try it and see what happens. Keep in mind that it's also important to consult with your gastroenterologist and dietitian before you start a new food program. To find a registered dietitian, visit *http://www.eatright.org/find.html*.

The following sections describe the most common diets or dietary changes that people with Crohn's and ulcerative colitis use to help manage their condition.

Clear liquid diet

The clear liquid diet is generally used for brief periods. You shouldn't stay on it for more than a few days because it doesn't provide all the nutrients you need. A clear liquid diet is typically used to

- Give your bowel a couple days of rest from solid food.
- Be a stepping-stone toward getting back on a regular diet after surgery.
- Clear the colon before a colonoscopy.

A clear diet is used for extended periods of time only if you are also receiving IV feeding or are supplementing your liquids with an elemental diet formula.

The clear liquid diet is very limited. It mainly consists of gelatin, broth, popsicles, and clear juices, such as apple or white grape. Sometimes cranberry juice, lemonade, fruit punch, lemon-lime sodas, or similar drinks are allowed.

Stacy has used clear liquid diets extensively to help control her disease:

> During the years I was really sick, clear liquid diets worked quite well for me. If a low-residue diet didn't work, I'd have to back-pedal another step to clear liquids. Sometimes I'd only need to do it for a few days. But other times I'd be on it for two to four weeks. I had the option of TPN, but my doctor said it was okay to try the clear liquid diet for an extended period, as long as I drank plenty of Vivonex, an elemental supplement drink. This combination really helped control my symptoms. On liquids, I functioned well and could still even go to work.
>
> I have to admit, however, that when you're only eating—or drinking—liquids, it gets old fast. There's not much variety when you can only have gelatin, juice, broth, and popsicles. I haven't been sick in several years. But even to this day, I can't stand gelatin—there are just too many bad memories associated with it.

Cheryl found it a challenge to go on clear liquids:

> There were a few times it got to the point where I couldn't eat anything but liquids for a few days. It's difficult though since there's not much for me to choose from. I try to eat pure foods; so commercial gelatin was out since it's so artificial. I'd pretty much stick to health

food store broth, organic apple juice, and herbal teas. Clear liquids
didn't solve my problems, but at least they helped a little to calm my
bowel.

Dairy-free diet

Some people with IBD are sensitive to milk and other dairy products. Lactose, the sugar found in milk, is sometimes the reason. Many people, including those without Crohn's or ulcerative colitis, can't properly digest lactose. As a result, abdominal discomfort and excess gas can occur. If you suspect you are lactose intolerant, your doctor can prescribe a lactose tolerance test. Or, more commonly, he may simply suggest you avoid lactose-containing foods, to see what happens. If it turns out you're sensitive to lactose, and you still wish to consume dairy products, you can buy lactase (the enzyme that digests lactose) over the counter. Some milk products are fortified with it, so you don't have to buy an extra supplement.

People can have other problems with dairy. Milk proteins, for example, are a common allergen. Also, some people with IBD have difficulty digesting dairy fats. Lastly, some people find that milk products just don't agree with them. If you are unsure whether dairy products irritate your GI tract, consider trying an elimination diet, discussed later in this section.

Cheryl found that dairy products don't agree with her:

> *I'm not able to eat dairy products without consequences. If I do,*
> *pain, cramping, and diarrhea are inevitable. I tried Lactaid, but it*
> *didn't help. My nutritionist said it's probably casein, the protein in*
> *milk, which causes me problems. I also tried eating goat cheese since*
> *some people can handle that better. But that didn't work either. So I*
> *have accepted the fact that I need to avoid all kinds of dairy products.*

Stacy does well with dairy products:

> *In my experience with support groups, it seems as though the first*
> *thing doctors tell people when they are diagnosed is to avoid dairy*
> *products. I understand that some people may truly have a sensitivity*
> *to milk. It certainly makes sense to try eliminating it to see what*
> *happens. But if it doesn't make a difference, I don't see any reason*
> *why people should avoid it. In my case, dairy has never been a*
> *problem. I'm not lactose intolerant. In fact, I've found that cheese*
> *especially helps with diarrhea.*

Elemental diet

An elemental diet consists of the most basic nutrients available. It provides complete nutrition in a liquid formula. Some kinds you can drink, but others are so unpalatable you need to use a feeding tube. Elemental diets are discussed in great detail in Chapter 8, *Alternative Forms of Feeding*.

Elimination diets

Elimination diets help you determine which foods agree and disagree with your system. There are a number of variations on this approach, so it's best to work with a knowledgeable dietitian or physician when trying an elimination diet. Probably the best way to determine your food sensitivities is to start with an elemental diet for about two weeks, or as long as it takes for all or most your symptoms to clear. Then gradually resume normal eating by adding one new food at a time every two or three days. Each time you add something new, you can see how your body reacts. If a food causes symptoms, then you know to avoid it in the future. If not, you know it's okay to eat.

If you don't want to start with an elemental diet, you can begin with a simple diet that is usually nonallergenic. It might consist of rice, lamb, and a few different fruits and vegetables, such as pears, carrots, or zucchini. The disadvantage of this approach is that you may have sensitivities to the foods you are starting with.

Another method is to simply begin eliminating foods one by one from your current diet. It's not the most organized approach, especially if you have multiple sensitivities. However, it might still help you identify foods that can trigger your disease. For more information on elimination diets, visit the following web site: *http://www.positivehealth. com/permit/Articles/Allergy/gamlin.htm.*

Cheryl shares her experience:

> *Elimination diets were very useful in helping me determine which foods I was sensitive to. I started by eliminating the foods that are often typical culprits: dairy, chocolate, spices, gluten, citrus, nightshade vegetables, and processed sugar. I also kept a food journal. Whenever I added a new food, I'd record it and note how I was feeling for the next 24 to 72 hours. Sometimes I'd react right away to something, but other times it could take up to three days. I realize not everyone needs to be as disciplined and organized about their eating. But this system worked for me.*

Gluten-free diet

Gluten is a protein found in grains such as wheat, barley, rye, and oats. Individuals with celiac disease cannot eat foods containing gluten without suffering gastrointestinal symptoms, some of which are similar to symptoms of IBD. A few researchers have hypothesized that people with Crohn's and ulcerative colitis—even if they don't have celiac disease—may be sensitive to gluten. However, no compelling evidence suggests a gluten-free diet can improve IBD symptoms. That said, some individuals have found a gluten-free diet helpful.

Following a gluten-free diet is not easy for most people, especially those living in industrialized countries where breads, pastas, and other flour products are dietary staples. Traces of wheat are found in many processed foods. However, there is a small, but reliable market for gluten-free products, and food manufacturers have responded. The best places to find them are health and natural food stores.

For more information, Shelley Case's book, *Gluten-Free Diet: A Comprehensive Resource Guide,* provides lots of valuable information. A good web site on this topic is *http://www.celiac.com/.*

Gluten-free diets didn't work for Richard:

> *I've tried gluten-free diets a few times over the years. The first time, when I was in college, my doctor suggested it. I was willing to try anything. However, at that point in my life it is was not easy, especially since I lived in the dorm. However, I'm disciplined and can do just about any diet. I tried it for several months, but I didn't notice any difference. It was such a relief to go back to a regular diet. I was actually kind of glad it didn't work. It's amazing how much our society revolves around wheat products.*
>
> *When I was older I tried it again. It was much easier this time since I was now used to preparing all kinds of different foods for myself. I really wanted it to work, but it still didn't. When I went back to eating gluten, I noticed I'd sometimes get a little tired after eating wheat, but I never noticed that it caused any kind of bowel symptoms.*

Cheryl finds value in a gluten-free diet:

> *Although a blood test indicated that I'm likely gluten-intolerant, I've never been officially diagnosed with celiac disease. However, my mother and her two sisters actually do have this illness. But it doesn't really*

matter if I'm diagnosed. I know my body well, and know that I feel much
better without gluten.

Low-residue diet

A low-residue diet is one that is low in fiber. Although healthcare professionals generally recommend people consume more fiber-rich foods, such as whole grains, fruits, and vegetables, there are times when such foods are not appropriate for people with IBD. If your gut is severely inflamed or narrowed, high-fiber foods can irritate the lining of the intestine or can contribute to a blockage in constricted areas of bowel. Once inflammation subsides, many people can once again tolerate high-roughage foods.

If you must temporarily avoid high-fiber foods, you may have concerns about how healthy your diet is. Here are some suggestions for getting the nutrients you need on a low-fiber diet:

- **Use a juicer.** You can juice fresh fruits and vegetables, such as carrots, celery, leafy greens, and apples, if you have a quality juicer. Juice generally has little fiber and retains many of the nutrients found in the whole vegetable or fruit. Also, most grocery stores now carry a variety of fresh juices that are flash-pasteurized.

- **Blend your food.** A high-powered blender can turn just about any food into something with a pudding-like consistency. Although fiber is not removed, some people find they can tolerate whole fruits and vegetables—and even nuts and seeds—if they are completely pulverized into a smoothie. It's a good idea to try a very small amount at first to make sure it agrees with you.

- **Steam or bake fruits and vegetables.** Some people find that these methods of preparing fresh foods are enough to help break down the fiber for easier digestion.

- **Take supplements.** If you feel you're not able to eat a balanced diet, consult with your doctor, nutritionist, or dietitian. They may suggest supplements that can partially compensate for nutrients lacking in your diet.

- **Eat baby food.** Baby food is a convenient way to get a variety of nutritious foods that are easily digestible. The small jars are ideal for snacks or small meals whether you are at or away from home.

Craig used to eat a lot of baby food:

> *There were times when baby food was a major part of my diet. It was a*
> *good way for me to get my fruits and vegetables. It was always so funny*

when I'd buy multiple jars at the grocery store. Little did the checkout clerks know that they were all for me.

I haven't had to eat baby food in years. Interestingly, my knowledge and experience with it paid off recently at a baby shower. For a contest, they had several jars of baby food and everyone had to guess what each one was. I, of course, won the prize!

Specific carbohydrate diet

The specific carbohydrate diet, outlined in Elaine Gottschall's book, *Breaking the Vicious Cycle,* is becoming better known among people with IBD. The diet is based on a theory that those with ulcerative colitis, Crohn's, and other bowel problems have difficulty digesting specific types of carbohydrates. When these undigested carbohydrates reach the lower small bowel and colon, they then support the growth of the wrong kinds of intestinal microbes. The overgrowth of these microbes, along with the toxins they produce, are thought to cause intestinal injury. By eliminating the offending carbohydrates, the bad microbes are starved of their food source. Over time, the bowel can come back into balance.

It's important to keep in mind, however, that no formal, well-designed studies on the specific carbohydrate diet have been performed on people with IBD. The theory is supported mainly by anecdotal evidence. It's not proven to induce remission or cure IBD.

The specific carbohydrate diet goes well beyond the gluten-free diet. Absolutely no grains are allowed, not even rice. Potatoes, sweet potatoes, and soy are not permitted either. You can have lactose-free dairy products, such as certain cheeses and butter, but not those containing milk sugar. Table sugar and corn syrup are forbidden, because they are more difficult to digest, but any kind of fruit or honey is allowed, because they are easier to digest. Most vegetables are allowed as well.

A major staple of the diet is almond or other nut flours that are used to make a variety of grain-free breads and muffins. Eggs and meat are fine, except for processed meats such as hot dogs or sausage, which may contain added sugars. It's suggested that if you notice improvement within the first month, you should stay on the diet for at least a year before you add any previously forbidden foods. If you find no improvement after a month, it's likely that diet won't work for you.

Trish has had some success with this diet:

For the first year, I followed the specific carbohydrate diet very strictly. I kept with it that long because it seemed to work. It actually stopped a flare of my colitis and I didn't need to go on prednisone. I found, however, that the impact dwindled over time. I eventually had another flare, and the diet didn't stop it.

I finally went to an allergy elimination professional (a nutritionist with other special training in alternative medicine) which has helped me tremendously.

The diet didn't work for Richard:

I followed the diet very strictly for several months. It was hard to tell if it was working, because I started it right after I had just gotten to a symptom-free state. I was hoping it would keep me that way. But about three months later, I had another major flare and landed in the hospital.

The one thing I've taken from this diet is the discovery of almond flour. It's been about six years since I went off the diet, but to this day I continue to make the almond flour muffins. They are absolutely delicious and nutritious.

Sugar-free diet

Several studies have linked a high intake of refined sugar to IBD, particularly Crohn's disease. However, these studies are questionable, because they are retrospective, meaning they try to assess people's pre-illness diets after they are already diagnosed. The problem is that people may not accurately recall exactly what they ate. Moreover, in the months before diagnosis, others may have changed their diet in response to symptoms from emerging IBD. Thus, it's difficult to draw any meaningful conclusions from these studies.

It's also unclear what role sugar intake plays in people who already have Crohn's disease or ulcerative colitis. Controlled studies that evaluate the effect of a low-sugar diet on IBD are rare. One group of researchers, however, examined this topic by dividing 352 people with mild or inactive Crohn's disease into two groups. They put one group on a diet low in fiber with unrestricted sugar. The other group was on a diet low in sugar but high in fiber-rich foods. The researchers found no clear difference in the course of disease between the two groups.[1] A recent review article on this topic found that the relationship between Crohn's disease and sugar is inconsistent and concluded there's currently no evidence low-sugar diets can help people with Crohn's.[2] More research is needed to clarify exactly how refined sugar affects IBD.

Karen found that refined sugar does not agree with her GI tract:

> *My system doesn't tolerate refined sugar very well. The natural*
> *sugars in fruit are fine. I can eat as much fruit as I want, but*
> *processed sweets cause my old symptoms to return. If I have just one*
> *little sweet treat on one day, I can usually get away with it. However,*
> *if I go beyond this occasional indulgence, the abdominal cramps and*
> *diarrhea will remind me that I need to get back on track.*

Vegetarian diets

No studies have examined how a vegetarian diet might influence the course of IBD. This is not to say a meatless diet high in fruits and vegetables can't help you. Like other diets, people have a wide range of responses. Some people do well with meat, and some don't.

There are many variations of vegetarianism. Following are descriptions of the most common types:

- **Lacto-ovo vegetarians.** Most vegetarians fall into this category. Lacto-ovo vegetarians avoid animal flesh, but still include other animal products in their diet, such as dairy products and eggs.

- **Semivegetarians.** Semivegetarians are those who consume some types of animal flesh, but not others. A typical example is someone who avoids red meat but eats fish or poultry. Of course, some people would say those who follow this type of diet are not vegetarians.

- **Vegans.** A small percentage of vegetarians are vegans, who consume a 100 percent plant-based diet. They consume no animal products.

If you choose to try a vegetarian diet, work closely with your dietitian or other knowledgeable healthcare provider. Although most vegetarian diets are healthy, some vegetarians—particularly vegans—need vitamin B_{12} supplements. Other nutrients, such as protein, calcium, or iron, are also sometimes lacking.

Carla found vegetarianism has not affected her IBD symptoms:

> *I've been a lacto-ovo vegetarian since I was 19. I chose this*
> *diet primarily for spiritual reasons, not health ones. Since I've had*
> *flare-ups of ulcerative colitis before and after changing my diet,*
> *I'd have to say that vegetarianism really hasn't affected my illness*
> *either way.*

Karen has had great success with a vegetarian diet:

> I suffered from Crohn's in my colon for about a year. It was in my rectum, so it was always very painful when going to the bathroom. Besides diarrhea and cramping, I also had mucus and blood in my stool.
>
> After a year, a healthcare provider suggested I try a vegan diet, where no animal products—not even dairy or eggs—are eaten. I figured I had nothing to lose since none of the drugs did much good. It turned out this was the best thing for me. After a brief, but medically supervised fast, I began on the vegan diet. It was like a miracle. For the first time in so long, I could go to the bathroom in complete comfort. I felt like sending out a press release! The bleeding, diarrhea, and cramping went away, too.
>
> I now eat mostly fruits, vegetables, legumes, whole grains (except wheat), soy products, nuts, and seeds—including flax for my omega-3s. If I stray too far from the vegan diet, I get symptomatic reminders. So I'm quite motivated to follow it strictly. I'm by no means saying this diet is for everybody. I know IBD is different for everyone. But for me, this is what has worked to restore my health.

Cheryl found that taking extra protein has helped her:

> I strongly believe that some people do not get enough protein. My nutritionist suggested I significantly increase my intake. She explained that this is especially important for someone with IBD, as it helps repair damaged tissue. I was amazed by how much better I felt after making this simple change in my diet. I know everyone's body is different, but I'm sure there are others like me who can also benefit from extra protein.

Supplements

Certain dietary supplements may help improve your condition. Although the vast majority of studies on treatment for IBD focus on pharmaceuticals, there is some research on nutritional supplements. The most promising ones are described next.

Fish oil

Fish oil may benefit people with IBD. It is a rich source of omega-3 fatty acids, which are a type of fat that may reduce your body's production of chemicals that promote inflammation. Some doctors therefore prescribe omega-3 fatty acids for people with inflammatory illnesses such as IBD or rheumatoid arthritis.

Research on fish oil for IBD is mixed. Some studies found it can slightly reduce symptoms or prevent relapse, but others have found no significant effect.[3] If you wish to try fish oil, ask your doctor how much you should take. You can also get a significant amount of omega-3s from eating fatty fish, such as salmon, herring, tuna, or mackerel. Flax seeds (which can be ground in a coffee bean grinder into a fine powder and sprinkled on just about anything) and walnuts provide some omega-3s, but they are not as good sources as fish.

Cheryl comments:

> *I have tried fish oil, but I can't say I noticed a difference. It may have been that I was just so sick at the time that nothing would have done much good. Perhaps if I had tried it early on when my symptoms were milder it could have helped. I've been reading a lot about it lately, though, and it sounds like it's something that can be good for almost everyone's overall health.*

Glutamine

Glutamine is one of the most common amino acids (building blocks of protein) in the human body. It's a major fuel source for the cells that line your small bowel. It helps keep these intestinal cells strong and healthy so they can maintain a proper barrier between bowel contents and the rest of your body.

Glutamine is considered a nonessential amino acid, because you generally don't need it in your diet. Your body makes it from other proteins you consume. However, when your body is under severe stress—from an illness such as IBD—your body may not be able to make enough.

Animal studies of IBD have revealed that supplementation with glutamine can reduce intestinal damage, weight loss, and overall disease activity. However, two small studies on humans did not reveal any positive effects.[4,5] More research is needed to see if supplemental glutamine has therapeutic value for those with IBD.

Probiotics

Your intestines are filled with bacteria. Some estimate there are up to 100 trillion microorganisms in your bowels. Although people often think of bacteria as harmful, many are beneficial to your body. These helpful bacteria, especially when in supplemental form, are sometimes called probiotics.

Doctors do not fully understand the complex balance among various intestinal microbes and how they influence health. However, they know your friendly bacteria play an important role in preventing unhealthy microorganisms from dominating your intestinal tract. Some researchers believe harmful bacteria are possibly linked to Crohn's and ulcerative colitis and think probiotics might have therapeutic potential for treating IBD. One recent review article on probiotics states they may help maintain remission in ulcerative colitis, prevent the return of pouchitis (see Chapter 6, *Surgical Treatments*), and prevent postoperative recurrence in Crohn's disease.[6]

Common strains of probiotics, including *Lactobacillus acidophilus* and *Bifidobacterium bifidum*, are frequently added to commercially prepared yogurt. If you do not consume dairy products, they are also sold as supplements. You usually need to keep them in the refrigerator to maintain their potency.

Cheryl's experience with probiotics is similar to what she experienced with fish oil:

> *I've taken acidophilus and bifidum, but it's difficult to say if they did anything. As with fish oil, I didn't start taking them until my symptoms were already quite severe. However, I think it's quite significant that my gastroenterologist prescribes them now to his IBD patients. He's more from the old school in terms of his thinking, so I find it interesting that he recommends probiotics.*

Ann feels probiotics have helped her and her son a lot:

> *Both my son and I have IBD. We take a number of supplements, but one I feel that has been an integral part of our return to health is probiotics. I feel they play a major role in keeping our symptoms under control. Fortunately, we both have doctors now who concur and support us in our use of such complementary therapies.*

Vitamin and mineral supplements

People with Crohn's disease and ulcerative colitis sometimes have difficulty eating enough or have certain dietary restrictions. It's therefore very important to work with a healthcare professional who is knowledgeable about nutritional needs. Because everyone's situation is unique, there are no standard recommendations for which vitamin and mineral supplements people should take. A common recommendation, however, is to take a multivitamin and mineral supplement as basic insurance. So many different ones are on the market that you should work with your doctor, dietitian, or nutritionist to help you choose the right one for you. Depending on circumstances, some people may require additional nutrients, such as extra iron, calcium, vitamin D, folic acid, or vitamin B_{12}. Your healthcare team can help you determine what you need.

Complementary therapies

Complementary therapies consist of treatments that aren't a regular part of traditional Western—sometimes called allopathic—medicine. Although some people commonly refer to these therapies as alternative, many individuals use them as complements to the therapies prescribed by their doctors. In general, complementary therapies include treatments that are either nondrug or nonsurgical. Many people commonly lump dietary and nutritional therapy in the complementary medicine category, too.

People have different preferences for the terminology describing these types of treatments. In addition to terms such as "complementary," "alternative," or "adjunctive," some people prefer to call them "integrative" or "holistic."

Whatever you decide to call them, many people with Crohn's disease and ulcerative colitis have an interest in these treatments. Indeed, an international survey of those with IBD at four major medical centers in North America and Europe found 51 percent use some form of complementary medicine.[7] Another study of children and young adults found a rate of 41 percent.[8]

Cautions

Many complementary medical practitioners are legitimate businessmen and women who truly want to help people achieve good health. However, some out there prey on sick people who are desperate for a miracle cure. At best, their products or services do nothing, other than make you lose money. At worst, their products or services can cause you significant harm. If a practitioner does any of the following, beware:

- Promises a cure for your disease
- Talks of conspiracy or major cover-ups by those in the medical establishment
- Insists you stop all other treatment before trying his
- Encourages you to sever communication with your doctor
- Tells you to inject an alternative product into your IV line
- Suggests anything else that goes against your common sense

Working with your complementary practitioner

Working with your complementary practitioner is often similar to working with your physician. For detailed information on this topic, see Chapter 9, *Working with Your Doctor.* Here are some tips to help you receive the most benefit from your complementary healthcare professional:

- **Ask about costs up front.** Although things are slowly changing, most insurance companies do not cover complementary therapies or office visits. By inquiring about all costs up front, you can avoid unplanned expenses down the road.

- **Check credentials.** It's a good idea to ask your practitioner what school she has attended and specifically what training and credentials she has. Many complementary healthcare specialties, such as chiropractic, have professional organizations that you can contact for verification. If you have difficulty finding this information, try calling several practitioners from the field in question and simply ask what their major professional organizations are.

- **Question and research recommendations.** If your practitioner advises specific therapies, ask her to provide objective research on its benefits for IBD. Inquire as well about how many times he's seen it help others with Crohn's or ulcerative colitis. If he's unable to provide sufficient information, ask a librarian at your local medical library to help you research your question. You can also hire an independent medical information researcher as well to research any medical topic. Please see the *Resources* appendix for more information.

- **Consult the National Institutes of Health's (NIH's) National Center for Complementary and Alternative Medicine.** This government organization also provides information—including the latest research—on many complementary therapies your practitioner might suggest. You can call this agency at (888) 644-6226, or visit the web site at *http://nccam.nih.gov/.*

- **Keep your physician informed.** Keeping your gastroenterologist informed of other therapies you are using or considering is very important. Potentially negative interactions between complementary treatments and Western medicine are possible. Although not all doctors are educated in this area, more are becoming aware of the latest research on these interactions. It's also a good idea to consult with a knowledgeable pharmacist. Most now have up-to-date databases that can spot a potentially harmful mix of treatments.

- **Consider seeing a physician who uses an integrative approach.** Many physicians are now enhancing their practices by becoming more knowledgeable about complementary therapies. Thus, you might consider making an appointment with a doctor who also specializes in another approach that interests you. For example, some doctors offer expertise in acupuncture, herbs, or nutritional medicine.

Craig felt comfortable consulting a physician familiar with complementary therapies:

> For a year or two I read everything I could about natural therapies for IBD. I wanted to consult a practitioner, but was unsure who would be the best person. I heard from an acquaintance about a physician who was very knowledgeable about alternative therapies. This made me feel comfortable because I felt I had the best of both worlds—someone familiar with both conventional and alternative medicine. He was only about 30 miles away so I decided to make an appointment. Seeing him was very helpful since he actually had experience using complementary therapies that I had only read about. His recommendations helped me feel much more confident about specific therapies, such as essential fatty acids, probiotics, and other nutritional supplements.

Specific therapies

Many people with IBD have found adjunct therapies useful. Research is scant on how the complementary therapies discussed next affect Crohn's disease and ulcerative colitis. With careful planning by you and your doctor, however, they are sometimes a useful part of an integrative approach for treating IBD.

Acupuncture

Acupuncture is an ancient Chinese practice. It involves the insertion of very thin needles at specific locations on the body. It's based on the idea that life force and energy flow through the body along certain pathways. If the flow of energy somehow becomes blocked or imbalanced, health problems can result. The goal of acupuncture is to re-establish your natural flow of energy and life force.

Acupuncture is generally painless. Needles are usually left in place anywhere from a few minutes to a half hour. Some people feel better immediately, whereas others require a series of treatments. Some individuals experience no discernible benefit.

Research published in a Chinese medical journal has reported some beneficial effects for people with ulcerative colitis.[9] Few data exist on using acupuncture for Crohn's.

People with IBD may perhaps benefit from acupuncture's analgesic effects. Although no research has specifically focused on the pain associated with IBD, other studies report acupuncture may have value for managing chronic pain.[10]

Cheryl found acupuncture somewhat helpful:

> I went to a physician who specialized in acupuncture. He also happened to know a lot about Crohn's. I felt his treatments helped me. The biggest thing I noticed was a change in sensation in my abdomen. It really helped my pain and cramping. However, I didn't notice much effect on my other symptoms. Unfortunately, we moved, and I have not found another acupuncturist with whom I get as good results. I've seen a couple others, but they haven't been able to provide me the benefit that the first doctor did.

Chiropractic

Chiropractors are among the most commonly used complementary healthcare practitioners. Chiropractic treatment is generally recognized for its ability to help back and neck pain. Whether it can help illnesses such as IBD is unknown. Most chiropractors believe misalignments in the spine can interfere with neural communication between the central nervous system (brain and spinal cord) and other organs, including the small and large intestine. They feel properly aligned vertebrae—which they achieve through spinal manipulation—allow the body to function optimally. This then gives the body the best chance to regain and maintain good health. However, research is lacking on whether chiropractic care can improve IBD symptoms.

Herbal medicine

Herbs have been used for thousands of years to treat various maladies. With the emergence of the pharmaceutical industry in the early 1900s, however, herbal medicine became less popular in Western, industrialized countries. Trends have shifted again recently, though, as there is now a renewed interest in these natural, plant-based therapies. Some practitioners, particularly complementary ones such as acupuncturists, use them frequently in their practices.

Research on herbal treatments for IBD is very limited. These two herbs may be helpful:

- **Aloe.** Aloe vera is best known for its skin-soothing properties. Some have hypothesized that it might work just as well internally as externally. In fact, acemannan, a complex carbohydrate derived from aloe vera, is under study as a potential therapy for IBD. If you wish to try aloe vera juice, consult with your gastroenterologist first. If the two of you decide it's worth a try, you can find it at any health or natural food store.

- **Peppermint oil.** Peppermint can help with pain and cramping in the GI tract. Although no research has examined peppermint's influence on IBD, researchers have studied its impact on irritable bowel syndrome (IBS). A major review article notes that most studies found peppermint oil helps reduce IBS symptoms.[11] However, the authors of this review article thought there might be flaws in the studies they reviewed. A more recent study reported 75 percent of children with IBS receiving peppermint oil experienced less pain after two weeks.[12] Check with your gastroenterologist before trying peppermint oil. If you take it, make sure you purchase the enteric-coated variety so that it doesn't dissolve in your stomach. Otherwise it may cause heartburn. Ask your doctor how much you should take and then do not exceed the recommended dosage.

Homeopathy

Homeopathy is a therapy developed in the late 1700s. It is based on the law of similars, which states that if a large amount of a substance causes symptoms in a healthy person, then a small amount of the same substance—taken by a sick person—will stimulate immunity and help him overcome illness.

No studies have assessed homeopathy's effect on IBD. Research on other illnesses has yielded mixed results, with some finding homeopathy works better than a placebo and some not. Because the remedies are so dilute, homeopathy rarely causes side effects. But it's still a good idea to discuss homeopathy with your physician before trying it.

Mind–body therapies

Many people with IBD highly value mind–body therapies such as meditation and guided imagery. These techniques are described in detail in Chapter 17, *Emotions and Coping*.

Cheryl, who has a lot of experience using complementary therapies, sums up her feelings on the subject:

> *I wanted so badly to heal my Crohn's naturally. After all, since nature made me, I thought there must be something natural out there that could heal my body, or at least help my body heal itself. Perhaps there is, but I wasn't able to find it before I absolutely had to have my*

surgery. My personal feeling is that if I had started all these natural therapies within the first year I had the disease, they would have had a better chance of helping. I think that if you get to a point where your symptoms are very severe, it often takes something dramatic, such as powerful drugs or surgery, to help get the body back on track. And this is nothing to feel bad about. We are fortunate to be living in a time where we have so many options. We have to take advantage of the best from both conventional and alternative medicine.

Stacy, who was a support group facilitator for many years, expresses her views on the variety of diets and complementary therapies available to those with IBD:

I've gotten to know many people with IBD over the years. And if there is one thing I've learned, it's that you've got to keep trying different things to see what works for you. Likewise, when you find something that works, you need to keep with it. Whether it's medications, diet, or an alternative therapy, what works for one person does not always work for another. I wish there was more consistency so we'd know the answer. But we don't. In the meantime, we have more options now than ever before. People just need to do what works for them and not worry about what works or doesn't work for someone else.

CHAPTER 8

Alternative Forms of Feeding

EATING IS A pleasure many people take for granted. Most people with Crohn's disease and ulcerative colitis, however, are consciously thankful for the ability to enjoy a meal, especially those who have lived for weeks, months, or longer on tube or intravenous (IV) feeding. Unfortunately, people with IBD can become so sick they are unable to eat or digest their food properly. This can happen during severe flares, after surgery, or if one develops a bowel obstruction. As a result, other ways to obtain adequate nourishment are necessary to prevent or treat malnutrition.

This chapter begins by defining enteral and parenteral nutrition—the two options for alternative nourishment. It then covers ways to determine which form of alternative feeding is right for you. The chapter also discusses how to cope with daily life if you need a feeding tube or intravenous nutrition for an extended period.

Tube and IV feeding

Alternative forms of feeding fall into two categories: enteral and parenteral. Enteral feeding uses the small intestine. Technically, eating regular food is a form of enteral feeding, because the small bowel absorbs nutrients from the food when it arrives there. When people talk about enteral feeding, however, they are referring to specialized liquid diets that are taken by mouth or through a feeding tube. These diets are often used to supplement or completely replace regular eating.

Parenteral feeding is the intake of nourishment that does not pass through the intestines. Instead, nutrition is given intravenously (through a vein).

Enteral feeding

The decision to undertake a course of enteral feeding is best made with the help of your physician. Although the use of enteral nutrition in IBD is much less controversial than the use of parenteral, the decision is not always an easy one, especially if you're facing the prospect of a feeding tube for an extended period (see section "Coping with a feeding tube" later in this chapter). Following is a list of reasons why you might benefit from enteral feeding:

- **You cannot tolerate regular food.** Enteral feeding is not used as first-line treatment for mild disease. It's generally something your doctor may suggest if your bowel can't handle a normal diet. For example, if you cannot eat enough regular food to sustain yourself, or if food causes your IBD symptoms to get out of control (excessive diarrhea, cramping, or bleeding), enteral feeding is worth a try.

- **You have severe Crohn's disease.** Research has shown that enteral feeding is more effective for people with Crohn's disease than for those with ulcerative colitis. In fact, enteral nutrition is considered a primary therapy (main treatment) for small-bowel Crohn's disease,[1] but not for ulcerative colitis. One review article reports that whereas remission rates for those with Crohn's on enteral feeding can reach 80 percent, only 25 percent of people with ulcerative colitis experience a remission.[2] Not all gastroenterologists use enteral feeding as a primary therapy, however. Those who do generally reserve it for people with severe Crohn's disease.

- **You have corticosteroid resistance or dependence.** Researchers have found that an elemental diet (one form of enteral nutrition discussed later in this chapter) is effective for people with Crohn's who are either dependent on or resistant to corticosteroid treatment.[3] In fact, some research suggests elemental diets are just as effective as corticosteroids in treating active Crohn's disease.[4,5] Others conclude that although enteral nutrition is effective for treating acute cases of Crohn's, it is not as effective as this type of drug treatment.[6,7]

- **You are a child or adolescent.** Perhaps the least controversial use of enteral feeding is for children and adolescents. Enteral nutrition promotes growth in children with IBD and avoids corticosteroid side effects. Several studies have found that total enteral nutrition (consuming nothing but an enteral formula) induces remission in children with Crohn's. Supplementing a normal diet with enteral nutrition after a course of total enteral nutrition can also prolong remission and improve growth rates of children with Crohn's disease.[8]

Enteral feeding is generally supplied by two basic types of formulas: elemental or polymeric. Each can play an important role in the treatment of IBD depending on individual circumstances. Discuss the advantages and disadvantages of each with your doctor to determine if either is right for you.

Elemental formulas

An elemental formula consists of the simplest, most basic forms of nutrients available. Although the nutrients are not literally broken down into single atoms, as the name might suggest, they are provided in the form of relatively small, simple molecules that require either minimal or no digestion. For example, carbohydrates are provided by glucose, the simplest form of sugar. Individual amino acids (or very short chains of them) supply protein. Medium-chain triglycerides are often used as an easily digestible source of fat. Essential vitamins, minerals, and trace elements are then added to complete the formula.

The major advantage of an elemental diet is that nutrients are absorbed easily in the upper small intestine, and virtually no residue remains for the lower gastrointestinal tract. The downside is that the formulas are expensive, although not as expensive as parenteral nutrition. In fact, most insurance plans do not cover the cost of elemental diets if your diagnosis is ulcerative colitis, but they may if you have Crohn's disease. The other major disadvantage is that most people dislike the taste. Some find semi-elemental formulas, such as Peptamen and Optimental, more palatable. They come in a variety of flavors. Still, if you have to drink six to twelve cans every day for weeks or months (depending on your caloric requirements), this option may not be ideal, either.

If you can't drink formula, another way to get it down is through a feeding tube. The tube goes through the nose, down the esophagus, and into the stomach. This option works for some people.

David had tube feeding once in the hospital:

> To be honest, I found tube feeding just miserable. The plastic irritates your nose and throat, and it feels really invasive to have the tube hanging out of your nose. I only had it for a week and it was just the pits. Fortunately, it really didn't work well for me. Instead, they had to put in a central line so I could get IV feeding. IV feeding might have more risks, but for me, it's easier to live with.

Richard has experienced enteral feeding several times:

> My dietitian told me she knew of only one patient who could actually drink the stuff. He would heat it up and drink it as a broth. I decided not to try that. Thus, the tube was my only choice.

The worst part about a feeding tube is getting it in—there's no way to get around your gag reflex. However, I did adapt to it once it was in a while. Yes, having a plastic tube up your nose and down your throat is not the most pleasant thing. But it really did help me—so it was worth having.

Some people are put on tube feeding for several weeks. However, others—especially growing children who can still eat a little bit—can benefit from nightly tube feedings. The tube is inserted every night before bedtime and then taken out every morning before going to school or work. Although it may initially seem unthinkable to have insert and take out a feeding tube every day, many adults and children adapt well to this regimen. Often, a thousand calories or more can be infused overnight, which can make a significant difference, particularly for growing children and adolescents.

One other option for receiving enteral nourishment is through a gastrostomy—an opening into the stomach. Prior to the early 1980s, gastrostomies were performed in the operating room under general anesthesia. Since that time, a different type of gastrostomy—called a percutaneous endoscopic gastrostomy (PEG)—is usually done. During this procedure, a flexible scope (endoscope) is inserted down your mouth and throat to view the inside of your stomach (see Chapter 3, *Diagnostic Procedures*). This is necessary to determine the proper incision site for your PEG. The gastroenterologist then makes a small puncture through the skin on your abdomen so she can insert a thin tube into the stomach. The tube is then sutured in place so it doesn't slip out.

When you need to "eat," a feeding tube can attach to the end of the tube coming out of your stomach. During feedings, you are hooked up to a pump with a hanging bag, much the same way that you are with a nose tube. The difference is that when you are finished "eating," you are completely free of tubes—you simply unhook the tubing from your PEG, cover it, and you are free. Depending on your caloric requirements, you will likely have many hours during the day when you can go about doing your normal activities completely untethered. When you are disconnected from your feeding pump, no one will know you are undergoing any treatment. This contrasts sharply with a traditional feeding tube: Even when you are unhooked from your pump, your tube is visibly hanging out of your nose.

One major disadvantage of the PEG is that installing it requires a minor surgical procedure, and surgery always involves risks. Because a small puncture is made in your

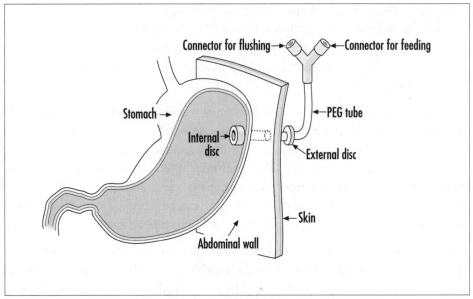

Figure 8-1. Percutaneous endoscopic gastrostomy (PEG)

abdomen, infection around the site of the PEG is possible. Contents from inside your stomach can also leak out and irritate your skin. And lastly, although rare, other problems can occur, such as accidental colon puncture or peritonitis (infection in the abdominal cavity). Thus, it doesn't make sense to agree to a PEG unless you and your physician determine you will need enteral feedings for an extended period of time.

Craig describes his experience:

> I had never had a feeding tube before and decided that I never wanted one. My doctor had determined that I really needed to give enteral feeding a try, but how could I without the tube? I let one nurse try to insert one, but after a half-hour of gagging and tears, we could not get it in. I decided I wanted the PEG until another doctor asked me why I wanted to put myself at risk when I didn't even know yet if enteral feeding would help. He explained that as awful as it is to have a tube up your nose, it's relatively safe. He assured me that with enough drugs and the right technique, we could get it in. Not only was he right, but after a few days, I could barely notice the tube in my throat! Although not an ideal situation, it wasn't nearly as bad as I had imagined.

Gastrostomies are generally safe and well tolerated by children with Crohn's. They are often recommended for children who cannot tolerate nose tubes, because nutrition is such an important factor for growth and development.

Polymeric formulas

Polymeric formulas contain whole proteins, such as casein, found in milk. Carbohydrates are often supplied by inexpensive sweeteners such as corn syrup. The fat content of these formulas is generally higher than that of the elemental ones and is commonly provided by corn oil or other inexpensive sources of fat. Vitamins, minerals, and sometimes fiber are added to make the products a complete source of nutrition. Unlike elemental diets, polymeric ones require digestion and leave residue for the lower gastrointestinal tract.

Although most people have never heard of a polymeric diet, you are probably familiar with some polymeric formulas available on the market, such as Ensure, Boost, or Sustacal. These types of products come in handy for people who need extra calories to maintain their nutritional status and weight. In addition, they are frequently helpful for children who need extra calories to support their physical growth and development.

Larry has needed to supplement his diet with polymeric formulas:

> *Of course, I'd prefer to just eat normal food. However, supplements such as Ensure have helped me quite a bit over the years. Drinking only two cans a day can make quite a difference in my caloric intake. It's helped a lot to keep my weight up when I needed it. When I use it, I drink the Ensure Plus, which has even more calories than the regular. The vanilla flavor is my favorite—it's almost like having a milkshake.*

The major advantages of polymeric diets are that they are inexpensive and are easily bought over the counter at almost any supermarket or drugstore. They also usually taste much better than elemental formulas. Because they are conveniently accessible for a reasonable price, they are a logical choice if you simply need to supplement your diet when you can't eat enough regular food. Many different polymeric products are on the market, so you can probably find one you like.

Choosing between elemental and polymeric diets

The research is mixed on which form of enteral feeding is best for treating IBD. Some studies indicate polymeric and elemental diets are equally effective.[9,10] Other researchers report elemental diets work better.[11] Until further research can clarify the matter, it seems best to discuss the pros and cons of each with your physician. It's probably reasonable to first try a polymeric formula, which is cheaper, more accessible, more palatable, and less likely to require a feeding tube. If, after a reasonable amount of time, you find it's not working, you might discuss an elemental diet with your doctor.

Coping with a feeding tube

If you temporarily need a feeding tube, you can take a few steps to make the procedure more comfortable.

- **Ask for a small tube.** Feeding tubes come in various sizes. Ask your doctor to order the smallest tube possible (given your feeding requirements). Even if you are an adult, one made for a child may be appropriate. However, if your formula is relatively thick, a larger one may work better.

- **Use sedation.** Ask if you can have a mild sedative before the tube is inserted, especially if this is the first time you are undergoing this procedure. If you are taking the sedative orally, make sure to take it at least a half hour ahead of time so it has time to take effect. Versed, a short-acting tranquilizer, is sometimes used for feeding tube insertions. If the tube is inserted at bedtime, a short-acting sleeping pill can be used the first few times until you get used to the regimen.

- **Get it in while you're out.** If you are undergoing surgery and will need a feeding tube afterward, have it inserted while you are anesthetized. If you are undergoing any other procedures around the time you'll need your tube (such as a colonoscopy), have it placed while you are still sedated.

- **Lay back at about a 45-degree angle.** If you're awake during the procedure, it's often difficult to get the tube down if you are sitting upright. The tube will slide down more easily if you are lying at a 45-degree angle.

- **Sip water.** Have a glass of water on hand with a straw right in front of you during the procedure. As the tube is inserted, take small sips and swallow so the tube goes smoothly down your esophagus.

- **Have a companion with you.** It may help to have a friend or nurse beside you during the procedure, for moral support. This person can hold the glass and straw in front of you with one hand and hold on to one of your hands with the other (you may want something to squeeze).

- **Relax.** Although it's easier said than done, know that you have the power to calm yourself. By relaxing, you'll find the procedure will go more smoothly, quickly, and easily. See Chapter 17, *Emotions and Coping,* for information on relaxation techniques, including meditation and guided imagery.

Once the tube is in place, you will need to adapt to having a long piece of plastic down your throat and dangling out of your nose. For the first few days, your throat may feel sore from the insertion of the tube. In time, your throat will adapt, and you'll hardly notice it, even when you swallow. Although feeding tubes are technically nasogastric tubes (ones that go from your nose to stomach, often called NG tubes), ones made just for feeding are generally softer, smaller, and more flexible than the traditional NG tubes that are made to suction contents out of the stomach. As a result, they are surprisingly comfortable once in place. Here are some tips that can help you deal with various aspects of having a feeding tube:

- Use an over-the-counter anesthetic throat spray (such as Chloraseptic) if your throat is bothering you. Lozenges can also ease throat discomfort.

- Tape your tube securely to your nose. If it's loose, the tube can slip up and down, irritating your throat and increasing gagging. Change the tape as needed, and periodically clean the skin on your nose with alcohol to eliminate oil so your tape jobs will last longer.

- Be careful around pets and small children. They may want to play with your dangling tube and may accidentally pull it out.

- Flush your tube with water at least every four to six hours to prevent blockages. If your tube won't flush, call your doctor or nurse immediately.

- Consider inserting your tube every night and taking it out every morning. This works well if you are using enteral feeding as a supplement to your diet. You can receive adequate nutrition while you sleep, and then be tube free during the day.

- Be comfortable with yourself. Yes, it's awkward to have a tube coming out of your nose. But if you can learn to accept yourself in this situation, others will have an easier time accepting you. Most people have good intentions, but they may avoid you for fear of reacting the "wrong" way. By demonstrating your comfort with yourself, you'll set the tone for your interactions with others. The artificial barriers between you and other people that you thought the tube created will likely disappear.

Richard, who has spent several months at various times on tube feeding, explains how he dealt with the awkwardness and stigma of having a tube hang from his nose.

> *The first few days I had my tube, I was miserable. I didn't want to see anyone, I didn't want to talk to anyone, and I certainly didn't want to see myself in the mirror. I realized, however, that I was getting better. And if I needed to stay on this for six weeks, I certainly didn't want to keep feeling miserable.*
>
> *I realized I had a choice when it came to my feelings. I could choose to feel sorry for myself, or I could choose to make the best of the situation.*
>
> *I always had an interest in how people react to different situations, so I decided to make it a game. I stopped worrying about how I looked and turned the whole thing into a big psychology experiment.*
>
> *I found it was kind of fun to observe people's reactions to me. Some would smile, some would turn away and pretend not to notice, and some would be startled if I appeared suddenly in front of them. I'll never forget how the UPS man practically jumped out of his shoes when I answered the door. I began to look forward to going out places because I couldn't wait to stir up more reactions! It got to a point where I could truly laugh at myself and other people's responses.*
>
> *After a few weeks of distracting myself with my game, I realized I didn't care anymore how I looked. I was still me, and I could relate to people the same way I always had. The tube didn't change who I was.*

Parenteral feeding

Parenteral feeding, as mentioned earlier, is nutrition received intravenously (through a vein). People with severe cases of IBD can sustain themselves for weeks, months, or even longer without ever ingesting any nourishment by mouth. The development of parenteral nutrition is truly a major accomplishment of modern medicine.

The most common form of parenteral feeding is called total parenteral nutrition (TPN). TPN, first used in the late 1960s, is a synthetic form of complete nutrition that is delivered intravenously. It consists of a combination of all essential nutrients, including proteins, fats, and carbohydrates that are mixed together to form a sterile and usually calorie-rich solution. Many years ago, the fat emulsion part of TPN was given separately from the protein and carbohydrate components. Today, all three can be combined into one IV bag. Essential trace minerals (except iron) and an IV multivitamin solution are then added to the mixture.

Before TPN, the only major IV nutritional support that existed was a 10 percent dextrose solution that could only provide a few hundred calories of carbohydrate per day. Today, whether a patient requires 1,000 calories or 4,000 calories, TPN can provide it.

TPN is sometimes given through a peripheral vein (a regular vein in your arm or hand). However, the concentration of fats and carbohydrates must be adjusted because it can damage these small veins. More commonly, TPN is usually infused into a central vein—one that is large and near the heart. Central veins are much less susceptible to the irritation that a high dextrose concentration can cause, because the large volume of blood flowing by will dilute it.

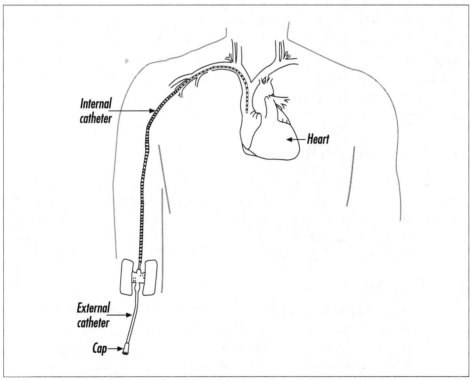

Figure 8-2. Peripherally inserted central catheter (PICC)

TPN given for a relatively short time (two to four weeks) is often infused through a peripherally inserted central catheter (PICC line). In this procedure, a specially trained nurse or doctor inserts the catheter into a vein in the crook of your arm (opposite your elbow). He threads it up your arm and around into your upper chest so that the end of the line sits in a large vein just above your heart. No anesthesia is needed other than a local injection to numb the area opposite the elbow. The procedure is generally performed right in your hospital room as you lie still in your bed with your arm stretched out. At one point during the procedure, the nurse or doctor may ask you turn your head or neck a certain direction to prevent the catheter from going the wrong way. Once the line is in place, an x-ray is taken to confirm its position. If necessary, the line can be easily adjusted to a better position.

If your doctor feels you will need TPN for months or longer, a different type of tube, such as a Hickman or Broviac, is recommended. Such lines are placed directly into your chest. Under anesthesia, a special technique is used so that the tube can remain in place for years, if necessary.

A second form of parenteral feeding is called partial parenteral nutrition (PPN). PPN is generally used when a week or two of IV feeding is necessary. PPN is just like TPN except its dextrose concentration does not exceed 10 percent. Thus, a peripheral vein in your arm or hand is suitable. No central line is required. Be aware, however, that PPN is often quite irritating. IVs running PPN generally don't last long and are often changed more frequently.

Deciding when you need it

As with enteral feeding, the decision to take a course of parenteral feeding is definitely best made with the guidance of your physician. Although TPN has been used as a primary treatment for acute episodes of IBD, most doctors recommend it's best used to support yourself nutritionally while on another course of treatment, such as IV corticosteroids, during severe flares.

Stacy describes her experience:

> I've only been on TPN while in the hospital. The last time, for example, I needed it because I only weighed 98 pounds and needed surgery. I was too weak to undergo an operation. I was also on corticosteroids at the time. A couple weeks on TPN were helpful because it allowed me to gain a little weight and increase my strength. Once I was more stable, I had the surgery and everything worked out fine.

Parenteral feeding is generally not as helpful a therapy for ulcerative colitis as it is for Crohn's. One study found that after three weeks on TPN, people with ulcerative colitis showed no significant improvements in their condition compared to others with ulcerative colitis who ate regular hospital food. In contrast, the same study reports that in people with Crohn's, TPN resulted in reduced inflammation and a disappearance of symptoms.[12] However, TPN can improve or sustain the nutritional status of those with severe ulcerative colitis while they are undergoing other treatments or preparing for surgery.

Parenteral nutrition has disadvantages that enteral doesn't, such as costing more and causing atrophy of the gut. When someone is on TPN and bowel rest, the intestines aren't being used. The person therefore loses muscular tone, and atrophy results. When eating resumes, normal intestinal tone and digestive function return, but it takes longer than if enteral feeding were used. Another downside is that parenteral feeding is riskier. On TPN, you have a slight risk of infection because you receive it intravenously. Any infection in someone with a central line is taken very seriously, because it can affect the heart or cause a blood infection. Blood clots are also a possibility on IV feeding.

Despite the disadvantages, at times parenteral feeding is advisable. Here are some factors that may indicate you could benefit from parenteral feeding:

- **You have short bowel syndrome.** This rare condition, often caused by repeated surgeries for Crohn's disease, is probably the least controversial use for parenteral feeding. Patients with less than 50 cm of small bowel often require TPN for life. Those who have less than 100 cm of small intestine may require at least some parenteral nutritional support. For more information on short bowel syndrome, see Chapter 4, *Complications*.

- **You have a fistula.** A fistula occurs when inflammation burrows its way through the intestinal wall, creating a tubelike structure between the bowel and another organ. Although enteral feeding also may help heal fistulas, researchers have found that total parenteral nutrition can play a role in closing them up as well.[13]

- **You have a bowel obstruction.** If your intestinal pathway is either significantly narrowed or completely blocked, anything through mouth, nose, or gastrostomy is not a good idea. Therefore, parenteral feeding is the logical choice for nutritional support in this situation.

- **You cannot tolerate enteral feeding.** If you don't want a nose tube or gastrostomy, parenteral feeding is your other option for nutritional support. Also, if enteral feeding gives you diarrhea or other side effects, parenteral feeding may be your best choice.

Craig, who has spent significant time on both TPN and enteral feeding, describes his sudden intolerance to tube feeding:

> I previously had much success with the nose tube feedings. Then, once while hospitalized, they put me on it again before I went home. Much to everyone's surprise, I couldn't tolerate it. It was the same elemental diet formula I had always used. But as soon as we started it, I had a sharp increase in diarrhea and bleeding. We backed off it for a few days, but upon resuming, the same thing happened, even with a very slow infusion rate. Since then, I have always had to use TPN as my nutritional support during flares.

Coping with TPN for extended periods

If you and your physician have agreed that a course of TPN for an extended period will benefit you, he'll arrange instruction on how to manage your IV feedings at home. This can be a scary prospect, but thousands of people with IBD have managed it successfully.

Richard describes his experience:

> I was afraid to go home on my TPN. I was fine with an IV in the hospital but it seemed like too much responsibility at home. I was resolved to go to a skilled nursing facility until my doctor had a talk with me. He felt that the nursing facility was not the right place for a young person like me. Of all people, he thought I was the ideal candidate for home TPN since I am educated and good with detail. He assured me that he wouldn't make me leave the hospital until I felt adequately trained and emphasized that I would have a lot of support from a home health nurse. He also said that in some ways, TPN at home is actually safer since hospitals are a host to some pretty bad germs.
>
> I decided to take a chance on going home. I soon found he was right. I had underestimated my abilities. Within a week or two, I was very comfortable managing my IV care at home.

With only a few exceptions, having TPN at home is actually not much different from having it in the hospital. You generally receive a week's supply of TPN bags you store in your refrigerator. Each day, about an hour before you start a new bag, you take it out and allow it to warm up so it won't be too cold when you begin your infusion. The tubing is slightly different from the kind you had at the hospital, because it's connecting to a different type of pump, such as the CADD-TPN, which is both portable and electronically controlled. Once you get yourself connected, the TPN bag and pump are generally placed in a backpack. This way, if you need to go out while hooked up, you won't need to drag an IV pole around with you. If the backpack is too heavy (especially in the hours after starting a new bag), you can try Richard's innovative idea:

> Since my metabolism was so fast, I always required at least 4,000 calories a day while on TPN, which is twice as much as most people get. As a result, my TPN bags were big and heavy. As I usually lost about twenty pounds when I flared, my muscles would be quite weakened—so the backpack was too heavy during certain hours of the day. To solve the problem, I strapped my backpack onto a luggage roller. After starting a new bag, I could roll it around everywhere very quickly.

Unlike Richard, most people on TPN don't need to be on it around the clock. Most only require approximately 10 to 12 hours of infusion per 24-hour period. Thus, the logical choice is to run it at night while you are sleeping.

David was fortunate he didn't need to be on TPN during the day:

> My doctor was able to set up a system where I only needed to be on TPN at night when I was sleeping. When I got up in the morning, it was time to unhook it and I didn't need to start it again till the evening. This made it very convenient during the day. I didn't have to drag my bag around with me everywhere. I was able to get out a little during the day and take a short walk. My wife and I would even go out to dinner. I'd always order my favorite: ice water!

Whether you are on home TPN for the first time or the tenth time, the following tips can help you avoid problems, cope with the TPN, and perhaps even improve your quality of life during this time:

- **Get trained properly before you go home.** It's stressful to be at home on TPN and not know what you are doing. Ask for as much coaching as you need before you leave the hospital. If possible, have a friend or family member attend training with you so you have a back-up person.

- **Have enough supplies for at least three days.** Like toilet paper, IV supplies are not the kinds of things you wait till the last minute to buy. Shipments can be delayed, or a natural disaster such as an earthquake or hurricane may occur. Being prepared can bring peace of mind.

- **Create a convenient schedule.** The best thing about home healthcare is that you have the freedom to set a schedule that's more convenient for you—there's no hospital schedule to worry about. If you have several hours a day during which you don't need your pump, time it so you can make the most of your untethered moments. If you are on your pump 24 hours a day, you may want to change your bag in the early evening so you'll have a lighter load to carry the next day.

- **Keep your pump fully charged.** Although your pump can go for many hours unplugged, why tempt fate? When you can plug it in somewhere, take advantage of the opportunity. Also, remember to keep extra 9-volt batteries around the house, and bring a few with you whenever you leave home.

- **Set your backpack in a plastic tub.** In case your bag springs a leak, place your backpack in a little plastic tub before setting it down anywhere.

- **Check your tubing periodically.** Leaks can occur in IV tubing, especially at connector points. Inspect your tubing every few hours during the day and before you go to bed. Check for both tears and leaks. In addition to keeping your connector points tightened, wrap some tape around them as well. Also, make sure your tubing is staying in place and not slipping at the insertion site.

- **Watch for other problems.** Report any of the following problems to your doctor or nurse and soon as you notice them: pain near the area where the tube is in your body, unusual swelling, fever, or chills.

- **Keep clean.** You or your home health nurse will change your IV dressing once a week. You can also do your part by avoiding situations where you might soil your dressing. If you inadvertently get your IV dressing or catheter site dirty, call your nurse immediately.

- **Find your own way to manage without food.** Although a few people on TPN are permitted to eat, chances are you won't be. Not eating is probably one of the most difficult aspects of total parenteral feeding. Everywhere you turn, it seems you are bombarded by images of food you can't have. Until you go on TPN, you probably won't notice how much food is shown on TV. There's no right or wrong way to deal with this situation. Some people cope by avoiding food as much as possible. For example, they change the channel when seeing food on TV, or they disappear during family mealtimes. Others, like Jamie, do just the opposite:

> *At mealtimes, I gladly sit with my family and watch them eat. They feel bad and tell me I shouldn't torture myself, but really, I want to see them eat so I can at least experience it vicariously.*
>
> *I'm already into recipe books and cooking shows. But when I'm on TPN, I really can't get enough of them. I'll never forget the time I was flipping the TV channels and I came across a cooking show in a foreign language. I had to stop and watch it! It didn't matter that I couldn't understand the words—whatever they were cooking looked delicious!*
>
> *In my free time, I'd write lists of what I wanted to eat once I was given permission. It's amazing how obsessed you can get about food if you can't have it for an extended period.*

- **Resume as active a lifestyle as you can.** You may not have the energy to run laps around the track, but you probably can engage in milder forms of exercise such as walking. Perhaps you can return to work or school at least part time. If you do need to take some time off and stay at home, make an effort to maintain social contacts via telephone and email. If you can't get out to visit people, invite them to visit you. You may feel different from everyone else, but the way you receive your nourishment doesn't change who you are.

Jamie, who's had Crohn's for ten years, explains:

> *When I was on TPN and managing all my tubes, sometimes I would suddenly see myself from a different perspective—as if I were observing myself from a distance. I would see this woman going through all these steps, coping, and getting through this difficult time. But then I found myself asking, "How has it come to this point?" I would then find myself feeling very remote and removed from other "normal" people. Yet despite these mixed feelings I had about myself, I could somehow always find my way back. Yeah, this TPN thing is sure something else. But I realized that through it all, I was still me.*

CHAPTER 9

Working with Your Doctor

PEOPLE WITH IBD have more than their fair share of interactions with various doctors. As a result, finding the right physician and creating an atmosphere of respect and trust is vital. Your doctor will play an active role in your care, so it is important to develop a good working relationship. And because you probably won't resort to putting a personal ad in the newspaper to find your ideal candidate, it's helpful to invest some time and energy in finding a good match.

This chapter can help you achieve this goal. You'll read about different ways to view your relationship with your physician. You'll also learn ways to evaluate the characteristics you want in a doctor. The chapter then discusses good communication and gives suggestions for conflict prevention and resolution. Next, it covers how and when to seek a second opinion. Last, it discusses changing doctors, and how to do so if it becomes necessary.

Models of the doctor–patient relationship

There are several ways in which people interact with their doctor. In the traditional model, the doctor takes the responsibility for making the major medical decisions. Another style of relating is the interactive partnership, where joint decisions are made about one's care. And yet another model is the "doctor as consultant" style, where the individual takes a more dominant role in determining the course of her treatment.

It's true that the doctor–patient relationship is shifting in our country, with more people moving towards the interactive styles. However, there is no right or wrong way to interact with your doctor. The different ways of relating described next are just that— different ways in which people choose to develop relationships with their doctors. There's no need to conform to any model. The styles of interaction only represent different places on a continuum. You can place yourself anywhere on the spectrum that feels right for you. The point is to evaluate where you are and ask yourself if that is where you want to be.

The traditional model

The traditional model is one in which the physician is primarily in charge of making medical decisions. The person who is ill doesn't research the latest treatments or question the doctor's recommendations. He trusts the doctor knows what's best for him. The major advantage of this type of relationship is that people don't need to worry about options or research, which is overwhelming for some people. With the doctor collecting information and making medical decisions, this frees the individual to focus on the nonmedical aspects of healing.

This particular approach is not necessarily passive. It often works quite well for people, especially in emergency situations or if one is new to IBD. Some people don't want the stress of helping to manage their own disease, or are simply not comfortable in participating in the medical aspects of their care.

The major disadvantage of this style of interaction is that sometimes doctors can make errors. They also may make decisions with which the ill person is not comfortable. If communication is also lacking in these cases, compliance to treatment may then suffer. Thus, if you choose to defer medical decisions to your doctor, it's probably wise to invest time in finding a very well qualified person to make these decisions for you.

The interactive model

The interactive model is one in which a person and his doctor are partners, although the doctor generally still plays a greater role in determining the ultimate treatment. The patient, however, takes a much more active role than in the traditional model. For example, she will let her doctor know what issues are important to her regarding her care. She will question the rationale behind her therapies and may make suggestions based on information she has read and researched. She makes joint decisions with the doctor on the best course of treatment.

The main advantage of partnering in decision-making is that individuals have more control in choices about their medical care. Also, because the style is interactive, the amount of communication between doctors and their clients is increased. As a result, joint decisions are often reached that both parties are comfortable and happy with.

Cathy, who's had a severe case of Crohn's for many years, exemplifies this model:

> *I'm the kind of patient who is always on the lookout for new treatments. If I hear or read about something, I always bring it to the attention of my doctor. For example, I had heard about*

*budesonide as an alternative to prednisone. I mentioned it to my
doctor, and he agreed that it would be a good thing for me to try. I still
rely on my doctor to make the ultimate call on treatment issues, but I
do my part in trying to find new things to help myself.*

The consultation model

Some people with chronic disease view their physicians as consultants. The doctor
and patient are still partners, but the patient takes a more active role in determining
his course of treatment than in the interactive model. Most people with IBD don't start
here. However, because these illnesses are chronic in nature, some people become
experts on their own disease. They usually arrive at this point after many years of battling Crohn's or colitis. Indeed, the person who uses this style of interaction generally
has had his condition for a long time and knows his disease and his body very well.
He knows his preferences for treatments. He knows what works for him and what
doesn't. He is always up on the latest research and discusses all treatment options
with his doctor.

People who manage their own care still maintain a close working relationship with
their physicians. While working together, the doctor is supportive of his patient and
lets him take the initiative in steering the course of his treatment. The doctor lets his
patient lead the way but makes sure he stays on course.

Richard, who's now healthy after many years of severe IBD, explains:

*I wasn't always the type of patient who basically managed his own
case. And I'm not recommending that everyone should do so. But it
just got to the point where I'd been through this so many times that
it just made sense for me to do so. I'm not in any way saying that
I ignored my doctors or just did whatever I wanted without consulting
them. On the contrary, I kept in close contact with my physicians and
let them know what I was doing and what I wanted to do. Plus,
whenever I was hospitalized, they would have to be the ones who
prescribed things for me. Fortunately, we were usually on the same
wavelength. And certainly, when things came up that were out of my
area of expertise, of course I relied on them for assistance.*

*What I'm trying to say is that there came a point when I realized
that the only person responsible for me is me—not my doctor, not
other family members—just me. I decided that I had to take control,*

take responsibility for my health, and not leave this to anyone else.
I truly feel this realization played a major role in my ability to finally
attain a good state of health.

After reviewing these models, think again about where you'd place yourself among them, and ask yourself if this is where you wish to remain. Only you can determine the mode of interaction with your physician that best suits you and your unique needs. If you find you are unhappy with the way you interact with your doctor, consider using the information in the rest of this chapter to help improve your relationship.

Choosing your doctor(s)

Most people have at least some choice of physicians. Unless you live in a rural area where there is only one doctor or one specialist (such as a gastroenterologist or GI surgeon) within reasonable driving distance, you'll probably have at least some ability to choose your physicians, even if your insurance (or lack of it) may limit your options. It's generally a good idea to make an active choice (if you have one) and to not leave the matchmaking process to chance.

The best time to choose your doctor is when you are healthy. If you are already sick, you may not have the strength and energy to search and properly evaluate your options. For some people with IBD, it isn't always possible to have the right doctor lined up before becoming ill. Crohn's and ulcerative colitis can strike quite suddenly. Or the onset can come on so gradually people may not pay much attention to it until symptoms have gotten somewhat out of control.

Most people are diagnosed with IBD in their teens and twenties. Individuals in this age group are generally healthy and don't think to establish a partnership with a regular doctor. And in most cases, there would never be a reason to already have a relationship with a gastroenterologist. If you do find yourself in a situation where you are very sick and need immediate help, you'll probably just work with the doctor or doctors assigned to you and postpone your search until you're feeling better.

The ideal situation, however, is to find a physician who suits your unique needs. Because IBD is generally chronic, most people with it will have at least some periods between flare-ups when their health is fairly stable. This is the perfect time for you to research available physicians. The time you invest in this process will pay off quite handsomely for years to come. Having a doctor whom you trust and are completely comfortable will bring you tremendous peace of mind. The following sections offer some tips on selecting a doctor.

Types of doctors

Most people with IBD have both a primary care physician as well as a second doctor specializing in gastroenterology. Primary care doctors are generally those who specialize in internal medicine, family practice, or pediatrics. They can handle your general medical concerns, and ideally should be working very closely with your gastroenterologist—who treats disorders of the GI tract, such as IBD. Your GI doctor has also specialized in either internal medicine or pediatrics, but he has also spent an additional three years studying gastroenterology. Thus, he is the doctor who will help you manage your Crohn's or ulcerative colitis. Sometimes people with IBD are working so closely with a gastroenterologist that they use him as a primary care doctor as well. In addition, some people with IBD require a third type of doctor—a surgeon.

Defining the characteristics you want

Once you determine the specialty of the doctor you need, it's time to identify what traits are most important to you in a physician. What's ideal for one individual can be a nightmare for another. Ruth, who was frustrated in her search for the perfect doctor, once wrote a want ad:

> *WANTED: Doctor. Must have all-encompassing knowledge of every disease, condition, disorder, whether minor or life-threatening. Must be able to make accurate diagnosis every time. Must have up-to-the-minute information on all possible treatments, medications, research, including those from non-Western traditions. Must be able to unfailingly prescribe optimal plan for relief, recovery, cure. Must have extraordinary skills in perception of patients' physical/emotional/social/spiritual needs and be able to communicate with patients perfectly. Must be continuously available and ultimately affordable. Must be kind, gentle, wise. Must know top experts with all of the above qualities should referral to specialist be necessary. Please reply immediately. Otherwise I'm going to have to go to the bother of getting personally involved in my own health care.*

You might ask yourself a few questions before you begin your search. Here are some questions you might consider:

- Do I prefer a male or female doctor?

- Do I prefer an older doctor or a younger one?

- Do I care how many years experience he has treating IBD?

- Do I want someone to just tell me what to do?

- Do I want a doctor who will treat me as an equal partner in decisions regarding my health?

- Do I want a more formal, professional relationship or one in which my doctor is like a friend?

- Do I want someone who is knowledgeable about alternative medicines and uses them in his practice?

- Do I care where she went to school?

- Do I want a doctor who is more liberal in handing out prescription drugs, or one who is more cautious in doing so?

- Do I want a doctor who's quick to refer patients to surgery, or one who isn't?

- Do I want a doctor who's open to new, experimental treatments, or one who's more committed to established ones?

- Do I want a doctor who is always on time, brief, and to the point, or one who will spend more time talking and listening (even if it means waiting longer for him during office visits)?

- Do I want a doctor who personally returns my calls, or would I prefer communicating through a nurse?

After you've asked yourself these questions, continue to write down other characteristics important to you. The more you identify what you want, the greater the chance you'll find what you're looking for. You may reach a point where you have so many specific requirements and standards it becomes difficult to find a good match. In these cases, you might consider making some compromises or ranking your needs. In other words, try to decide which traits are most important, and which are somewhat negotiable.

Cathy, who's had IBD a long time, explains what's important to her:

> *The characteristic I find most important in a doctor is the ability to really listen and understand what's going on with me. Of course, I want my doctor to be sharp and know what he is doing, but for me, a doctor who is compassionate is just as important.*

Referrals

One of the best ways to find a doctor is through the personal recommendations from people you trust. Try to elicit substantial information, such as a person explaining, "I've been a patient of Dr. XYZ for five years and he's always taken the time to answer all my questions." This type of information is generally more helpful than someone telling you, "She's a really nice person," or "I went to medical school with him." You can get referrals from a variety of sources. Here are a few suggestions:

- **Your current doctor.** If you are looking for a gastroenterologist, talking with your primary care doctor is a good place to start. Again, make sure you ask for specifics instead of settling for general, noninformative answers. Likewise, if you need surgery, you can ask your gastroenterologist for a recommendation.

Craig, who has had a number of surgeries over the years, describes how he got referrals from others:

> *During the years that I was in and out of the hospital with flares,*
> *I realized that at some point I might need surgery. So I started early in*
> *terms of figuring out who would be the best surgeon. I received*
> *recommendations from others with IBD, but I also greatly valued the*
> *opinions of my doctors. My GI and primary care doc had both spoken*
> *highly of a particular surgeon. And on top of that, another surgeon*
> *who I had seen for another problem also advised that this same*
> *surgeon was the best for GI surgery. When the time came, I decided*
> *on the doctor everyone recommended and it all worked out fine.*

- **Other medical professionals.** If you know any other medical professionals, you can ask them to recommend doctors. Nurses are generally a good resource. They often work directly with physicians on a daily basis in stressful environments. They are in a unique position to observe doctors in a variety of situations, so their opinions are worth considering.

- **Other people with IBD.** Perhaps one of the best places to receive a referral is from other people with Crohn's or ulcerative colitis in your local area. If you know no one near you with IBD, attend a support group meeting. As you get to know people, you can ask them for their opinions. Call your local Crohn's and Colitis Foundation of America (CCFA) chapter for information on meetings.

Jamie explains how helpful it was for her to receive referrals from others with IBD:

> *Other IBD patients were a great resource for me when I needed*
> *to find a new surgeon. I was diagnosed with Crohn's when I was*

suddenly very ill. I needed surgery right away and just had to go with
who was available at the time. Although my first surgeon always
made sound medical decisions, I didn't particularly care for her
bedside manner and how she interacted with me. When I recovered, it
occurred to me that I might face a similar situation again. So I started
talking to lots of other people with IBD whom I met through support
groups. Several people specifically mentioned another surgeon. It
meant a lot to me to get the recommendations from other IBD folks
since they had undergone similar operations themselves.

- **Crohn's and Colitis Foundation of America.** Your local CCFA office is another resource if you are looking for a doctor. Chapters are allowed to provide two or more names of leading IBD specialists who primarily treat Crohn's disease and ulcerative colitis. In addition, the "Find-a-Doctor" feature on the CCFA web site (*http://www.ccfa.org/medcentral/roster/*) lists healthcare professionals who are members of CCFA. Chapters also organize patient education meetings that frequently include IBD specialists. However, understand that CCFA cannot guarantee the competence of any doctor. It's up to you to make contact and determine whether a doctor is a good match.

Interviews

If you were hiring a business consultant for your company, you'd probably interview several candidates before making a final decision. Wouldn't hiring a doctor to help manage your health be just as—if not more—important? When making interview appointments, be candid. Explain that you are looking for a new physician and that it is very important to find someone compatible, because you highly value the doctor–patient relationship. At your interview appointment, have respect for the doctor's time. Come prepared with a list of your most important questions. Usually after spending fifteen minutes talking, you'll have a sense of whether or not you are compatible.

Richard, who had been with the same gastroenterologist for seven years, explains what happened when he learned his doctor was moving away:

When my doctor was moving out of town, he gave me three names
of people he thought would be good choices for me. I immediately
made an appointment with one of them. When I arrived, I made it
clear the first thing that I was doctor shopping, and that it was really
important for me to find someone who'd be an ideal match. She was
completely comfortable with my approach, and gave me all the time

I needed to ask my questions. At the end of the appointment, she expressed that she would enjoy working with me, but encouraged me to take the time I needed to interview other doctors. I had planned to call up the other two and set up appointments, but by the time I got home, I knew in my heart that she was the doctor for me. I signed on with her, and to this day we still have a great relationship.

Credentials

It's generally a good idea to confirm a doctor's credentials before making your final choice. Although a doctor should not practice without proper certification in an area outside his area of expertise, it does happen.

Training

When you are evaluating credentials, it helps to have a basic understanding of physician training. After earning a four-year college degree, a doctor must complete four years of medical school. At this point, he is not licensed to practice. He then moves on to a residency to specialize in a particular field of medicine. Residency generally lasts from three to seven years. For example, a physician must complete a three-year residency in internal medicine before he can practice in this field. To become a gastroenterologist, one must finish a residency in internal medicine or pediatrics and then complete a three-year fellowship in gastroenterology.

Board certification

The American Board of Medical Specialties (ABMS) is the major organization that grants board certification to physicians in 24 different areas of medicine, such as internal medicine, surgery, radiology, psychiatry, or pediatrics. To acquire ABMS certification, a doctor must complete all his years of training in his chosen field and pass a series of written and oral exams.

A physician, once he is board certified, can later become a subspecialist by obtaining further training (through a fellowship, for example). The options for subspecialties depend on the field of medicine in which the physician is board certified. For example, if someone has earned board certification in internal medicine, he has sixteen choices for subspecialties certified through the ABMS. Among others, the choices include geriatric medicine, hematology, pulmonary disease, or gastroenterology. Pediatrics, which has seventeen subspecialty certifications, is the only other field of medicine that offers a subspecialty in gastroenterology besides internal medicine.

It's generally a good idea to choose a doctor who is board certified in her specialty. ABMS certification will not guarantee that your doctor will always know the right thing to do, but it does mean she meets one of the highest standards within her field. Of course, many good physicians are not board certified. These doctors are often called board eligible. This simply means that for whatever reason, they haven't taken the tests yet, chose not to take the tests, or took the tests but didn't pass.

Jamie, who has taken the time to research her doctors, explains her feelings on the matter:

> I'm so glad I have the ability to do all this research so easily on my own computer. I actually didn't do my research until after I had been seeing my doctors for some time. It's reassuring to know that my doctors are who they say they are.
>
> Board certification isn't everything to me. All of my doctors are, except one, and I'm okay with that. There are other factors to consider, including my impression of his knowledge and how we interact.

Checking credentials

Checking a doctor's credentials is easy, especially in the Internet age. You can ask a doctor about his professional qualifications or do a little background check on your own. It's as easy as a few keystrokes and mouse clicks on your computer. If you don't have a computer or Internet access, you can go to your local library. And if you're too sick to make it to the library, you can call any library and ask a reference librarian to check for you. Here are some resources you can use to check an MD's credentials:

- **The American Medical Association.** The American Medical Association (AMA) offers a service on its web site called Physician Select. Using this feature, you can acquire basic information on just about every doctor of medicine (MD) and doctor of osteopathy (DO) in the United States and its possessions. A physician's listing does not depend on whether he or she is a member of the AMA.

  The database, which includes more than 690,000 listings, is searchable by a physician's name and state, or by medical specialty and state. The AMA web site address is *http://www.ama-assn.org/*. At the top of the home page, click on Doctor Finder. This link will take you to Physician Select. The database provides useful information, including where the doctor went to medical school, where he did his residency training, and what certifications he has.

If you don't have Internet access, the AMA publishes the *American Medical Association Directory of Physicians in the US*. This directory alphabetically lists every physician in the United States, and you can find the same information found on the web site. Most public libraries keep this directory in their reference section.

- **The American Board of Medical Specialties (ABMS).** The organization that grants board certification is also a useful resource when you want to check on a doctor's credentials. The ABMS has an online database you can access on the Internet at *http://www.abms.org/*. From the home page, click on the "Who's Certified" button on the left side of your screen. To use this system, you register by providing your name and email address. They then email a password you use, with your email address, to log on to the system. You can search by physician name or by a specific certification and location. The ABMS also publishes annually the *Official ABMS Directory of Board Certified Medical Specialists*. This four-volume directory provides a brief biography on over 535,000 physicians in the United States and Canada, focusing on medical education, training, and board certifications. It's found at many medical and public libraries and is also available on CD-ROM. The ABMS has a toll-free phone number: (866) 275-2267.

- **Other professional medical groups.** Many medical specialties have their own professional organizations. You can use these groups to find information on MDs as well. For example, the American Board of Internal Medicine (ABIM) has information most people with IBD would find useful, because any gastroenterologist treating adults is licensed in internal medicine. If you go to *http://www.abim.org/* you can click on Certification, and then on ABIM On-Line Directory of Diplomats. For information on pediatric gastroenterologists, visit *http:/www.abp.org/*.

- **State medical licensing boards.** Your state medical licensing board is a resource if you have concerns about a doctor's licensing, inappropriate conduct, or disciplinary actions taken against her. From *http://www.doh.wa.gov/medical/med_web.htm*, you can click on any US state to get to its medical board web site.

- **Public Citizen.** Public Citizen is a national nonprofit consumer-advocacy group founded by Ralph Nader in 1971. The organization currently publishes a book titled *20,125 Questionable Doctors* that provides information on doctors who have been disciplined. For $20, you can purchase one of eighteen regional directories covering your state. For several hundred dollars, you can also buy a national directory covering every state in either print or CD-ROM format. For the latest information, go to *http://www.citizen.org/*, click on publications, type "questionable doctors" in the keyword field, and then click Search.

Decisions

After you've identified the type of doctor you want, asked for referrals, interviewed physicians, and checked credentials, you'll have all the information you need to make an informed decision. Although you should take enough time to make a proper evaluation, it's usually best to decide relatively quickly, because you want to be under a physician's care as soon as possible. If this relationship doesn't work out, you can always go through the process again and choose another doctor at a later time. By following these steps, you'll have a good chance of finding a doctor with excellent credentials, a comforting manner, and a philosophy in harmony with yours.

Communicating with your physician

Your relationship with your doctor is valuable. It's therefore to your advantage to nurture and fortify the alliance. One of the best ways to do this is through clear, open, and honest communication.

Communication is the lifeblood of any relationship. If people have problems communicating with each other, the partnership is sure to suffer. In contrast, a relationship often flourishes if both parties can express themselves and listen to each other. The doctor–patient relationship is no exception to this rule. The following are some suggestions to help you facilitate open communication with your doctor:

- **Ask questions.** Doctors cannot read your mind. If you have questions concerning your treatment, simply ask. Sometimes people may feel their questions are dumb or embarrassing, but your doctor will probably be glad to explain anything you don't understand. Most doctors want to create a safe, comfortable environment for questions and answers.

- **Be organized.** You'll get the most out of your interactions with your doctor if you are organized before appointments or phone consultations. Make a list of all your questions and concerns and take it with you to your appointment. During the appointment, take notes when talking to your doctor. If you prefer, bring someone with you to take notes and provide support. You might even want to use a tape recorder when consulting with your doctor. Just get her permission before you start recording.

Brenda, who has had Crohn's disease for over ten years, explains how she handles her doctor appointments:

> When I go to the doctor, I come with a written list of questions.
> Otherwise, I might forget something important in the midst of the

*appointment. On top of this, I like to bring my husband with me as
well. It helps to have a second person listening in case I happen to
miss something.*

- **Be conscious of time.** If you always have a lot of questions and take longer than average, let the doctor's assistant know this when scheduling your appointment. If appointments are generally fifteen minutes, ask for either a 30-minute consultation or two consecutive fifteen-minute appointments.

Craig is someone who often needs more than the average amount of time with his doctor:

> *I'm the kind of person who has a ton of questions. Fortunately, my
> doctors understand this and give me the time that I need. Before I had
> my surgery, I told my surgeon that I'd probably need more than just
> the standard appointment. So he told the woman who makes the
> appointments to schedule me for a double so that we'd have plenty of
> time to discuss everything.*

- **Tell your doctor what you want to know.** You may be the kind of person who wants to know everything regarding your case, or you may not be. It helps to tell your doctor how much you want to know, so you remain comfortable with your level of knowledge.

- **Express your needs.** It helps to share any needs you have. For example, you may want to tell your doctor you want her to accept you as an equal partner in the management of your case.

Richard, who was very sick for many years but is now well, tells what he asked of his doctor:

> *Although I had been very ill for so many years, I knew that some
> day I would be healthy again. It was important for me to work with a
> doctor who actually believed that I could be healthy and drug-free—
> quite a stretch from where I had been for the previous twelve years. I
> didn't need the negativity of a doctor who would make the assumption
> that I'd be sick and on prescription drugs the rest of my life in order to
> control the disease. When I started with a new doctor, I told her that
> although I didn't expect her to cure me, I really needed her to believe
> in my ability to be well. She understood my request and why it was
> important to me. Within two years, I achieved my goal of being well*

again. I can't prove that it had anything to do with my doctor's beliefs,
but I know in my heart that her optimism and encouragement played
a role.

- **Ask what your doctor needs of you.** Likewise, it's a good idea to ask your doctor what she needs and expects of you. For example, an internist likes her patients to check with her before trying any alternative remedies.

    I confess that I don't know that much about alternative medicine,
    but I do like my patients to tell me what other medications they might
    be taking. Sometimes, patients just say "I'm taking vitamins," but
    often it turns out that it is more than just that. I want to know
    specifically what are in the supplements they are taking so we can
    avoid any harmful interactions.

- **Communicate about what's going on with your body.** It's also important to clearly communicate to your doctor all your symptoms, medication side effects, and any other concerns about your health.

    Cathy explains:

    I think it's so important to always tell your doctor what's going on.
    You have to keep in contact, because if you don't tell him things, he's
    not going to automatically know. I find it so strange that some people
    are always complaining about their health to everyone but their
    doctor. Yet if you don't communicate your concerns to him, he's just
    going to assume that you are doing fine, and nothing is going to
    change. Doctors are not psychic. They can't read your mind. And on
    top of that they have a lot of other patients who are communicating
    with them. So I say, speak up, be heard, and make sure your doctor
    understands what's going on with you.

- **Iron out contact details.** It's important that you and your doctor agree on how to contact each other. For example, is it okay for you to call her voice mail? Or should you always leave a message through her nurse or answering service? How long does it generally take for her to return calls? Is she available to page on weekends or holidays? Would she prefer to communicate via email? Share with your doctor whether it's okay to call you at work, leave detailed messages on your answering machine, or only talk directly with you.

Jamie, who has a good relationship with her gastroenterologist, explains how she contacts her doctor:

> I'm fortunate that my doctor has a voice mail specifically for his patients that only he checks. It makes me feel more secure knowing that I have direct access to him and don't have to go through anyone else who might not quite convey my full message. I try to be careful not to abuse this gift. One time, when I had a message that wasn't too urgent, I thought I'd just call his nurse and leave the message with her. So I did. When he called me back, the first thing he said was, "Don't you have my voice mail number?" I guess I'm one of the lucky ones!

- **Listen.** Communication is a two-way street. If you want something, such as being listened to carefully, you often have to give it first. When your doctor is speaking to you, listen and pay attention. Resist impulses to interrupt or finish her sentences.

- **Express complaints with care.** Express any complaints in a diplomatic manner. If possible, offer potential solutions to the problem.

Jamie, who's had a variety of doctors over the years who have helped treat her Crohn's, explains how she once handled a complaint:

> I had one issue come up with a doctor that really bothered me. In the midst of it, I didn't know quite what I was feeling. About a month or so after, I did, and so I decided to send a very diplomatic but honest letter to my doctor confidentially. I think I handled it well by providing specific examples of what hurt me and what could have been done to avoid that. I also made sure to mention a few positive things. For me, this was the best way to communicate my complaint.

Resolving conflicts

Living with an illness such as IBD can create a lot of stress. When your life, health, or comfort is on the line, problems can quickly escalate into crises. Doctors are often under extraordinary levels of stress that simply come with their job. Thus, it's not uncommon for people to experience conflict with their doctor now and then, given the nature of medical settings. Trying to avert serious disharmony in the first place is often helpful. But if a conflict has already developed between you and your doctor, identifying and fixing the disagreement quickly can help preserve and even strengthen your relationship with him. Quick conflict resolution can also save you much needed energy that you'd probably prefer to save for fighting your disease rather than your doctor. Here are some suggestions to help you both avoid and resolve conflicts with your physician:

- **Treat her respectfully.** There's perhaps no better way to maintain good relations with anyone than to show respect.

  Jamie, who has worked well with her doctor for many years, explains:

  > I think it's very important to respect my doctor, but at the same time, he needs to respect me. I think it's best to think of your doctor as just any other human being. Sometimes we tend to elevate doctors to another level, and I don't think that this is right. My doctor and I are both human beings and we deserve equal respect.

- **Have empathy.** As stressful as IBD is for you, realize that your doctor is under a great deal of stress, too, trying to help you and others who are ill. Take a moment and try to imagine yourself in her shoes. By making an effort to understand her perspective, you'll likely have a greater appreciation of her point of view.

  Brenda, who has had IBD for many years, nicely demonstrates how her empathy toward her doctor has enhanced her relationship with him:

  > I'm fortunate I have a good relationship with my doctor, and I definitely empathize with him. In fact, I think about him and his work a lot. I can only imagine what it's like doing colonoscopies all day long! I know he is stressed and overworked. Yet he's still so kind and gentle. I don't know how he does it.

- Show appreciation. Almost everyone needs to feel appreciated, and doctors are no exception. Thank your doctor for the little things as well as the big ones.

  Richard, who gets along well with his doctors, shares how expressing appreciation has enhanced his relationships with them:

  > I am very fortunate that I have had some really good doctors over the years. It's easy to just take them for granted, but I decided many years ago not to do that. In support group, I've heard a few stories about people having problems with their doctors. This made me realize how lucky I was. I now make a point to tell my doctors how much I appreciate them. I feel that over the years this has enhanced my relationship with them, especially in terms of the comfort level in

*the relationship. When you have an illness like IBD, it can sometimes
be difficult to find things to be thankful for—but at least this is one
thing I can always put on my list.*

- **Manage negative emotions.** It's only natural for you to have feelings of anger, fear, and frustration when dealing your IBD. However, this doesn't give you the right to take your negative emotions out on your doctor. Some creative ways to release your ill feelings are pounding inanimate objects, doing artwork, or by emphatic housecleaning. Or seek help from a mental health professional.

Journal writing has helped Brenda:

> *I'm not always very good with expressing myself verbally. So I often
> just write out my feelings about what's going on with me and that
> helps get it all out. Sometimes I even let my doctor read what I write.
> He appreciates this as it gives him a better insight into what's going on
> with me.*

- **Use "I" phrases.** If you need to express something to your doctor, it helps to start by saying, "I'm feeling . . ." rather than "You're making me feel . . ." No one can "make" you feel anything. "I" messages help to communicate your thoughts and feelings without creating additional friction.

- **Make use of staff social workers and psychologists.** Many hospitals and large medical centers have mental health professionals on staff. Not only can they help you deal with your own concerns, but they can often act as mediators between you and staff.

- **Invest in the relationship.** If you want to create and maintain a good relationship with your doctor, it helps to invest some time and energy in it, just as you would in any other kind of relationship.

Brenda, a mother of two who has Crohn's, explains:

> *I have a great partnership with my doctor, and I feel much of it is
> due to the fact that I have invested a lot in the relationship over the
> years. I always take a personal interest in what's going on with him.
> I ask him how he is doing. I take him baked goodies. When each of my
> children was born, I brought them in so he could see them. I've
> invested a lot, and gotten a lot in return. He always goes the extra
> mile for me.*

Getting a second opinion

Seeking a second opinion is a smart thing to do whenever you are facing a serious medical condition such as IBD. Fortunately, most doctors feel just the same way. In fact, it's common for doctors to consult their colleagues when dealing with difficult cases.

An internist, who works in a group with four other physicians, explains:

> *I have no hesitation in consulting my colleague if I need another opinion. Sometimes, it just feels good to bounce ideas off someone else whose opinion I value.*
>
> *I also respect the patient's decision to get a second opinion and I would not be insulted by it. I want to make sure my patients are informed and comfortable with their course of treatment.*

Some people feel that by asking for a second opinion, they may hurt their doctor's feelings or imply they don't trust him. However, getting a second opinion is a common practice. Many insurance companies require them prior to beginning treatment or having surgery.

It's a good idea to let your doctor know what you are doing. He'll likely support your decision and even provide a list of referrals for you to choose from. Any doctor who has a genuine concern for his patient will respect this decision. However, it helps to try and handle the request as respectfully as you can. When bringing the subject up, you can say something like "I really value your opinion on my options, but I'm considering whether I should get another opinion. Do you think this would be a good idea?" Or you might say something like "I really value our relationship that we've had over the years, but I think I owe it to myself and family to seek another opinion. Do you have any recommendations?"

Choosing the doctor who gives you a second opinion is something you can do on your own or with the help of your current doctor. If possible, it's usually a good idea to pick a doctor who is not part of the same group as your current one. An independent specialist at another medical facility is a good option. Your physician can usually help you make an appropriate choice. If he is unable or unwilling to assist, you can call your local CCFA office and ask them to provide you with the names of a few of specialists in your area. You might also seek out IBD support groups. Other people with IBD are often good resources if you need help finding another opinion.

Jamie, who has obtained second opinions, shares her experience on this topic:

> *I think getting a second opinion is a good thing, and every patient should have a right to one. It's important that people don't see it as a lack of confidence in their current doctor. In my case, I fully trust my doctor, but realize that he is just one person. He can't know everything. I see nothing wrong with checking in with someone else who has a different perspective.*
>
> *I had to do this one time when I had a complication with my liver. One doctor recommended that I should undergo a procedure to scope my bile ducts. I then consulted with another specialist who would do the procedure, but he didn't think I should have it. I didn't know what to do, so I decided to talk to my surgeon who performed my resection. He thought it made sense in my case. So I went ahead with it. It was a good thing I did because they found and removed a gallstone that had probably been there a long time. The pain I had for so long finally went away, and was not part of a Crohn's flare.*

Whether you are deciding to have surgery, a particular procedure, or are considering a new medication, two opinions from independent specialists (and sometimes three) are usually enough. However, if you find yourself running from doctor to doctor in search of a particular answer you want to hear, recognize that this behavior may not be in your best interest. True, it may be hard to accept your diagnosis or the prospect of treatment. However, consider that you may jeopardize your health by delaying your treatment during the time you're seeing that fifth doctor for the "final" word.

In the rare case that you have a physician who does not support your decision in seeking another opinion, you might consider finding another doctor. Your health is too important to leave in the hands of just one medical professional. Although some cases of IBD are mild, others are life threatening. You have the right to a second opinion—so why not work with a doctor who respects this right?

Changing doctors

The thought of changing doctors is often uncomfortable. It's generally something most people would prefer not to do. However, if you've spent a reasonable amount of time and effort trying to enhance your relationship with your physician, and you still feel you are not getting what you need, it's time to consider switching doctors.

Some people become distressed with the idea of changing doctors. Understandably, you've already invested much in the relationship, and it is often overwhelming to think of having to start all over again with someone new who is not familiar with your situation. Even if you are unhappy or frustrated, it's sometimes easier to just continue in the relationship, because change is uncomfortable (especially when you're sick). There is certainly some stress involved with switching doctors, but ask yourself if it's costing you more to stay with a doctor with whom you're unhappy.

Larry faced with this dilemma several years ago:

> For years I had a doctor I wasn't happy with. I've had a very severe and unusual course of Crohn's that never fit the classic textbook case. Yet the doctor I had at the time never listened and instead had preconceived notions of what was wrong with me. As a result, I suffered needlessly under his care.
>
> It was stressful at first after making the change, especially since my new doctor was one of his partners. But I've never regretted my decision. Although it took some time, I have a doctor now who is empathetic and truly understands my unique case.

If you do decide to switch, there are various ways to handle the transition. You don't have to confront your doctor face to face and tell him you're leaving. You may, though, want to send a brief personal note. If you do, keep the tone positive. Explain that you feel your new physician is a better fit, and you need to do what you feel is best for you.

The other item you need to do when changing doctors is transfer your records. You can make this request in writing, or you can pick up the records yourself from the doctor by signing a medical records transfer form. It shouldn't be a big deal, as most doctors' offices are used to receiving these types of requests. Keep in mind that doctors are required by law to transfer your records if your request is made in writing.

Different people have different needs when it comes to working with a doctor. The important thing is that you find a doctor whose style works well for you. If you're unhappy with your current physician, you owe it to yourself to try to find one better suited to you and your needs. After all, your health and life are at stake.

Craig, who has dealt with Crohn's for a long time, explains it best:

> I've had to switch doctors several times. The first time was when I began college. I wanted to have a doctor on campus familiar with

my case. I didn't know anyone, so I just went along with whom they assigned to me. I only had one appointment with him, after which I immediately knew I couldn't stay with him. He knew what Crohn's was, but he had not even heard of one of the drugs I was on, 6-MP. He was asking me what it was and why I was taking it. Kinda scary. He was also of the old school, where the doctor tells the patient what to do and the patient is just expected to follow orders. Needless to say, none of this went over very well with me, so I never returned to him. I couldn't afford to stay with someone like that.

The second time occurred when it was time to move on from my pediatric physicians, who had followed me since I was a young teen. I initially chose an adult GI doctor that one of my friends had recommended. At first, he seemed like a good doctor for me, as he was both educated and personable. However, once I started having some problems, I began to question whether I should remain with him. When I would call with questions, he would take a week to get back to me. Not that it was anything that was an emergency, but a one-week response time was not acceptable to me.

At appointments, I began to realize that he really wasn't listening to what I was saying, much less understanding. It became very frustrating, and I was becoming concerned about how I'd be able to deal with him if I were having severe problems with my Crohn's. Fortunately, I had the courage to switch. And it was a good thing, too. About a year later, I became severely ill. My new doctor was very good at helping me manage my condition—and it would have been a mess with the old one. I'm so thankful I made the change, as I seriously believe I would have jeopardized my health by staying with my previous doctor.

CHAPTER 10

Going to the Hospital

SOME PEOPLE WITH IBD never need to go to the hospital to treat their Crohn's disease or ulcerative colitis. Their condition is mild enough that the disease is easily managed on an outpatient basis. For others, hospitalization is necessary from time to time to bring severe flare-ups under control. Some may only go to the hospital once or twice in their lifetime, whereas others require repeated hospitalizations over many years.

Hospitalization has the potential to be one of life's more unpleasant ordeals. However, you can do many things to make your hospital stay a healing—and possibly even pleasant—experience. Knowing what to expect, educating yourself about all your treatment regimens, having an inquisitive attitude, and being diplomatic when expressing your needs can all go a long way in making your hospital more bearable.

This chapter begins with a discussion on how to tell if you need hospitalization. It then explains how to best prepare for your stay. The importance of a private room, as well as your relationships with key hospital personnel is then addressed. Next, it gives some tips on how to reduce the risk of medical errors during your visit. The chapter concludes with how to prepare for discharge.

Deciding when to enter the hospital

Many people with IBD who have endured repeated hospitalizations seem to know intuitively when it is time to go. But for those without much hospital experience, it's often difficult to gauge.

Craig, a Crohn's veteran, gained confidence in making the choice over time:

> The first few times I was hospitalized, I really had to rely on my doctor
> to help me decide whether I needed to be admitted. I didn't have the
> experience to make a good judgment. I had many fears about being in
> a hospital and didn't know what to expect or how it could help me.
>
> After a while, however, it got to the point where I knew exactly when
> I needed to go. When I became so weak that I would essentially just lie in

bed until my next run to the bathroom, I knew it was time. So after a
while, I'd call up my doctor and say, "You know, it's time again," and he'd
make the arrangements without even asking me many questions.

Monitoring your symptoms

It's important to keep in close contact with your doctor during a significant flare-up. Although only a physician can admit you to the hospital, you can play a vital role in the process. You know your body best. When your symptoms have gotten out of control and you are not getting better with outpatient treatments, it is time to tell your doctor, so he can make arrangements.

People sometimes wonder what it means to say that symptoms are out of control. It can certainly vary from person to person, but the following indications may suggest it is time to talk to your doctor about hospitalization.

*   Persistent nausea and vomiting
*   Significant, unusual weight loss
*   Inability to drink significant amount of fluids; dehydration
*   Excessive amounts of blood in the stool
*   Unusual number of bowel movements
*   Severe pain and cramping
*   Persistent high fever
*   Symptoms that don't respond to treatments that have normally worked in the past
*   Symptoms that keep you away from work, school, or other daily routine for an extended period

Experiencing any of these symptoms doesn't necessarily mean you require hospitalization. When in doubt, call your physician. If you cannot contact her and you feel it is an emergency, go to the nearest emergency room.

Stacy comments:

I've probably been in the hospital about 25 times. Over the years, I've
learned to know my body and when it's time to go. My advice though is
that when you're in doubt, go earlier rather than later. I can think of two
times when I waited too long. I was lucky I didn't die. I think one of the

problems is that people with IBD often have a very high threshold for pain. Since they are used to being in so much pain, they don't always take it so seriously and think they can handle it. But I always tell people it's better to err on the side of caution and get to the hospital. It's not worth risking your life.

Avoiding unnecessary hospitalization

If you and your physician are contemplating hospitalization, ask him to explain the pros and cons. Sometimes changes in your outpatient treatments can resolve your flare-up. Although the treatments available in hospitals often save lives, staying in the hospital also poses risks. This is potentially a serious concern for people with IBD, whose immune systems are often compromised by corticosteroids and other immunosuppressive drugs.

You have no doubt read stories in the news about antibiotic-resistant bugs spreading to vulnerable people in the hospital. Such stories are backed up by evidence. For example, the US government's Centers for Disease Control and Prevention estimates that about 2 million people every year contract an infection while receiving care in a hospital.[1] Even more disturbing, a growing number of these infections are becoming resistant to antibiotics each year.[2]

Moreover, mistakes are sometimes made in hospitals, such as hospital personnel administering the wrong drug or the wrong dosage of a drug. Even without counting errors in drug administration, one study reported in the *Journal of the American Medical Association* that an estimated 2.2 million people in 1994 alone had adverse drug reactions while hospitalized, and approximately 100,000 of these persons died.[3]

These statistics are not intended to scare you away from hospital treatment when you need it. Instead, they are meant to educate you so you are armed with the facts when making decisions regarding your treatment.

It is reasonable to ask your doctor if the benefits of hospitalization outweigh the risks. Here are some questions you might ask:

- What specific treatments will I undergo in the hospital that can't be done at home with the help of a home health nurse?

- Is there evidence to suggest these in-hospital treatments will improve my condition?

- Has the hospital to which you're admitting me had problems with antibiotic-resistant infections?

- What is the hospital doing to prevent resistant infections? Does it have a program in place?

You may surprise your doctor if you ask these kinds of questions. However, you can tell her you are concerned about getting an infection in the hospital. You can then ask if she has any suggestions for ways to avoid potential problems if the two of you agree hospitalization is necessary.

Estimating the length of your stay

How long you are hospitalized depends on your condition and why you were admitted. Ask your doctor how long he expects you to stay. People with Crohn's or ulcerative colitis may remain only a day or as long as several weeks. For example, if you are dehydrated you may get IV fluids for a day or two and then go home. If you need major surgery, you'll probably stay in the hospital for at least a week or two, although some people who recover quickly may get out sooner. For severe inflammation in the intestines that is not responding to outpatient treatment, length of time in the hospital depends on how quickly you respond to your inpatient therapies. If you have concerns, ask your doctor what goals you need to reach (for example, a pattern of weight gain, or ability to eat sufficient calories) before he'll discharge you.

Hospital stays are shorter now because of the need to reduce healthcare costs. However, shorter stays do not necessarily imply reduced care. Often, what used to be done in the hospital is now done at an assisted care facility or at home with the help of a home health nurse.

Richard, who has Crohn's disease, explains:

> Many years ago, it wasn't uncommon for me to be in the hospital for four or five weeks at a time. I would need to be on TPN and bowel rest, and it sometimes took this long for my gut to heal before I could eat again. Now they would never keep me that long. Once I'm basically stable on IV feeding for a few days, they send me home with my IV. It's great to be able to go home so soon.

Preparing for hospitalization

Preparing for your hospital stay can make your visit there more comfortable. Preparation also eliminates the need for your family and friends to rush back and forth bringing you clothes and other items.

During an emergency, don't worry about getting ready to go to the hospital—just head for the nearest emergency room. If you are unable to drive yourself safely, have a friend or family member take you. If no one is available to drive you, call for an ambulance. Don't be ashamed or embarrassed to do so. Your taxes support emergency services—so use them if you need them.

If, however, you've been in touch with your doctor and the two of you have decided there is time to enter through the admitting department, you may want to take a little time to become organized before you go if you are feeling up to it.

Packing for your stay

As a general rule, pack lightly. You probably won't have a lot of space for your belongings. You can always have friends or family bring more later if space permits. Some people with severe IBD prefer to have a hospital bag always ready to go in case there's little time to pack. Another option is to keep a list of items so either you or a loved one can quickly gather what you need before you go.

Here are a few suggestions of things you may want to bring:

- **A pillow.** Hospital pillows are notorious for being stiff and uncomfortable. Bring your own pillow in a pillowcase that is colored or has a design so the nursing aides won't get your pillow mixed up with hospital pillows when changing your bed. Your own decorative pillowcase can also add some color and warmth to an otherwise drab hospital room.

- **Earplugs.** Hospitals are often noisy at all hours of the day and night. Earplugs won't eliminate all noise, but they may muffle things enough to allow you more peace and rest.

- **Hand sanitizer or hand wipes.** Hospitals are full of germs. Because it is not always convenient for you to get out of bed and wash your hands, it's a good idea to keep some liquid hand sanitizer or antibacterial hand wipes nearby. Use them every time before you eat or touch your face.

- **Comfortable clothes.** Although most people wear hospital gowns, there is usually no reason you have to. If you are undergoing surgery or other procedures, it may make sense to wear the gown most of the time. But if you are primarily in the hospital for IVs or tube feedings, you may prefer to wear your own clothes. Short-sleeved shirts make IVs more convenient, and sweat pants or shorts are really comfortable. Another option is to where a robe over your gown. Lastly, don't forget your underwear, socks, slippers, and shower sandals.

Larry expresses his views on hospital gowns:

> Hospital gowns are not for me. I don't like them and I generally don't wear them. There's just something about them that's very unappealing. Maybe it has to do with them being open in the back! I've always brought my own pajamas. They're more comfortable, and the hospital has never had any problems with my wearing them.

- **A tape player/radio with headphones.** With your own tape player or radio, you can listen to your favorite music or inspirational tapes without bothering anyone else.

- **Reading material.** If you are very sick, you may not want to read. But if you enjoy reading, bring some favorite books or magazines with you for the times you feel up to it.

David comments:

> I never brought books with me to the hospital. I was so weak that I couldn't really focus on anything that intellectual. However, I always had my Walkman with me. I used it to listen to music. It often helped me fall asleep.

- **Address book.** It soothes the spirit to keep in touch with friends and family. Call people you know who are supportive and a joy to be with. Avoid people who are emotionally draining or are unable to handle your being sick.

- **Laptop computer.** If you have a laptop and are feeling well enough, surfing the Internet is an enjoyable and productive way to spend your time. Let your friends and family know you would like to receive email and will try your best to respond. Before you leave for the hospital, however, make sure your room is equipped to handle it. If you have a laptop security device, bring that, too, so your laptop won't be stolen while you're out getting x-rays.

- **Other personal hygiene products.** Don't forget to bring a comb, hairbrush, toothpaste, toothbrush, shampoo, mouthwash, hand cream, deodorant, lip balm, throat lozenges, and soap. Hospitals usually provide some of these items, but most people prefer their favorite brands or types. Avoid bringing products with strong scents (such as perfumes or colognes), as others in the hospital may have sensitivities to strong smells.

- **Toilet paper.** Yes, toilet paper. Hospital toilet paper is not known for its softness. Rough toilet paper is the last thing people with Crohn's and ulcerative colitis need when they are running back and forth to the bathroom many times a day. Bring a four-pack of your favorite brand with you. When you start running low, have a friend or family member bring more when they visit you.

- **Medications, vitamins, and other supplements, both prescription and over-the-counter.** Generally, once you are admitted, the hospital staff doesn't want you to use your own medications or supplements. However, in case the hospital doesn't have what you need, it's best to have everything with you. Ask your doctor to make a note in your chart that it's okay for you to take your vitamins or other supplements at certain times of the day.

- **A TV program schedule.** Let's face it—you may spend a lot of time watching television. Get a local cable channel conversion guide so you can identify the channels.

- **Shaving gear.** Plugging in an electric razor may be against hospital policy. Check ahead of time, or bring a shaver that has a fully charged battery.

- **For women, sanitary products.** If your period might start while in the hospital, bring your own sanitary napkins or tampons. Most hospitals have pads, but they are usually the big, bulky kind that you'll probably not want to use.

- **Makeup.** Many people say that when they feel they are looking their best, they feel better, too. For some women, this means wearing makeup; for others, it's the last thing they want to think about in the hospital.

Making other preparations

Besides packing, there are a few other matters you may want to deal with before you leave:

- **Take care of any outstanding bills.** If you are well enough to pay these now, it will save you much stress later. It's no fun to come home from the hospital and have to face overdue bills. If you are unable to pay the bills before your admission, have a trusted friend or family member take care of them if you feel this is appropriate.

- **Cancel any upcoming appointments.** Check your calendar to see if you have anything coming up such as a dentist appointment or plans with a friend. Although being hospitalized is a pretty good excuse for standing someone up, people will appreciate your letting them know of your need to cancel.

- **Contact your employer or school.** Call as soon as possible so that your boss, coworkers, or teachers can work around your absence. Try to give an idea of when you will return, but make clear that the exact timing is unpredictable. If you are in school, contact each of your instructors directly so you know they are informed about your situation.

- **Hold deliveries.** If you live alone, contact your post office and newspaper and tell them to stop your deliveries. Or, if you have trustworthy neighbors, have one of them pick up your mail and paper.

- **Get your hair cut.** If you have the time and feel up to it, you might as well get it done. If you end up stuck in the hospital for a long time, it'll give you a boost every time you look in the mirror and can say, "Well, at least my hair looks good."

- **Other responsibilities.** If you are the caregiver for children or elderly parents, or you have pets, make alternative arrangements with a responsible relative or friend. Be sure to leave written instructions and important phone numbers.

Preparing her children was not easy for Stacy:

> I have two daughters. Although they knew I had Crohn's, they never saw me when I was really ill. I had been severely ill years before, but that was well before they came along.
>
> There was really no good way to prepare them when I had to be hospitalized. At the time, they were 10 and 6. My husband and I explained what was happening, but it still didn't fully prepare them for what was to come. Fortunately, we had a lot of support from friends, family, and neighbors. They helped with meals, housework, and taking care of the children while I was away. One friend even made my daughter a costume for a school play. We would have never managed without everyone's help.

Avoiding emergency admissions

There are two ways to arrive at the hospital: through the emergency department or through the admitting department. Arriving through the admitting department is definitely the better way to go.

Admission through an emergency department is often a very long and painstaking process. You would think—because you arrived in an emergency situation—that the process ought to go quickly. This is not often the case. Emergency waiting rooms are generally full, and unless your situation is life threatening, you have to wait your turn. Mention any rectal bleeding when you register, as this symptom may bump you up to a higher priority.

If you can't sit up, stay in the car and have the person who drove you go in to ask for a gurney. It helps to have some place to lie down while waiting. After you have registered, a triage nurse will assess your condition and determine your priority. At this point, all you can do is wait.

Sometimes you must wait hours in the exam room until an emergency physician sees you. When she comes, she will ask you many detailed questions about your symptoms. She'll also conduct a brief physical exam, which may include a digital rectal exam. If you are having extreme rectal pain already, you can decline. Anytime you don't think an exam or a procedure is in your best interest, explain your reasoning to the doctor. Then listen to what he says. Unless you are unconscious or a threat to others, you have the right to refuse any treatment.

The doctor may order some blood work, and maybe even some x-rays if she thinks they are indicated. If you are showing signs of dehydration, a nurse will start an IV as well. If you haven't been able to eat and have lost a lot of weight, ask the physician if she can hang an IV bag that has either a 5 or 10 percent concentration of dextrose (as opposed to only normal saline). This way, you can at least get a few calories into your system. If the doctor thinks admission is likely, she'll call the hospital doctor on duty, who will come and assess you as well.

If the doctor decides to admit you, the admitting department will pay you a visit and ask you another round of questions. When your bed is ready, an attendant will wheel you up to your room. If you're lucky, you can get through this process in less than four hours, but it can take over twelve.

Jamie, who's had to go to the emergency room many times over the years, shares her feelings on the subject:

> Patience definitely comes in handy around the emergency room. I've generally had pretty good luck when it comes to the waiting room—they usually get to me fairly quickly. The exam room is another story. One time I was held up for eighteen hours before they could admit me! Although it's frustrating for me, I realize that, for the most part, everyone is doing his best. When you're sick and hurting, it's easy to forget that it can take a while to figure out what's going on. Blood work, x-rays, waiting for the right specialist, finding out what's wrong—it all takes time. There's certainly room for improvement in the system, but when it comes down to it, I know they care about my well-being.

In contrast, arriving directly through the admitting department is a breeze. When making arrangements ahead of time, your doctor has the admitting department call you and let you know when to arrive. When you show up at the appointed time, the interview process often takes less than a half hour, especially if you've previously been admitted to the same hospital. This half-hour process sure beats the lengthy routine in the emergency department.

Asking for a private room

People without hospital experience sometimes don't know they can request a private room. Chances are you can get one, although the ultimate decision is based on a combination of availability, staffing, your medical needs, and your insurance coverage. If you are admitted in an emergency situation and no other rooms are available, a shared room (also known as semiprivate) is certainly better than no room at all. Some insurance plans only cover the cost of semiprivate rooms. If your insurance covers a private room, or if you are willing to pay, it certainly can't hurt to request one.

Larry illustrates this point:

> I'd say I usually get a private room about half the time. One time though they put me in a room that holds four people. It was really bad. One guy in the room was screaming constantly. I couldn't get any sleep or rest. I asked my nurse if I could move. She agreed it would be a good idea for me to do so. It took a day or two before they could do

it, but I eventually got out of there. But if I hadn't said something, they probably would have just kept me where I was.

Simply having IBD doesn't necessarily constitute a medical need for a private room. However, certain complications of the disease are sometimes very good reasons for having one. For example, if you are running back and forth to the bathroom fifteen or twenty times a day, it may not be fair for someone else to have to share a room—or especially a bathroom—with you. Also, if you have a fistula on your bottom (a connection from your intestine to the skin on your rear, which is considered an open wound), you should never share a toilet. Discuss with your doctor any concerns you have regarding medical reasons for needing your own room or bathroom.

David always got a private room:

> *My case was very severe, and fortunately the hospital staff had the sense to always give me my own room. I'm sure part of it was that I used to smell up the room so bad. I had fistulas coming out all over my abdomen—so it was very difficult to control all the fecal matter draining from me. Every time the nurses came in, they'd have to spray some air freshener. Besides the odor, I was in general a very high maintenance patient. Hospital staff was always coming in and out. It was a very disruptive environment. It would not have been fair for anyone to have to share a room with me.*

Of course, you might be someone who wants to have a roommate. Sharing a room can be companionable. If you happen to get paired up with someone with whom you are compatible, and this person is also respectful of your needs, then the semiprivate room experience can be a very pleasant and beneficial one.

Richard shares his story about one of his roommates during his first hospitalization:

> *Although I certainly prefer a private room, I'll admit that sometimes having a roommate can be a valuable experience. The first time I was hospitalized in a children's hospital as a teen, I shared a large room with three other kids, two of whom also had IBD. One of these was a little boy, about 5 years old. He had a very severe case of Crohn's for almost his whole life. He had almost no intestine and always had to be on IV feeding. He had been constantly in and out of the hospital for most of his life. He was a wonderful little boy, and one of his parents was always there with him. His parents shared with me*

some of their story and what they've been through as a family. I was touched by what they shared, and I was amazed at how well they managed through such difficulty. It also made me realize that regardless of how sick I was at the time, my case was not that bad. I found that despite all that was going on with me, I still had much to be thankful for.

Working smoothly with hospital staff

You'll interact with a wide variety of hospital personnel during your stay. Although it is their job to care for you, they have many others to tend to as well. Hospitals are often high-stress environments, and this atmosphere can take its toll on employees.

Hospitals aim to provide excellent care for all people—even the difficult, unpleasant ones. But a combination of diplomacy, courtesy, and a gently assertive style can help you receive the top-notch care you deserve and can help build valuable relationships with your hospital's staff.

Here are a few suggestions to enhance relationships with the people providing your care:

- **Communicate clearly and diplomatically.** If you aren't getting what you need or want, ask courteously how to improve the situation. People who bark out demands and orders may temporarily get attention but are unlikely to solve any problems.

- **Have respect and empathy.** You may think this is a suggestion for hospital staff when interacting with hospital patrons, rather than vice versa. But it works both ways. When you show respect and empathy to those caring for you, you'll soon find you receive plenty of the same.

- **Express appreciation.** Never hesitate to compliment someone on a job well done. By expressing a thankful attitude, you'll open yourself up to receive even more. Hospital employees may go the extra mile for you without your having to request it.

Craig, who has always made an effort to invest in his relationships with people at his hospital, demonstrates how these suggestions can pay off:

I've been in and out of the same hospital for many years, and I have always made an effort to treat the staff with much love and respect. Over the years, I've developed some solid relationships with a large

cross section of the hospital staff. I think that I was touched the most
one time after I had some surgery. When I woke up in my room, the
unit assistant on the floor came in to see how I was doing. She said,
"When I came in this evening, I noticed that someone had assigned
you to a double room. I know you value your privacy so I switched
you to a private one." I didn't know what to say, other than to thank
her. It made me realize how important it is to truly cherish the
relationships I have with people at this wonderful place.

Nurses

One of the most important relationships you will have in the hospital is with your nurses, because they provide most of your care. Although you may think of your nurse primarily as someone who gives you your medications, nurses can provide much more.

Larry, who has had Crohn's for many years, describes his view on nurses:

I think nurses are probably the most important of all the different
hospital personnel. Whereas doctors generally don't have a lot of time
to spend with patients, nurses are likely to have a little more time. In
fact, many times over the last few years I've found my nurses to be
my best advocates, especially when I had a difficult time
communicating with my doctors.

Your nurse is your primary link to everyone else in the hospital. If you are too weak to be your own advocate, ask your nurse to help you get what you need from other hospital personnel.

In addition to patient advocacy, your nurse can make your stay more pleasant by remembering what most people would call the "little things." For instance, ask her about the timing of your medication. Although your doctor is the one who orders when your medications are given, depending on the drug, the nurse can give it a half-hour to one hour early or late. Ask your nurse to adjust this timing to maximize your sleep.

David developed good relationships with his nurses:

There was one time when I was in hospital for months. It was a
really terrible situation. I was so ill. I don't know what I would have
done without some of my nurses. They were fabulous. They'd come in
on their days off to visit me, call me from home to check in on me, and

*even have lunch with me in my room. They didn't tell me this at the
time, but later several of them said they were always afraid that the
next time they came to work, I'd be dead. I really appreciated all their
personalized care.*

Lastly, you can help your nurse by taking a proactive approach to your health care. Although you don't need to start your own IVs or insert your own feeding tubes, probably you can do some things to help yourself. For example, you can keep track of your input and output (including the color, consistency, and frequency of your bowel movements), learn some of the basics of your IV pump, or help out with your bathing.

Physicians

Your interaction with physicians depends largely on the type of hospital to which you are admitted. If you are admitted to a private or community hospital, there is a good chance your own primary care physician or gastroenterologist will be in charge of your care. Sometimes these hospitals have in-house staff physicians, and you will work with one of them instead. However, because the treatment of IBD generally requires a specialist, the in-house physician will probably work closely with either your own gastroenterologist or another one who is part of the same group.

If you are in a teaching hospital, care is provided by a variety of physicians. In fact, there are so many it can become thoroughly confusing. Here's a list to help clarify their roles:

- **Medical students.** Although not physicians yet, these students are either in their third or fourth year of medical school. They won't be treating you, but they will accompany your attending physician on rounds. Make good use of your medical student if one is assigned to you. Students are often eager to provide information, explain what you want to know, or just listen if you need an ear.

- **Residents.** Residents have graduated from medical school and are in the process of acquiring their postgraduate training in a particular field such as internal medicine, pediatrics, or surgery. Residency programs last from three to seven years, depending on the specialty. First-year residents are called interns, and those in their later years are called residents.

- **Fellows.** A fellow has completed his residency but has decided to undertake an additional three years of training (called a fellowship) in another specialty, such as gastroenterology or pulmonary medicine. Gastroenterologists specialize in either internal medicine or pediatrics in their residency, and then gastroenterology in their fellowship.

- **Attending physician.** This doctor has the highest authority when it comes to managing your care. Your attending physician is permanently employed by the teaching hospital and most likely is a professor at the hospital's affiliated medical school.

The exposure to all these levels of physicians in a teaching hospital has its advantages and disadvantages. The major disadvantage is that you will have many doctors coming to visit you at all hours of the day, which, especially in the beginning, is very exhausting. They'll ask you the same questions over and over, and they'll all probably want to poke around your belly and do rectal exams on you. Remember, you can always refuse any test or exam (especially if you just had an identical one a few hours earlier). The major advantage, however, is that you will have access to a wide range of doctors positioned on the cutting edge of medicine. You'll thus have the opportunity to get a variety of opinions on your suggested and prescribed treatments.

For information on how to enhance your relationship with your physicians (whether in the hospital or out), see Chapter 9, *Working with Your Doctor.*

Social workers

Hospitalization is often stressful. Fortunately, the staff at most medical centers recognize this fact and provide social workers to those in need. Many people are unsure of exactly what role hospital social workers can play. They can assist you in many ways:

- Helping you adapt to the hospital environment
- Helping you cope with your IBD
- Referring you to mental health professionals once you are discharged
- Referring you to other resources outside the hospital that can help you
- Being an advocate for you if you are having difficulty communicating with any members of your medical team

Cheryl was thankful that a hospital social worker was available:

> At first, I didn't quite understand the role of hospital social workers. It wasn't until a week before one of my surgeries that another patient suggested I contact the one at my hospital. The social worker asked me many questions about what the hospital could do to make my stay more

pleasant, including things as diverse as what my food preferences were, whether I needed help with my medical insurance, or if I'd like to watch videos in my hospital room. She made it clear that she was someone who would be consistently there to act as a coordinator or intermediary between me and the rest of the staff.

Phlebotomists

"Phlebotomist" is the technical name for the laboratory technician who draws your blood. You'll probably have a lot of contact with phlebotomists during your hospital stay.

When the phlebotomist comes to draw your blood, make sure he puts on a new pair of gloves. If you find a phlebotomist who consistently draws your blood well, you can request that this person always be the one to draw your blood when he is on duty. Likewise, if one can never get it right the first time, politely request another technician. Your veins are very important while you are in the hospital. There is no point in becoming an experimental pincushion.

Another way you can help protect your veins is to work with your phlebotomist when choosing the appropriate needle to draw your blood. If you are an adult, phlebotomists usually use an adult needle. In some situations, this is the best choice. In others, a children's or butterfly needle may make more sense, because smaller punctures can help preserve your veins over time. Most phlebotomists will gladly honor your request. If you are unclear about what needle is best for you, discuss the issue with your doctor and have him write a standing order for it.

If you have difficult veins, it also sometimes helps to apply a warm compress before your blood draw. This helps increase blood flow to the area and may make increase your chances of a successful poke.

David worked closely with his phlebotomists:

> *I don't have good veins. As a result, the phlebotomists had a very difficult time drawing my blood. Over time, we learned that the pediatric butterfly needle worked the best for me. I'd give someone three chances. If they couldn't get it, I'd request that an anesthesiologist come and do it.*

When you are first admitted, it is not uncommon for your doctor to order frequent blood tests. If you feel your blood is drawn more times than seems reasonable, politely ask your doctor about the reason for all the tests. Ask him to coordinate blood draws so you can have multiple tests drawn all at once, if possible. Keep in mind that if your hemoglobin is already low and you are still losing blood with your bowel movements, it is necessary to monitor your blood quite frequently. In general, however, twice-weekly draws are usually sufficient unless you have significant blood loss, infection, liver concerns, or electrolyte imbalances (such as sodium or potassium).

If you are in doubt about your multiple blood draws, speak up, as Craig—who used to lose a lot of blood during his flare-ups—describes:

> *My hemoglobin had fallen down to about 9, which is low but still above the point where they would transfuse me. There was also no doubt that I still had blood with my bowel movements. But my condition had stabilized, and the frequency of my bowel movements was much less. I understand that they wanted to keep a watchful eye on my hemoglobin, but really, the blood draws four times a day were getting ridiculous. Since my hemoglobin was not trending lower, I asked my doctor to switch me to a once-a-day draw. He agreed to give it a try.*

Dietitians

Nutritional support during your hospital stay is an integral part of your treatment and will help you recover quickly. Thus, it's to your advantage to cultivate a solid partnership with your hospital dietitian. Your dietitian will have either a bachelor's or master's degree and hold the title of registered dietitian (RD). Some even subspecialize in IBD therapy.

If you have concerns about your dietary or nutritional needs, seek assistance from a dietitian. Your doctor is the only one who can prescribe an alternative form of feeding, but your dietitian can play an important role in determining your need for it. Although a dietitian should automatically evaluate your nutritional needs if you've been on bowel rest for more than a day or two without any nutritional support, you can make sure to request an evaluation if one doesn't occur. If you are unable to eat and require another form of nourishment, read Chapter 8, *Alternative Forms of Feeding*.

If you are able to eat, your dietitian will help you make the best food choices based on what kind of diet your doctor has prescribed for you (or what kind of diet you and your doctor have agreed is best for you). Ask your dietitian to bring a list of all the foods available to you in the hospital so you know all the in-house options. You can have friends and family bring food if you feel the hospital food is inadequate.

Hospital food

Hospital food is notorious for being unpalatable and of poor quality. In some cases, this reputation is justified. In others, it's not. There are hospitals out there that have good food. Somewhere.

Many hospitals contract with the same companies that provide food to airlines. The entrees are generally heavily processed, frozen, and then microwaved before serving. From a food safety perspective, as well as an economics perspective, this approach makes sense. It's convenient, efficient, and—assuming the food was originally prepared properly—there is little chance of someone contracting food poisoning.

But what's safe for the short term, is not necessarily nutritionally sound for the long haul, especially for people whose ability to absorb nutrients may be compromised.

Richard, who is very nutrition conscious, describes his first days of eating in the hospital after a long bowel rest:

> I had been in the hospital for four weeks on TPN and was so excited about being able to eat. I thoroughly enjoyed the food I ate those first few days, but I questioned the rationale of the food they gave me. For breakfast, they would give me things like white flour pancakes with margarine and artificial syrup along with deep-fried potatoes. Lunch and dinner would consist of goopy entrees that were very salty and heavily processed. The vegetables in these entrees were pale in color and certainly devoid of nutrients. For dessert they would give me artificial puddings and pound cake that had a list of ingredients even a chemist would have a hard time deciphering.
>
> I tried to work with the dietitian to pick healthy foods, but everything they had on the soft food diet was the same heavily processed stuff. I told my doctor and dietitian it was such a shame that we live in a country with access to so many high-quality, nutritious health foods, yet the hospital serves the most processed, unhealthy food you can buy. Even my doctor admitted that the food quality was poor and that if I could I should have someone bring me food. Fortunately, once I was able to eat for a couple of days, I got to go home and could then prepare nutritious food for myself.

You might luck out, like Stacy, and rarely have to eat hospital food:

> *I've been in the hospital so many times, but I've never really had to deal with the food. By the time I can, they're already sending me home. But if it's anything like the broth they serve, I'm thankful I get to avoid the hospital meals.*

Assuming you do have to deal with hospital food that is not to your liking, what can you do? Following are a few suggestions:

- Work with your dietitian to find items on the menu that meet your needs. Realize that you won't be in the hospital forever and that soon you'll go home and have access to better-quality food.

  David worked out a plan:

  > *The food at my hospital was just terrible. I couldn't eat it. However, the hospital cafeteria food wasn't bad. I worked out an arrangement where they opened the cafeteria menu to me. You would think that the quality of food they give to patients would be at least as good as what they serve in the cafeteria. But that wasn't the case.*

- Complain nicely to your dietitian. Appeal to her sense of reasoning, nutritional awareness, and taste buds. Acknowledge that you are sure she is doing the best she can with what she has to work with, but that she should try to convince higher powers at the hospital to invest in higher-quality, more nutritious food.

- Write a letter to the head of the dietary department that expresses your concerns in a friendly manner. Again, hospitals are businesses, and they want to please their customers. If enough people demand better food, improvements may occur.

- If you can't find enough wholesome food in the hospital, have friends or family bring your favorite snacks or meals. Make arrangements ahead of time with the nursing staff if you'll need refrigerator space. Of course, be reasonable—you can live without watermelon and a whole roasted turkey while in the hospital. Also, you might try to spread the burden among family and friends so just one person is not responsible for bringing food to you.

- Order take-out food and have it delivered. If you don't want to trouble anyone and you can afford it, this may be a good option. Many restaurants and gourmet shops are happy to deliver meals if you are willing to pay the price. However, check with your doctor or nurse first. Some hospitals have policies against their patrons ordering take-out food.

- Try taking a different attitude toward the food provided to you. Be thankful for it and the fact that you are able to eat it. Sometimes people can become so obsessive about what they eat that it becomes unhealthy (even if the food itself is healthy).

Watching out for yourself

Nowhere is it more imperative to watch out for yourself than in the hospital. As mentioned earlier, hospital mishaps happen: Wrong medications are sometimes given, wrong dosages of the right medications are occasionally given, procedures may be performed incorrectly, and so forth. You certainly can't control everything going on around you, but with some vigilance you can help minimize the chances of becoming a victim of a hospital error.

Many people with IBD are mentally alert during much of their stay. Being vigilant to your surroundings can definitely work to your advantage:

> I tend to be one of those people who is hypervigilant about everything they do to me in the hospital. One evening, a nurse I knew well told me flat out that she thought I was being too neurotic. I had to admit she was right. After all, she knew my routine well—there was really no reason for me to check every little detail.
>
> I decided to kick back that night and just let everyone else take care of me. After my first few episodes of an I Love Lucy marathon, I couldn't help but glance at my TPN bag. I noticed that it was looking a little too empty for that time of the evening. Also, the bag itself looked smaller. Giving in to my natural tendency, I got up to examine my TPN bag. Everything looked fine except for the fact that it had someone else's name on it. The nurse had hung the wrong bag! She hung another patient's bag (which was much smaller) but was running it at my normal high rate. No wonder the bag was looking empty.
>
> Needless to say, my nurse was horrified that she could have done such a thing. She became very apologetic about criticizing my hypervigilance just hours earlier. "Maybe you should go back to being neurotic," she admitted.

If you are alert enough to look out for yourself, keep in mind you can drive yourself crazy scrutinizing every detail. At some point you'll have to trust that your medical team is competent and its members know what they are doing.

How do you know at what point to let go and trust? There is no easy answer to this question. A lot will depend on your condition and also the kind of person you are. If you don't want to participate in managing your own care (or are so sick that you are unable), then you're going to have to completely rely on others.

However, if you are alert enough to be involved (and you want to be involved), here are some tips to consider in your effort to achieve balance:

- Let your doctors and nurses know you want to participate in the management of your medical care. Explain you want to be involved in decisions regarding your treatments.

- Become familiar with the medications you receive during your stay. Know the dosages and how often you are receiving each medication. If there are too many to remember, write everything down. If you can't write them down yourself, have someone write them down for you. Some hospitals have a board on which they write all medications in large letters so people in bed can keep track of what they're getting.

- Confirm with your nurse what you are receiving when she gives you your medications. If she gives you a drug that's not on your list, or the dosage is not what you expect, kindly ask if any changes were made in your treatment. If you are uncomfortable or have questions about alterations made to your prescribed regimen, discuss them with your doctor.

- Become familiar with your hospital's protocol for sterile technique. Because the risk of hospital-acquired infection is significant, it's a good idea to take steps to protect yourself. For example, during a dressing change for a central IV line, if you notice someone is not performing a task correctly or you are unsure, diplomatically ask if his methods are part of hospital protocol. You can say you have noticed other people perform this task differently, and you want to know which is the proper way. If you are not satisfied with the answers, ask to speak to your floor's nursing supervisor.

You may want to ask friends and family who visit you frequently to help you handle these suggestions, especially if you are too ill to watch out for yourself.

Stacy's enlisted her family's help:

> I think it's very important to have a personal advocate or advocates when you're in the hospital. Even if you can do it yourself, it doesn't hurt to have someone else around most of the time. I can't tell you how many times that I've almost been given the wrong medicine. It's kind of scary.
>
> For the most part I can watch out for myself. But there have been times when I've been just so exhausted, or so sick, or under the influence of medications that I've needed someone else around. I usually had either my mom, dad, or husband to stand watch. It wasn't 24/7, but they were there a lot of the time and it really helped to have them with me.

Other tips

Whether you are in the hospital for one day, one week, or one month, you might as well make the best of it. Beyond the issues of arriving at the hospital, dealing with medical personnel, and watching out for yourself, other factors to consider also can help your mind, body, and spirit during this time. Here are a couple of additional tips:

- **Move around as much as possible.** Check with your doctors and nurses about recommended limitations given your condition. Usually healthcare providers want you to be as active as possible because it helps increase circulation, improve lung function, and may promote faster healing. If you can, go for frequent walks down the halls of your floor. If you have the energy, venture out to other areas of the hospital or take walks outside, weather permitting.

Richard explains:

> The hospital that I used to go to many years ago was right across the street from a large mall. I would have about six hours a day off my TPN, and the nurses would encourage me to take advantage of a day pass to go to the mall for an hour. More recently, the hospital I was at was also near a major shopping center, but I never actually got to go to it. But I would take long walks around the hospital and be gone for a long time. They would always ask me where I had been, and I would always joke with them about my adventures of dragging

my IV pole through the department stores. They of course knew I was
kidding, but after a while, whenever I'd be leaving for a walk, it
became an old joke to ask, "What do you want me to pick up for you
at Nordstrom's this time?"

Of course, you may barely be able to get out of bed, much less take a stroll over to the local mall when you are in the hospital. Nevertheless, it helps to move, even if it's only doing a few leg exercises in bed or lifting a water bottle.

- **Do your breathing exercises.** If you are walking around a lot, you won't need to worry so much about breathing exercises. But if you are mostly bedridden or have recently had surgery, it's necessary to perform these exercises to prevent pneumonia and other respiratory problems. Your hospital should provide you with a spirometer, a device that helps you expand your lungs while measuring the volume of your breaths. Use your spirometer at least once every few waking hours. You may also want to look into doing some other kinds of deep breathing exercises on your own. (See the *Resources* appendix for a book on breathing exercises.)

- **Decorate your room.** Hospital rooms often have a drab, sterile atmosphere. Therefore, there's much you can do to liven the place up. If you are going to be in for more than a day or two, you can ask friends and family to bring pictures, posters, flowers, plants, scented candles, and anything else that can help personalize your room.

A decorated room helped Stacy:

My room was filled with plants, flowers, and balloons. My kids also
drew pictures and they hung them on the walls. All and all, my room
had a festive atmosphere. It helped lift my spirits when I was going
through such a difficult time.

- **Have fun.** Although most people don't think of the hospital as a place to have fun, there's no reason you can't do things to help lighten the mood around the place. Many hospital rooms now have VCRs—so you can entertain yourself for hours watching funny videos. Also, have your friends or family bring your favorite games and comic or joke books. And don't hesitate to share the laughs with other around the hospital. Not only will you help yourself feel better, but the hospital staff will appreciate your humor as well.

Going home

Some may think discharge is the best part of a hospital stay, but not all people with IBD embrace it so enthusiastically. Although most people want to go home, many have concerns about being released either too soon or without the training necessary to take care of themselves at home.

Craig puts it this way:

> It's not that I didn't want to start eating and go home. Even though my symptoms had abated, I knew that my digestive system was not ready for solid food. I felt I needed at least a few more days on bowel rest. But my doctor said my reduction in symptoms indicated that I was ready to eat. So I went along with what he said. Within five days of going home, I had to go back to the hospital and resume bowel rest.

Remember, you know your own body best. If for any reason you feel you aren't ready to go home, express your concerns to your physician. It's not going to do you any good or save the insurance company any money if you have to return to the hospital within days or weeks of coming home.

When you and your physician determine your condition has improved enough for you to go home, you will receive a visit from a discharge nurse. If you are able to eat and walk and will not require any IV medications, the discharge process is very simple. Little planning is involved, other than arranging with the pharmacy for any medications you do not already have at home and making a follow-up appointment with your doctor. In addition, the discharge nurse will review with you activity restrictions you may need to follow temporarily, as well as any procedures you need to know to care for yourself if you've had surgery (see Chapter 6, *Surgical Treatments*, for more information on this topic).

If you are unable to eat when you go home, or you will require IV medications, the discharge process is more complicated. You and the hospital staff will need to make plans with a home health nursing agency. Your hospital may have its own or may contract with a local company. Generally, hospitals contract with medical equipment companies to provide you with the equipment you need, such as pumps for either IV or tube feedings. Also, the hospital staff will help make arrangements for other necessary medical supplies, such as tubing, syringes, saline, and so forth. The staff will also help you connect with a pharmacy to provide your IV medications as well as your TPN or elemental diet products. Sometimes the hospital outpatient pharmacy provides these supplies and medications, but some people may need to use a neighborhood pharmacy.

If several people are involved in home care, it helps to have one person coordinating services. A good discharge nurse will perform this function. There is, however, much you can do to make sure you have everything organized before you leave the hospital.

Richard, who has been hospitalized for IBD many times, explains:

> *Several years ago, I was going home on my TPN and IV corticosteroids. The discharge nurse had given me a bag of supplies to take home to carry me through till I would receive my delivery from the outpatient pharmacy.*
>
> *On my first night home, I realized she had not included any heparin in my bag, which was recommended to flush my central line. My father had to drive 30 miles at 11 P.M. back to the hospital to get some. The people at Emergency would not give him any, saying that it was a drug and thus he needed a prescription. There was no explaining that the hospital had forgotten to include it in my supplies and that I needed it ASAP so my line wouldn't clot. Finally, he went back to the floor where I had been staying, and one of my nurses had mercy on him and gave him a few bottles.*
>
> *Fortunately, he made it back in time. Since this experience, I make sure to check everything before leaving the hospital.*

The following tips can help make your discharge go smoothly if you are going home on IV feeding, tube feeding, or IV medications:

- Work closely with your discharge nurse. Explain any concerns about being on your own at home, and make sure you have everything organized before you leave the hospital.

- Get adequate training before you leave the hospital. This training should include operation of pumps, administration of IV drugs, flushing your lines, and anything else that's necessary for you to do at home. In addition to training with your discharge nurse, you can also ask your regular nurses to coach you the last day or two of your stay. Make certain you are comfortable with all procedures before you leave.

- Have a close friend or family member learn everything, too, so you can have a backup person on call. Make sure he or she is also comfortable with all procedures before you are discharged.

- Make sure you have all training instructions in writing. If the literature provided isn't well written or is just plain confusing, write up your own during a training session (or have your nurse or a friend help you write it).

- Ask for a list of phone numbers to call if you run into problems. Confirm that with these numbers you can reach a live person 24 hours a day, seven days a week.

- Before you leave, make sure you have all the supplies and medications you need (including TPN or elemental diet formula) to get you through at least two days at home, even if they say you will be receiving a delivery to your home within 24 hours. Have the discharge nurse make an itemized list of all your necessary supplies. Then go through the bag she gives you to make sure everything is there. If you need any assistance, ask the discharge nurse or one of your regular nurses to help you.

- Request that the pumps you will be on at home be delivered directly to your hospital room so your nurse can set you up on them before you leave. Don't go along with plans to be set up once you get home, because too many things can go wrong this way.

- Arrange to have your first visit with the home health nurse within 24 hours of going home. If you can, make the appointment for a time you'll need some help, such as the first time you must change your TPN bag at home.

Ask for an itemized bill before you leave the hospital. When you get a chance, go through everything and make sure the charges are valid. Be on the lookout for extra charges, such as meals you didn't order or medications you didn't take.

Last, remember to thank the staff. If too much is going on around the time of your discharge, you can always make thank-you calls or send notes of thanks once you've had time to recover some at home.

Jamie, who has experienced hospitalization on more than one occasion, shares her views on thanking the staff:

> *I feel very strongly about letting people know when they've made a difference in my life. In addition to four or five nurses who stood out among the rest, I found the orderlies to be a wonderful source of*

support, as well as being respectful and sensitive. Since they are probably the least recognized among hospital staff, I made a special effort to track them down and send thank-you cards. In addition to simply acknowledging what a difference they made in my stay, my hope is that my gratitude will stay with them so that they will have even more to give to future patients.

CHAPTER 11

Life with an Ostomy

AN OSTOMY IS the surgical creation of an abdominal opening that allows the elimination of either feces or urine. If the colon or bladder is severely diseased or damaged, an ostomy is often necessary so a person can excrete waste products.

Ostomies are frequently a major concern for people with ulcerative colitis or Crohn's disease of the colon. Although most people with IBD will never need ostomy surgery, many still worry that some day they might lose their large intestine and have to wear a bag the rest of their lives.

Ostomy surgery is definitely a major life event for those who undergo it. In most cases, it forever changes the way you eliminate waste products. But people with IBD who have the surgery go on to lead happy, healthy, normal, and productive lives. In fact, after they recover from surgery, most feel better than they have in years.

This chapter begins by discussing the different types of ostomies and when they are needed. It then explains how to care for one and what types of products are used. Next the chapter examines the personal experience of living with an ostomy and how to seek support if you need it. Throughout the chapter, people with IBD share their stories of what it's like to live with an ostomy.

Types of ostomies

Most types of ostomies include an opening on the skin called a stoma. Waste products empty from the body through this opening. The person, sometimes called an ostomate, usually needs to wear a pouch over her stoma to collect the feces or urine. People with ostomies generally have no control over when waste is eliminated through the stoma. Some types of ostomy procedures, however, allow a person to control elimination. Following are descriptions of the most common types of ostomies.

Colostomy

A colostomy is an ostomy in which part of the colon is brought to the surface of one's abdomen to eliminate stool. Colostomies are performed when someone has part of the large intestine—including the rectum, in most cases—removed. The remaining end of the colon is then brought to the surface of the skin to form a stoma. The draining stool is generally solid, because the person usually still has enough of his large bowel to absorb fluids back into the body.

It's unusual for someone with IBD to have a colostomy. When colon surgery is recommended for people with Crohn's or ulcerative colitis, doctors almost always advise removal of the entire colon. If only part of the large bowel is removed in people with IBD, chances are very high that disease will return in the remaining piece of large intestine. The person soon is just as sick as he was before the surgery. Colostomies are much more common in people who have had cancer of their lower colon, including their rectum (but no history of IBD), and in people with spinal cord injuries who have no bowel control.

Ileostomy

An ileostomy is similar to a colostomy, except that the end of the small intestine, the ileum, is brought through to the exterior side of the abdominal wall. A stoma is then made with the end of the ileum, allowing waste to exit the body. Drainage from an ileostomy is often more liquid, because the person no longer has a colon to absorb fluids from digested food.

An ileostomy is by far the most common ostomy procedure done on people with IBD. Removal of the entire colon with ileostomy is considered a cure for ulcerative colitis. Although Crohn's can occur anywhere in the GI tract, people who have only had it in the colon may remain disease free many years—and even for life—if they have the entire large bowel removed. For information on this surgical procedure, see Chapter 6, *Surgical Treatments*.

Stacy has had very good results with her ileostomy:

> *I developed Crohn's well over twenty years ago when I was in college. I suffered for many years. A few years ago, I had a complete colectomy with ileostomy. I know that technically it's not considered a cure as it is for ulcerative colitis. However, I have not had a recurrence of Crohn's since my surgery. It's given me a whole new life.*

J-pouch

A J-pouch is technically not an ostomy, because it involves no stoma. It's commonly performed on people with ulcerative colitis who have had their colon removed, including most of the rectum. However, surgery spares a small portion of the upper anal canal, as well as the anal sphincter muscles. Tissue from the end of the small intestine is then taken to create an internal J-shaped pouch. This pouch, which serves as a reservoir to hold waste products, is later attached to the anus so that elimination can occur normally.

The procedure is popular, because no external appliance is needed to catch waste. Other common names you might hear to describe the J-pouch include "ileal pouch–anal anastomosis" (IPAA) or "ileoanal pull-through." For more information on this procedure, see Chapter 6.

Krystal, who had ulcerative colitis for six years, describes her experience with the J-pouch:

> Since I had ulcerative colitis, I had other choices besides a standard ileostomy. I opted for the J-pouch, as I knew I didn't want to have a bag. My surgeon said he could do it in one operation, which sounded good to me. But when I awoke from surgery, I was shocked to discover that I had a temporary ileostomy. I was not prepared for that outcome. I now always tell others that even if the doctor says he can do it in one surgery, accept the fact that it may require two. Sometimes the surgeon really doesn't know until during the operation what's the best decision. Although I wasn't happy at the time, in retrospect I'm glad we did it in two steps. The three months in between allowed me to regain much of my strength so that I was better able to handle the second step.
>
> The J-pouch has worked very well for me. I now go to the bathroom seven or eight times a day. To some people that still seems like a lot. But I'm not sick and I feel great. Overall, I feel I have a very high quality of life.

Other continent ostomies

The J-pouch is now the standard for continent procedures. However, there are other surgical techniques that are occasionally used to create continent ostomies. Like the J-pouch, the following options are only performed on people with ulcerative colitis, not Crohn's.

Kock pouch

One well-known ostomy that allows a person to control elimination is the Kock pouch. After the colon is removed, the surgeon creates a reservoir from the end of the small intestine. But instead of connecting it to the anus, a valve is made and attached to a stoma that is flush with the abdominal surface. The individual with a Kock pouch does not need to wear a bag, but instead wears a small covering to protect the stoma. A catheter (drainage tube) is used to empty the reservoir several times a day.

Laura carefully researched her options and chose the Kock pouch:

> *The diarrhea caused by my ulcerative colitis was so bad that I was going twenty to thirty times a day. After speaking to others who had the J-pouch, I couldn't bear the thought of going through surgery only to still have soft or watery stool coming out my bottom multiple times a day. I also preferred not to have a bag at this point in my life. That left the Kock pouch option. I was originally told that it would probably only last about four years, but I've had it now for fourteen. I don't know anyone who has had theirs as long as I. Others have needed another surgery to get a standard ileostomy. I accept the fact that I will someday, too. But even if that happens tomorrow, I know I've made the right decision for myself. The Kock pouch gave me my life back. I've been able to do everything I want with it. I've even been able to have a baby. My quality of life has been great and I've never regretted my decision.*

Barnett continent ileal reservoir (BCIR)

The BCIR is a modified version of the Kock pouch procedure that's performed at a few hospital centers in the United States. The differences include changes in the internal reservoir design that aim to reduce valve problems and fistula development. Since 1988, over 1,300 people have undergone this surgery. To learn more about the BCIR, you can call the Continent Ostomy Centers at (800) 721-7989 or you can visit the web site at *http://www.ostomybcir.com/*.

Urostomy

A urostomy is a surgical creation of an opening in the abdomen that allows the elimination of urine. It's usually performed on people who have had their bladder removed because of cancer, or in people with spinal cord injuries who no longer can control their bladder function. Tissue from the small intestine is taken to form a channel that connects the ureters (the tubes that carry urine from the kidneys to the bladder) to the surface to the skin where a stoma is made. Urostomies are not common in people with IBD unless they have some other problem with their urinary tract.

When an ostomy is necessary

An ostomy is generally necessary for someone with IBD when his life is endangered by severe disease in the colon. For instance, toxic megacolon is immediately life-threatening and often requires surgical removal of the large intestine. The discovery of dysplasia or colorectal cancer is also another example. Most people facing these complications have little choice other than colectomy (complete removal of the colon) with a creation of an ostomy to save their lives.

Hollie was in a life-threatening situation when she was a young girl:

> *I was diagnosed with IBD when I was 11. It started out mild but gradually got worse over the next year. I developed what we later discovered was an abscess in my abdominal cavity. My doctor was treating me with antibiotics and prednisone at the time, neither of which seemed to be doing much good.*
>
> *One morning I woke up in the worst pain I could ever imagine. I could barely move or talk. My parents took me to the hospital, where they identified that I had an abscess. However, they didn't catch it in time, and it burst in my abdominal cavity. I had to have emergency surgery, and it was unsure whether I'd survive.*
>
> *I was told that during this surgery I came very close to dying. All they could do was clean out my abdominal cavity and insert various tubes so that the infection could drain out of me. I was much too weak for the colectomy at this point.*
>
> *It was touch and go following this surgery. I can recall in the days after it that many doctors and nurses who came into my room and saw me awake and sitting up, either cried or turned white as a sheet, since they didn't think I would live through the first night. However, I stabilized relatively quickly, and they were able to take me back to surgery to finish what they needed to do. Since my colon was so diseased and damaged, they had no choice but to give me an ostomy. Also, when the abscess burst, it severely damaged one of my kidneys*

and my bladder. They were able to rebuild my bladder, but I did lose the one kidney.

I don't know why I had to go through this at such a young age, but I must say that I am extremely grateful for my life. The ostomy took some adjustment, but I am very thankful for it because without it I wouldn't be alive.

When an ostomy is a choice

An ostomy is often chosen when a person with IBD and his doctor determine that quality of life will be better with one than without one. Making this judgment is not easy or clear-cut, because it depends on what an individual defines as quality living.

Laura discusses how she decided to have her colon removed:

I had ulcerative colitis for over four years. My case was a severe one, but it wasn't life threatening. Not that I would have wanted it to be, but sometimes I think it almost would have been easier if it were. Then I wouldn't have had to take the responsibility of making such a life-altering decision.

The years I was sick were difficult. I had a young daughter and was unable to do simple things with her like go to the park. I had too much diarrhea. The whole time I never really had a remission and was on a lot of medication. I knew surgery was an option, but it seemed like such an extreme solution.

At one point, for the first time in four years, it seemed like things were starting to get better. I was gradually decreasing my medication and thought I'd finally have some healthy time. But out of the blue one morning I was back to the horrible pain again. That was it. I called my doctor and said, "I'm done. Let's do it." I just couldn't take it anymore. I decided to take a chance, hoping my life could be better afterward. And sure enough, it was. I no longer have ulcerative colitis, and can live a normal life.

The "Elective surgeries" section in Chapter 6 describes several situations that examine IBD's impact on the quality and enjoyment of your life. If you see yourself in one of those examples—and if your disease is mainly in your colon—you might consider discussing an ostomy with your doctor. If after careful consideration you and your doctor determine that having an ostomy is a good choice, your next step is to meet with an enterostomal therapy (ET) nurse. An ET nurse specializes in ostomy management and can help you get ready for your operation. For information on specific surgical procedures—including preparing for and recovering from surgery—please see Chapter 6.

Characteristics of a stoma

The ileostomy is the standard and by far the most common ostomy for those with Crohn's or ulcerative colitis. Generally, the ileostomate's stoma is located in the lower right portion of the abdomen, just to the right of and below the navel. If your surgery is not an emergency situation, you'll have a chance to meet with both your surgeon and ET nurse to discuss and plan the specific location. Your ET nurse will examine how the skin on your abdomen folds while sitting, standing, bending, and moving in different positions.

Your presurgery appointments are also a good time to express your concerns about how your stoma's location may affect various aspects of your life, such as the clothes you like to wear and physical activities you enjoy. When a good location is identified, your ET nurse will mark the spot with a felt tip pen. Although your surgeon will do his best to accommodate the chosen position, he may have to override the decision during surgery if he deems another location will allow for a better functioning stoma.

The stoma is usually large and swollen after surgery. Over about eight weeks, it shrinks to its permanent size. Stomas can vary among ileostomates, but typically they protrude a $\frac{1}{2}$ to 1 inch above the skin surface. They are usually round, with a diameter ranging from $\frac{3}{4}$ to $1\frac{1}{4}$ inches. Some stomas have an oval shape.

Stomas are bright red. They are similar in color to the mucous membranes inside your mouth, and have their moist appearance as well. Stomas look this way because they are made from the inner lining of your digestive tract. Your surgeon brings out the end of your small intestine and folds it back on itself, revealing the mucosal lining of your small bowel. Because this is the region where digested food is normally absorbed into the bloodstream, the area contains many tiny blood vessels, making it appear red and moist. If your stoma ever appears dry or starts changing color, contact your doctor immediately, as this can mean the blood supply has been cut off.

Types of pouching systems

The pouching system used to collect waste is called an appliance. Several decades ago, people with ostomies had few choices of equipment. Today, osteomates have an abundance of products from which to choose. In fact, there are so many it is sometimes overwhelming. It's therefore a good idea to work closely with your ET nurse to find a system that works well for you. There are two basic categories of appliances: two-piece and one-piece systems.

Two-piece systems

A two-piece system consists of a faceplate and bag. The faceplate, sometimes called a wafer or barrier, has a special adhesive on its backing that sticks to your skin. A hole, the size and shape of the stoma, is cut in the middle of the wafer. (You can also buy wafers that are pre-cut to certain sizes.) This faceplate is then placed on the abdomen so the stoma protrudes through the hole. The front of the faceplate has a flange, or plastic ring around it, that attaches to the pouch. The bag and the flange snap when they are sealed, much like what happens when you close a Zip-Lock bag.

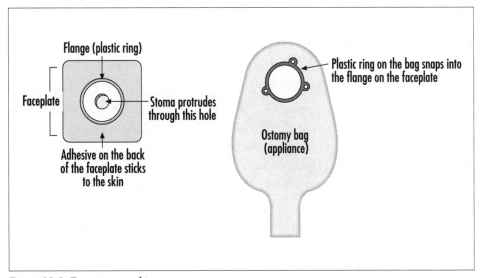

Figure 11-1. Two-piece pouching system

Pouches used with two-piece systems are either drainable or closed. Most people wear a drainable one for day-to-day use. They empty it by removing a special clamp at the base of the bag. There's no need to detach the pouch from the faceplate when eliminating waste. A closed bag is generally used during activities lasting no more than a few hours. For example, someone may take off the large, drainable pouch they normally wear and snap on a smaller, closed pouch for a romantic interlude. Closed pouches are usually thrown away after their one-time use, whereas drainable ones are typically used for approximately a week and then discarded.

Hollie, who had IBD as a child and now has an ileostomy, explains why she prefers a two-piece system:

> A two-piece pouching system works best for me. Although it's a little bulkier with the bag snapping into the flange, I feel like the pouch is more secure and supported this way. Also, the shape of the faceplate on my two-piece allows for a good seal on my abdomen, better than some of the one-pieces I've tried. And lastly, you can't beat the convenience of being able to snap a smaller sized bag on any time you want without having to pull the faceplate from your skin.

One-piece systems

A one-piece system comes with the pouch already bound to the faceplate. It works the same as a two-piece system just described, except you don't need to take the extra step of snapping on the bag, because it's already attached.

The main advantage of a one-piece is that it's a little quicker to put on and has a slightly lower profile under your clothing. The wafers are usually a little more flexible (because there is no flange), allowing the appliance to stay in place better on your skin as you move around. The main disadvantage is that you cannot snap different types of bags on and off as you can with a two-piece. If you want to change bags, you remove the whole appliance.

It's usually recommended that ileostomates who wear a one-piece pouching system use medium- to large-sized, drainable appliances. A closed bag can fill up within a few hours, and taking appliances on and off frequently can damage your skin. Also, if a bag is drainable but too small, you might not like having to empty it so frequently.

Craig describes why he likes wearing a one-piece:

> The main reason I wear a one-piece is that none of the two-piece systems I've tried hold for more than a day or two. I think this is

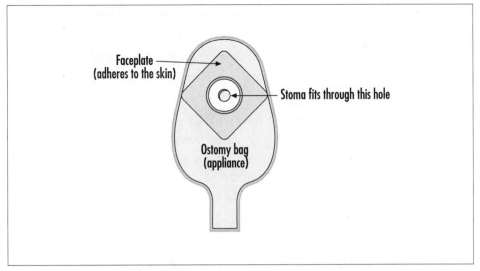

Figure 11-2. One-piece pouching system

because the faceplates are a little less flexible since they have the plastic ring on them. Within a few hours, they usually start peeling off right where the skin on my abdomen curves into my belly button. Others I know don't have this problem. So it just may have to do with the position of my stoma. Fortunately, one-piece bags are flexible enough that they remain adhered on my abdomen no matter how much I'm moving around. So I'll stick with my one-piece until I can find a two-piece that will actually stick to me.

Skin care

People with ostomies are at risk for skin problems around their stoma. The skin surrounding the stoma, called peristomal skin, is easily irritated, inflamed, or infected if exposed to waste products. This happens because effluent from the stoma contains many digestive enzymes. Your stoma, because it is made from the lining of your intestine, is accustomed to these chemicals. But the peristomal skin is not. If exposed for an extended period of time, the enzymes begin to break the skin down. This leaves the skin open to other problems, such as infection from the bacteria present in the ostomy drainage.

The peristomal skin is also vulnerable, because it is constantly exposed to adhesives. Over time, the skin can develop allergic reactions to these substances and become inflamed. In addition, the mechanical nature of repeatedly putting appliances on and taking them off can also irritate the skin.

Keeping the skin around your ostomy healthy is sometimes a challenge, but it is an attainable goal. Here are some tips to help you maintain or achieve good peristomal hygiene:

- **Keep skin clean.** It's usually best to use a mild soap or cleanser when washing your peristomal skin. Some prefer to clean the area when showering, whereas others use a soft cloth or paper towel while standing by a mirror and sink. Scrubbing vigorously or removing all the adhesive is not only unnecessary, but may do more harm because it irritates the skin.

  David, who has had his ileostomy for over ten years, shares how he cleans his skin:

  > I've found that using salt water works much better than any kind of soap. I actually don't even measure the amount of salt. I just pour some in a cup of warm water. The salt solution is not only good for your skin, but it is antibacterial as well. I haven't had any problems since I've been using it. My peristomal skin is very healthy.

- **Change the appliance at appropriate times.** There's no right amount of time to wait between appliance changes. It's good to keep your wafer attached to your abdomen for as long as possible so you avoid irritating your skin when removing the adhesive. However, don't leave it on so long that the barrier starts breaking down and effluent from the stoma contacts your skin. Over time, you'll learn what works well for you.

- **Use skin-protecting barriers.** There are products you can apply between your skin and the faceplate for extra protection. The most common are powders and pastes that not only help create a better seal but also can help protect the periostomal skin from repeated exposure to adhesives. These products, though, can sometimes cause more irritation than they prevent. Before using a particular product, test it on another area of your body first. You might also consider not using any extra barrier. Many people do fine without them, as David says:

  > When I first had my ostomy, I was told that I needed to use some extra type of skin barrier. The ET nurse recommended it and so did other ostomates that I spoke to. Everyone said it was the greatest thing to help protect your skin. I tried it for a while but it didn't work for

me. I found it actually irritated my skin more than anything else.
I stopped using it and my peristomal skin has been fine ever since.

- **Work closely with your ET nurse.** ET nurses have helped many people overcome persistent periostomal skin problems. They specialize in helping people cope with ostomies. Because they are familiar with the latest ostomy products, they can give you suggestions regarding different pouching systems and accessories that may help.

Stoma care

Your stoma actually requires very little care. It basically cleans itself, because it is continually producing mucus, a natural cleansing agent. However, soap and water in the shower doesn't harm it. Scrubbing your stoma, though, is unnecessary and not recommended.

It's important to protect your stoma from physical trauma. Although doctors usually encourage people with ostomies to engage in as much physical exercise as possible, it's a good idea to avoid contact sports or other activities where you might experience a blow to the abdomen. Heavy lifting is also discouraged, because it can cause a hernia near the stoma.

Emptying your appliance

People with ostomies vary on how frequently they need to empty their pouch. It depends on several factors, such as how much you eat, how much fluid you absorb, and how large your bag is. A good rule of thumb is to drain your pouch when it is approximately one-third full. You can let it fill up more, but the extra weight can contribute toward weakening the adhesive. Also, depending on your activities, you may decide to drain it when it's less full. Some people make a habit of emptying their bag, regardless of how full, before bedtime or before a long meeting. Overall though, most people with ileostomies discharge the contents of their appliance five to nine times over a 24-hour period, including once in the middle of the night.

People have different ways to empty their pouches. Some sit on the toilet, remove the tail clip at the base of the bag, and carefully drain the waste into the toilet between their legs. Others kneel in front of the toilet, and some people squat. There's no right or wrong way—people simply do what works best for them. Whichever method you use, it's usually a good idea to put a piece of toilet paper in the bowl first to help reduce splashing.

After emptying, most people use a few squares of toilet tissue to wipe the base of the pouch—both its outside and an inch up the inside. They then clamp the base of the bag, and usually wipe the small area below the tail clip one or two more time to make sure no feces remain. There's no need to wash the inside of the bag. Virtually all ileostomates today use air-tight, disposable pouches that last up to one week. As long as the adhesive around your stoma is intact and the clamp is on, no odor will escape.

Craig, who's had his ostomy for three years, describes how he empties his bag:

> *I have different ways of emptying my bag depending on where I am.*
> *At home, I keep a small chair in my bathroom. When I need to go,*
> *I bring it right in front of the toilet, sit on it facing the bowl, and*
> *empty the contents into the toilet. Away from home, I kneel. For the*
> *first year after my surgery, my knees weren't as strong, so I used to*
> *wear a thin but cushioned knee guard. No one could see it under my*
> *pants, and it made kneeling very comfortable on hard bathroom*
> *floors. My knees are pretty strong now so I don't use a knee protector*
> *anymore. And oh, if a restroom floor is really dirty, I never kneel.*
> *I just squat in front of the toilet.*
>
> *The best part about how I go to the bathroom though is that I never*
> *again for the rest of my life have to sit on a toilet! I figure I've already*
> *served all my time doing that before my surgery!*

Changing your appliance

How long people can go between appliance changes varies widely among people with ileostomies. Some need to attach a new pouch every three or four days, whereas others can go a week. A lot depends on your skin and the type of pouching system you use. A minority of people, however, have difficulty keeping their appliance on for more than a day or two. If this describes you, consult with your ET nurse to find a better system that lasts longer. Some people try to make their appliances last more than a week, but most ET nurses discourage this practice, because you may jeopardize the health of your peristomal skin.

People have different routines for changing their appliances. Some like to do it sitting in a chair, whereas others favor standing. Many also prefer to change it right after they take a shower. Like empting your bag, there's no right or wrong way. You'll eventually establish a system that works well for you. It's generally a good idea, though, to choose a time when your stoma is inactive.

Many people, like Hollie, find that early in the morning before breakfast is a good time:

> *I generally change my bag once a week on Saturdays. My stoma is usually quiet in the morning before I eat. This gives me a chance to remove my appliance and take a shower without having to worry about my stoma draining. Sometimes my peristomal skin gets a little itchy and I won't make it all the way till Saturday. It's no big deal to change it sooner. But for the most part, I can go for seven days and don't have to worry about it during the week.*

Odor

Some people with ostomies have concerns about odor. Although pouching systems from decades ago often did a poor job controlling unpleasant smells, appliances today are very effective at managing this potential problem. Pouches are airtight. If you smell a fecal odor, it usually means there is a leak and the appliance needs changing.

The smell of ileostomy gas and drainage is often less intense than the fecal smell of those who still have colons, but not always. If you have concerns, there are a number of different of ostomy deodorant products on the market. Some are tablets or drops that you put in your bag, and others are oral supplements that reduce odor throughout the body.

You can also control the smell of your waste products by carefully monitoring what you eat. Consuming foods such as fish, eggs, garlic, or onions can often create problems. Eating yogurt, parsley, or a few other green vegetables high in chlorophyll may help. If all else fails, keeping plenty of air freshener on hand when emptying your pouch is probably a good idea, especially if your bathroom is not well ventilated. Ostomy supply companies also sell tiny containers of odor eliminator spray. You can easily carry a little bottle with you if you have concerns away from home.

Hollie, who's had an ostomy for over twenty years, explains how she manages odor:

> *I only worry about odor when I'm emptying my bag or releasing gas. When my pouch is clamped, it's not an issue. I've found that eating roasted garlic creates the worst odor. But even when I haven't eaten any strong smelling foods, I still like to use a deodorant in my bag. The one I use works fairly well if I add a few drops every time*

*I empty my pouch. I'm hesitant to use the oral products since I have
concerns about taking a pill that might have other side effects. I tried
using one a long time ago, and it wasn't effective for me anyway. I'm
more comfortable just putting something in my bag.*

Gas

Excessive gas is sometimes a problem for people with ostomies. One advantage
ostomates have, though, is that nobody can immediately smell it, because the bag
traps the gas. However, excess gas can blow the pouch up like a balloon. This creates
a bulge under your clothing that may be noticeable. The solution is to check your
bag periodically and release the gas when you notice it's accumulating. When you are
asleep, however, monitoring your bag is much more difficult. The pressure from gas
can pull the appliance's adhesive from your skin without your even realizing it. Solid
or liquid waste from the bag can then leak out and create a mess. When awake, you
don't need to worry about this problem. You generally have plenty of time to release
the gas before it can cause the pouch to pull off.

Craig explains how he manages problems with gas:

> *It seems that no matter what I eat I have a lot of gas. It's not a
> major problem during the day since I can simply take a few extra
> trips to the bathroom to release it. At night though, the pressure from
> the gas sometimes pulls my appliance off my skin. I then awake to a
> big mess on myself and in my bed. After spending too many nights at
> 3 A.M. changing sheets and taking a shower, I started setting my alarm
> clock for two and a half hours after I go to bed. This has solved my
> problem. I get up, empty my bag, go back to sleep, and then don't
> have to worry about getting up another time before morning.*

One ostomy supply company has created a product that attaches to any pouch and
allows a person to release gas at his discretion. Unfortunately, this invention doesn't
work as well for people with ileostomies, because their drainage is generally more
liquid and can seep through the filter. It tends to work better for people with
colostomies, almost none of whom have IBD.

One option for releasing gas is simply to empty the bag in the toilet as described
earlier in this chapter. However, sometimes a person has minimal drainage and only
wants to release gas. The most common way to let air out of the bag is to lift up its
bottom to ensure that effluent from the stoma falls away from the end of the pouch.

Then carefully unclamp the end of the bag and push the air out slowly and gently. This is the only option for someone using a one-piece system. However, if you wear a two-piece appliance, you can release gas from the top of your bag by carefully detaching a segment of it from the flange. Press on the bag gently to expel the gas, and then make sure you snap the pouch securely back into the flange.

You can also help control the production of gas through your diet. You can usually figure out which foods are problematic through trial and error. Many people find that beans, dairy products, and cruciferous vegetables such as broccoli and cauliflower are major culprits. Others, like Laura, report that just about any food high in carbohydrates causes excess gas:

> It never had occurred to me that the reason I had so much gas was because I ate a lot of carbohydrates. Recently, I went on a low carbohydrate diet to help me lose weight. I was surprised to discover that the diet had a side benefit! I had significantly less gas. It amazes me that I still continue to learn things even years after having my surgery.

Living with an ostomy

An ostomy does not physically prevent you from enjoying your favorite hobbies or from having intimate relationships. Nevertheless, some people fear having an ostomy will prevent them from taking part in fun activities or cause their personal relationships to suffer. This section discusses ways to minimize the effect your ostomy has on activities you enjoy.

Activities

Activities you delighted in before your surgery are still possible for you to enjoy after your operation. In fact, many people who have had severe cases of IBD find they are able to participate in life much more fully with their ostomy. When they had their colons, some were so sick they were unable to take part in many of life's pleasures.

People with ostomies can work, swim, run marathons, and have an active sex life. There are very few limitations, except heavy lifting and contact sports. You can do just about anything you want in life with an ostomy, just as Hollie does:

> I think it's important that people know that you can live an active and normal life with an ostomy. I'm able to participate in just about

whatever I want, such as swimming, hiking, backpacking, and sailing.
I'm even taking advanced yoga now. Having an ostomy doesn't
interfere with the things I want to do.

Some people worry their appliance may not stay in place—or even fall off—if they are too physically active. In most cases, adhesives usually hold quite well, even in warm, humid weather. However, if you still have concerns, there are other options. For example, some people use a special ostomy tape for extra reinforcement or if they go swimming. An ostomy belt is also another option if you want extra security or support. It wraps around your waist and has a special attachment to hold your bag in place.

David, who has an ileostomy, explains why he uses one:

I suppose I really don't need to wear an ostomy belt. The appliance
I use sticks fairly well to my skin. But the belt provides extra support
so that I'm not totally dependent on the adhesive. I'm quite active, so
I feel much more secure this way.

Relationships

Many fear having an ostomy will interfere with their personal relationships. Understandably, people may have concerns about body image or worry how others might react if they know about or see the appliance. As either a new ostomate or someone facing ostomy surgery, you may have questions such as these:

- Will friends and family accept me?
- Will they treat me differently knowing I have an ostomy?
- Will my spouse/boyfriend/girlfriend reject me?
- Will I be able to have sex?
- Will anyone ever want to have sex with me, even if I'm able?

It's normal to have such questions. Probably every person with an ostomy has asked them at one time or another. Although some continue to struggle with self-acceptance and intimacy, many people with ostomies have found that over time, having an appliance has little, if any, impact on their relationships.

It's true that some people in the world might react negatively to you if you have an ostomy. But their reaction probably has more to do with them than you. Your friends and family love you for who you are, not for the way you go to the bathroom. It probably won't matter much to them that you eliminate your waste products a little differently.

David, who was already married when he had his ostomy surgery, explains:

> Having an ostomy has not had a negative impact on my marriage. If anything, it has brought my wife and me closer. She was very supportive during the time I was sick and going through my surgery. We now realize how fortunate we are to have each other.
>
> The ostomy doesn't interfere with our sex life. Of course, I need to make sure to empty the bag beforehand. I also always wear a soft cloth cover over the pouch. But having an ostomy has not been a hindrance to us enjoying intimacy.

Julie, who's had her ostomy since she was a teenager, has had mixed responses from people:

> I've experienced the gamut over the years. I've had a couple of boyfriends who were uncomfortable being in a relationship with me. It hurt, but that's just the way it was. For whatever reason, they couldn't handle it. But most have had no problem with my having an appliance. In fact, I think many times it's bothered me more than anyone else. Even after all these years, I guess I'm still in the process learning to accept myself with an ostomy.

Hollie, who is 30 and single, describes how having an ostomy has affected her relationships:

> I'd say that if anything, having an ostomy has enhanced my relationships with people. Everything I've been through has made me much more understanding and compassionate toward others, especially other friends who are going through health challenges.
>
> In terms of my relationships with men, having an ostomy has never been an issue. In fact, when one boyfriend first saw my appliance and scars on my abdomen, he said they were beautiful because they were the reason that I'm alive! It was an incredible thing to say, and it touched me very deeply.

Coping with an ostomy

Adjusting to an ostomy is difficult for some people. Having a surgical procedure that forever alters the way you go to the bathroom is a significant life change. So is living the rest of your life with a bag hanging from your abdomen. It's only normal that you need some time to adapt to your new way of eliminating. The following sections provide some ideas to help you deal with having an ostomy.

Seek support

A good way to adjust to your ostomy is to seek support from others. There are many people who can assist you during this transitional time, such as an understanding psychotherapist or others who have ostomies.

Other ostomates

New ostomates sometimes feel they are all alone and nobody else in their life could possibly understand how they are feeling. To a certain degree, this is true if none of your friends or family have an ostomy. However, plenty of people in the world do. You might consider bringing a few of them into your life. No one can understand your situation better than someone who has already "been there, done that."

The United Ostomy Association (UOA) is a wonderful resource for bringing people with ostomies together. You can call toll free at (800) 826-0826 to have a volunteer in your area call or visit you. The association can also provide information on nearby support groups. Support groups are a great place to meet a variety of people who are also learning how to deal with their ostomies. Support groups sponsored by the Crohn's and Colitis Foundation of America (CCFA) are another place to meet others with ostomies. Call your local CCFA chapter for support group information in your area, or (800) 932-2423 if you don't have your local chapter's phone number.

The UOA also has an annual conference where people from all over the United States and Canada gather to discuss a variety of ostomy topics. The program includes seminars, support sessions, a trade show, and plenty of social time to meet and talk to other people.

The UOA sponsors an annual youth rally as well, which is like an ostomy camp for kids age 11 to 17. The five-day event usually takes place in a university setting. It's often the first time a young person with an ostomy can meet other kids his age facing similar circumstances. The CCFA also sponsors summer camps across the United States for children with IBD. Although not all the kids at IBD camp have ostomies, most camps have handful of counselors and campers who do.

Hollie has had an ostomy since she was 11. She describes how the UOA Youth Rally affected her:

> After I got my ostomy, I wanted to meet others my age who went through the same thing. I went to a support group, but there were mostly older people at those meetings. The UOA Youth Rally was great for me because I was able to meet other kids my age dealing with same issues I was. Although I'm sure it's difficult at any age, when you're that young you feel really different from everyone else. I was able to find a peer group in which I truly fit. I'm so thankful for the Youth Rally as it played an important role in my life. I am still friends with and keep in touch with people I met there.

You can learn more about the UOA and CCFA by visiting their web sites at *http://www.uoa.org/* and *http://www.ccfa.org/*, respectively.

Psychotherapy

Psychotherapy is another tool you can use to help yourself. A compassionate therapist trained in adaptation to chronic illness may have the professional skills you need after your surgery. Your doctor, ET nurse, and people you meet through the UOA or CCFA are good sources for referrals.

Psychotherapy helped Cheryl adapt to her ileostomy:

> I had difficulty at first accepting myself with my ostomy. At the time, I hated how I looked with it. I struggled with the stoma, the scar, and the pouch. I didn't want to look at myself in the mirror and I dreaded every time I took a shower because I'd have to see it. Crohn's had already torn up the inside of my body, and now it had forever changed my external appearance.
>
> Although I did a lot of work on my own, my therapist played an important role in helping me get back to a place where I could love and accept myself. One thing that stands out in my mind the most was when she asked me how I would treat a small child who underwent ileostomy surgery. Would I think she was ugly? Would I turn her away and have nothing to do with her? Would I think of her

*as damaged and treat her differently? Of course I wouldn't. I'd do
everything I could to embrace and accept her and make her feel loved.
My therapist pointed out that if I would treat a child—or anyone else
for that matter—in such a positive way, why wouldn't I do the same
for myself? She had a good point. Sometimes people like me can be
their own worst enemies or critics.*

*It's been quite a process learning how to treat myself as I would
others. I've come a long way and am still learning. But today I can
say that I do accept myself with my ostomy.*

Attitude

Your attitude is perhaps one of your strongest assets when learning to adapt to an
ostomy. Although it's sometimes difficult to keep an upbeat frame of mind, many
people who are well adjusted to their ostomy have found their positive outlook on
life makes a big difference. Following are two methods some people use to help
themselves maintain a good attitude.

Use of humor

Having a sense of humor is often useful for people who are learning to deal with their
ostomy. It often helps when facing any new or unexpected challenges that arise.

Craig explains how a lighter attitude helped him when he had a mishap five months
after his surgery:

> *I've only had one major accident away from home since I've had
> my ostomy. On my way to visit a friend, I noticed my bag was filling
> up. I figured I'd just empty it when I got to her place, but decided to
> release some gas before walking up to the house. As I stood up to get
> out of my car, having a plant in one hand and a bag of muffins in the
> other, I felt a warm gush run down my leg. I knew it could only be one
> thing. My friend was already on her porch starting to come down to
> greet me when she could tell something was wrong. She knew about
> my ostomy, and I simply said that I had soiled myself. She
> immediately said she'd run in to get a paper towel, but I knew it was
> going to take much more than that to fix the problem. When she came
> back and saw the brown mess all over my light colored pants, she
> said, "Oh, when I heard you say 'soil' I assumed you had gotten a*

little soil on your pants from the plant. I wasn't thinking you meant this kind of soil."

Up till this point I was almost on the verge of tears standing out on the street covered by my stool. But at that moment, knowing that I was with someone who both cared for me and had a good sense of humor, I just started laughing. She began laughing, too, and invited me in. She suggested that we use her washing machine to clean my clothes and offered her shower facilities as well. During the time we were waiting for my clothes to finish washing and drying, the only thing she had for me to wear was one of her robes—with a leopard skin design! So there we were sitting in her living room talking and laughing about what had happened while I'm wearing this leopard-skin, woman's robe! Of course, I was extremely fortunate that this incident happened with someone like her. But I also learned that by not taking everything so seriously, I can step outside of myself and see the humor. This had the potential to be a nightmare, but by just shifting my attitude, it turned into something hilarious.

Perspective

Another method of coping is to try and keep all that has happened to you in perspective. As mentioned earlier, many people with ostomies because of IBD were very sick during the months and years prior to their surgery. It's not that having an ostomy isn't an adjustment for them. But compared to what their lives were like before, many find living with an appliance is a small price to pay for their renewed health and freedom.

David, who had a severe case of Crohn's before his ostomy surgery, explains:

I had one of the worst cases of Crohn's that my doctors had ever seen. At one point, I developed a blood infection and almost died. Having a colectomy with an ileostomy saved my life—there was no doubt about it.

I admit that it was difficult at first, especially during my recovery process. Often it was two steps forward, one step back. Adjusting to the appliance itself was also a big challenge. For a long time, I had to just hold on to the good days and get through the bad ones.

Once I was well, I began to see that having the bag wasn't so bad. In fact, I soon realized how fortunate I was. When you look at how

I was before my surgery compared to how I am now, it's like night and day. If not for my ostomy, I wouldn't be here. I'd be dead, and wouldn't be able to enjoy the wonderful life I'm living. I'm now in my late sixties and I'm able to do a lot more than a lot of people my age. My ostomy is truly a blessing.

CHAPTER 12

Coping with Prednisone

PREDNISONE IS a commonly used anti-inflammatory drug. Its release in the early 1950s radically changed treatment options for many chronic diseases, including IBD. Some compare the significance of its discovery to that of antibiotics.

Many people with Crohn's and ulcerative colitis take at least one short course of prednisone. Others with more severe disease may need to stay on the drug for months or years. Those who take it for extended periods may develop short- and long-term side effects.

This chapter begins with a discussion about prednisone and how it differs from other steroid drugs. Next, it covers the medication's physical and emotional side effects. Suggestions are offered for preventing as well as coping with prednisone's multitude of side effects.

Prednisone basics

Prednisone is a synthetic (made in a laboratory) hormone. A natural hormone is a chemical made by one of your organs or glands to help regulate the function of other cells in your body. Hormones can stimulate or slow life processes, such as growth, metabolism, sexual development, and emotions. Synthetic hormones have a similar impact on your body.

Corticosteroids are hormones produced by the adrenal glands, which sit on top of your kidneys. They fall under the broader category of steroids, a large family of chemical substances that include many drugs, hormones, and other compounds made by your body. Corticosteroids also include synthetically made hormones, such as prednisone, that either resemble or are equivalent to their natural counterparts.

There are three types of corticosteroids:

- Mineralcorticoids primarily regulate the concentration of electrolytes, such as sodium and potassium, in your cells.

- Androgens, such as testosterone, promote male characteristics such as facial hair and muscle growth.

- Glucocorticoids, such as cortisol, control what many people call the body's fight or flight—or stress—response. This includes increased blood sugar levels, the breakdown of proteins from bones and muscle for energy, and a dampening of the body's immune response.

Prednisone is a synthetic glucocorticoid. It very closely resembles the natural cortisol hormone that your adrenal glands make. In large doses, prednisone has a profound anti-inflammatory effect throughout the body. Thus, it is a useful drug for IBD and other inflammatory diseases, such as asthma and rheumatoid arthritis.

Other forms

Prednisone, which is taken orally, is the most commonly prescribed corticosteroid for IBD. Corticosteroids are sometimes administered through the anus, using a foam (Cortifoam) or liquid enema (Cortenema). This is a good choice if the inflammation is primarily limited to the end of the large bowel. Side effects, discussed later in this chapter, can occur from these uses, but they are usually less intense.

People with severe IBD who are hospitalized often receive their corticosteroids intra-venously. SoluMedrol is a commonly used IV drug. Once the disease is brought under control, the person can usually switch to oral prednisone.

Dosing

Doctors generally prescribe the lowest amount of prednisone they think is necessary to get disease under control. Some doctors, though, choose to start with a high dose for a brief period to extinguish inflammation as quickly as possible. Then they gradually reduce the dose to a lower level (this is called tapering). Following are commonly prescribed doses of prednisone for the average-sized adult:

- High dose: About 35 to 60 milligrams (mg) per day. Most doctors don't prescribe more than 60 mg of prednisone for people with IBD. If they do, it's usually for just a few days.

- Moderate dose: About 10 to 35 mg per day.

- Low dose: About 10 mg or less per day.

It's important to keep in mind that people respond differently to various doses of prednisone. For example, one person may have difficulty sleeping when taking 50 mg whereas another may be fine on that dose. Over time, you'll know what works best for you. However, tapering the dose is always necessary to avoid withdrawal symptoms (see the "Tapering off" section later in this chapter).

Stacy explains how she worked with her gastroenterologists:

> After years of experience, I became quite familiar with how to regulate my prednisone dosage. It was therefore important for me to work with a doctor who could trust my judgment. Some like to follow everything strictly by the book, but that never worked for me. Forty milligrams was my max. Anything above that caused me too many problems. I also had a good sense when it was okay to lower my dosage. Fortunately, over the years I've worked with good doctors who understand that I know my body best.

The steroid label

You might hear your doctor or other healthcare practitioners refer to you as "on steroids." Some people aren't comfortable with the term "steroid," because it has a negative connotation in Western society. Technically, the label is accurate: Prednisone is a steroid drug. However, when people mention this term in casual conversation, they are usually referring to the androgen hormones some athletes take (illegally in most countries) to improve their physical performance. This type of steroid has a masculinizing effect on the body and is often used to increase muscle mass. Prednisone, a glucocorticoid, is the last thing an aspiring athlete would want to take, because it can cause the breakdown of muscles.

Craig explains how he handled the terminology:

> When I was in high school and college, I was always very careful not to tell people that I took steroids. If the topic of my medication came up, I would specifically say that I take prednisone, and not even mention the S word. Unfortunately, though medically correct, I've never liked the term 'steroids' because I don't want uninformed people jumping to the conclusion that I am—or ever was—on the same stuff that some athletes take illegally. The few times that people asked me if prednisone was a steroid, I would say that it was but made sure to explain that it was a completely different kind.

Physical side effects

Prednisone has a profound effect all over your body. It effectively reduces IBD inflammation, and sometimes completely eliminates all symptoms within a few days. For many, it feels miraculous. Unfortunately, the miracle comes at a price, especially if you need to remain on the drug for more than a few weeks. Over time, prednisone can take a toll on eyes, bones, skin, and other organs. The following sections review the most common side effects of prednisone.

Bone loss

Prednisone can cause significant bone loss. This can lead to osteoporosis, a condition marked by thinning and demineralization of the bones. As a result, bones become brittle and fragile, increasing the chance of a fracture.

People who take prednisone long term should have their bones checked periodically. You can have this done by requesting a bone density scan, which is a low-dose x-ray that measures the mineral content of your bones. The cheap tests that only examine your ankle are not your best option. Ask your doctor to order a test that measures the bone density in your spine, hip, and hand. In addition, be sure the order is to scan the nondominant side of your body. In other words, if you're right-handed, the technician should scan your left hand, hip, and ankle.

Clarissa tells her story:

> I have been up and down on prednisone for 27 years. This is a very long time, but I need it to keep the disease under control. The lowest I can generally go is 10 mg, although I got down to 5 mg when I was pregnant.
>
> I have osteoporosis. I've been taking a calcitonin nasal spray for the last couple of years. I'm due for another bone scan soon, so we'll see how much it's helping. I have to confess I'm a bit scared. I'm only in my early 50s now. I often wonder what it's going to be like when I get older. I've already broken a bone in my hand. Fortunately, it healed—so that's a good sign. Hopefully, there will be better options to treat Crohn's in the near future so that I can get off prednisone.

Bone loss increases with the amount of prednisone you take, as well as how long you are on it. However, it's difficult to predict how much bone you'll lose while taking prednisone. Two people on the same dose for the same duration can have quite different rates of loss. Fortunately, you can take action to help preserve bone.

Diet

A diet rich in calcium and vitamin D helps prevent osteoporosis. Good sources of calcium include dairy products such as milk, yogurt, and cheese. Almonds and green leafy vegetables—especially kale and collard greens—also provide significant amounts of calcium. A good source of vitamin D is cold-water fish, such as salmon, herring, and mackerel. Vitamin D is also in egg yolks and milk. Moreover, a major osteoporosis study found that a diet filled with lots of fruits and vegetables, as well as an adequate amount of protein, helps maintain strong bones.[1]

Supplements

Not everyone with IBD can get enough calcium and vitamin D through diet. Thus, nutritional supplements can play an important role in preventing bone loss. If you feel you need supplements, work closely with your doctor and nutritionist. Most recommend a total intake of 1,500 mg calcium and 400 international units (IU) of vitamin D for people with IBD on prednisone. Many studies have found that taking these nutrients together helps preserve bone in people taking corticosteroids.[2]

Magnesium may also have value in preventing osteoporosis. A two-year study of menopausal women (not on corticosteroids) found that supplemental magnesium increased bone density and prevented fractures.[3] Before taking magnesium, discuss the pros and cons with your doctor. Too much of the mineral can cause diarrhea in some people.

Stacy was fortunate that she never developed any bone problems:

> I was on prednisone steadily from age 21 to 40. With the exception of a few three-month periods when I was off, I was mostly taking anywhere from 10 to 40 mg per day. I've had bone studies and there are no signs of osteoporosis. I attribute this to many factors. First, I have no family history of osteoporosis. Also, I've always stayed as active as possible, doing as much exercise as my body could handle. I've always eaten a healthy diet—at least when I could eat—and have taken calcium supplements for many years. I believe all these things really made a difference.

Exercise

Exercise is good for your bones. However, the kind of exercise you engage in makes a difference. To build and maintain strong bones, weight-bearing exercise, such as weight lifting, is essential. Daily walks, stair climbing, rowing, and even jumping jacks help bone density as well. Exercises such as swimming and stretching are good for you in other ways, but they don't help prevent osteoporosis.

Medications

Doctors generally reserve medications for people who have already lost significant amounts of bone. Because drugs have side effects, it is unusual for a physician to prescribe these medications simply because you are on prednisone.

Several drugs are available for reducing bone loss, including calcitonin and bisphosphonates such as Fosamax. Your physician can help you determine if these prescription drugs are necessary.

Race

Race can influence susceptibility to osteoporosis. People of African descent generally have greater bone density than Caucasians and are at lower risk of developing osteoporosis. Asians usually have less bone mass than Caucasians. Regardless of race, however, everyone who takes prednisone long-term is at risk of bone loss; hence, action should always be taken to preserve bone.

Sunshine exposure

Sunshine plays a key role in maintaining bone mass. When sunlight hits your skin, a chemical reaction occurs, causing your body to produce vitamin D, a nutrient important for bone health. Vitamin D can be taken orally, but a recent study found that commonly recommended amounts may not be enough if sunlight exposure is limited.[4] Another study involving elderly women living in northern New England reports similar information. Despite vitamin D supplementation, they were deficient in the nutrient and had decreased bone density.[5]

Sunbathing has risks. It's therefore important to consult with your doctor about the risks and benefits of sunlight before you expose yourself to potentially skin-damaging rays.

Eye problems

Taking prednisone is associated with two major eye problems: glaucoma and cataracts. Glaucoma is a condition marked by increased fluid pressure within the eye. Nerve damage can result, leading to either partial or complete blindness. It's therefore very important to periodically be examined by an eye doctor (opthalmologist) while on prednisone.

Trish explains:

> I can't emphasize enough how important it is see an eye doctor regularly while on prednisone. I recommend seeing an ophthalmologist over an optometrist. The ophthalmologist is a medical doctor and has other tests he can do besides the simple pressure test that the optometrist uses. In my case, I had borderline high pressure in one eye. After further testing, it was found I was in the very early stages of glaucoma. I hadn't noticed any problems with my eye, but it turns out I have a little loss in my peripheral vision. Fortunately, the drops I use now reduce my eye pressure to normal. The glaucoma is not progressing anymore. I'm glad we caught it early.

Cataracts are cloudy areas on the eye's lens. They usually form as people reach their 60s or 70s, but prednisone can cause them at any age. Dose and the duration of taking the drug do not consistently correlate with their development.

Trish also developed cataracts:

> I was on 5 to 40 mg of prednisone for eight years straight, with the exception of a one and a half year period and a few months here and there. Overall, I didn't have too many problems. I didn't have emotional side effects and my bones are fine. For some reason, my eyes were the target of the side effects. In addition to developing glaucoma, I've developed cataracts in both eyes. Cataracts runs in my family, but not at such an early age (40 years old). My right eye is not too bad. For now, my vision in that eye can be corrected. But my left eye was cloudy in the middle—so my vision was distorted. I had surgery on my left eye and can now see well. My eye doctor says I can probably go at least another two years till the right one needs surgery.

Sometimes cataracts aren't preventable. However, in some cases, steps can be taken to reduce your chance of developing them. Although the research on prevention is not specific to those on corticosteroids, it's possible the following suggestions can still help you:

- **Eat carotenoid-rich foods.** Carotenoids are red, yellow, and orange-pigmented substances commonly found in fruits and vegetables. A diet rich in them can help prevent cataracts. Researchers report that the ingestion of lutein and zeaxanthin—two carotenoids—are associated with a lower risk of cataracts.[6] Good food sources include broccoli, spinach, and egg yolks.

- **Protect your eyes.** Exposure to ultraviolet (UV) radiation from sunlight is associated with the development of cataracts.[7] You might consider wearing glasses that filter UV light.

- **Don't smoke.** Cigarette smokers have a higher chance of developing cataracts than nonsmokers. Former smokers still have an elevated risk, but it is less than the risk run by those who currently smoke.[8] Thus, although it's best to never have smoked in the first place, quitting can reduce your risk of cataracts.

Hyperglycemia

Hyperglycemia is a condition in which a person has an elevated amount of glucose (sugar) in the blood. Symptoms include excessive thirst, urination, fatigue, and hunger.

Prednisone can cause blood sugar levels to rise in susceptible individuals. As a result, people who are borderline diabetic may have to take insulin to keep their blood glucose level under control. Diabetics on the drug often need to increase their insulin dose. If you have diabetes, discuss your prednisone prescription with your endocrinologist (or the doctor you see for your diabetes) to work out a plan to manage your blood sugar level.

Hypertension

Some people develop hypertension (high blood pressure) on prednisone. The drug can further elevate blood pressure in those who already have the condition. Reducing your salt intake, practicing relaxation techniques, and exercising can help prevent this problem. Ask your doctor about the Dietary Approaches to Stopping Hypertension (DASH) diet. The DASH diet is a lowfat eating plan that emphasizes fruits, vegetables, and lowfat dairy products. For more information on how this diet can help lower blood pressure, see *http://www.nhlbi.nih.gov/health/public/heart/hbp/dash/*. If your blood pressure is still high, your doctor may recommend medication.

Infection

Prednisone reduces inflammation by effectively decreasing your immune response. Although this comes in handy for your inflamed gut, the effect is not specific to your bowel. Because your immunity is lowered, you are more susceptible to infections. Here are some suggestions to help you avoid infections:

- Stay away from sick people as much as possible.

- Wash your hands frequently, and especially before you eat or touch your face.

- Keep your skin clean to avoid local infections, such as boils.

- Eat a balanced diet. Consult your doctor, dietitian, or nutritionist about taking appropriate supplements if you think your diet is lacking in nutrients.

- Try to reduce stress, which can impair immunity.

Muscle loss and weakness

Loss of muscle mass is possible when you are taking prednisone. Unlike other steroids that help build muscle, prednisone breaks it down. Thus, it's important that you do everything you can to maintain your muscles while you're on the drug. This includes consuming adequate amounts of protein and calories, as well as engaging in as much physical exercise as you can handle. Weight lifting is excellent for counteracting prednisone's muscle-wasting effects. Cardiovascular exercise, such as walking, bike riding, and stair climbing, is good, too. The important thing is to try and stay as active as you can, given your condition. If you are unsure of your dietary needs or how to exercise safely or properly, consult a knowledgeable dietitian or exercise trainer.

Richard describes how he handled this side effect:

> Dealing with muscle loss was very difficult for me. Of course, it was sometimes hard to tell how much of it was the Crohn's and how much was the prednisone.
>
> Between major flares, I'd spend a lot of time at the gym trying to rebuild my strength. I'd make good progress, but then it was so sad how I could lose it all so quickly when I got sick and had to be on high doses of prednisone again. Although it was frustrating when I was heading down, I was always able to bounce back and rebuild my strength. It took a lot of discipline with exercise and diet, but the results were always well worth it.

Skin problems

Prednisone can cause thin skin. Weight gain and water retention (see next section) can also stretch your skin. As a result, you might develop stretch marks. Stretch marks can appear many different places, such as on your thighs, buttocks, and upper arms. They usually fade once you get off the drug, but sometimes they are permanent or can linger for years.

Acne is another side effect of prednisone. Hormonal changes caused by the drug are thought to contribute to this skin problem. Prednisone often makes the condition much worse for teenagers and others who are prone to acne. Acne, whether caused by prednisone or not, is sometimes difficult to treat. Here are a few suggestions to help you deal with it:

- **Keep your skin clean.** Washing with antibacterial soap helps, and so does using over-the-counter products containing benzoyl peroxide.
- **Avoid trigger foods.** No food has been proven to cause acne, but some people find eating certain things aggravates their problem.
- **Get enough zinc.** Although not quite as effective as prescription antibiotics, a recent study found zinc is an effective treatment for over 30 percent of people (from the general population) with acne.[9] Good dietary sources of zinc include red meat, shellfish, whole grains, legumes, and nuts. If you think your diet is not providing enough zinc, talk to your doctor, dietitian, or nutritionist before taking supplements.
- **Consult a dermatologist (skin doctor).** If you develop acne when on prednisone, consider seeking professional assistance. A dermatologist can prescribe treatments that may help you get the acne under control.

Weight gain and water retention

Many people gain weight on prednisone. Whereas this is sometimes welcome if you've been sick, unable to eat, or have lost a lot of weight, not everyone wants the extra pounds. Part of the weight gain is simply water, because the drug causes fluid retention. This disappears when you go off the medication. The other part is caused by prednisone's effect on appetite.

Laura's appetite increased significantly:

> *Before I started on prednisone, my doctor told me that it might increase my appetite a little. What an understatement! I couldn't believe how hungry I got. I recall one time my husband and I were eating with some*

friends. I literally ate a half a pan of lasagna. Our friends were shocked how much I could put away. So was I.

I tend to gain weight fairly easily anyway, and on prednisone, I gained rapidly. It sometimes got depressing, especially living in a society where thinness is so valued. It was also frustrating since none of my clothes fit me. There wasn't much I could do other than try to deal with it with my sense of humor and by seeking support from my friends in the IBD support group. This helped carry me through this difficult time.

Gina gained a lot of weight, too:

I once gained 40 pounds on prednisone. I had a big appetite and used to bake my own sweet treats. Sometimes I felt as though I had almost no self control when it came to food. When I was younger, I lost weight pretty quickly once I got off. However, as I got older, it became harder to lose the weight. I've been off prednisone for several years now and am still about ten or fifteen pound above my ideal weight.

Water retention is the other reason people gain weight on prednisone. You may notice swelling in any part of your body, but two common places are the belly and the face. So characteristic is the prednisone puffy face—sometimes described as a moon face—that once you know what it looks like, you can usually spot someone on prednisone almost anywhere.

Stacy describes her water retention:

I can generally spot people on prednisone at the mall, airport, or wherever. It's a certain look. I know it all too well with all the years I was on it. I generally didn't gain too much weight on prednisone other than in my face. Even when I weighed 105 pounds, my face looked like I weighed at least 150.

The moon face was very difficult for me to deal with. I didn't like the way I looked and I felt embarrassed. When I'd visit home, people I grew up with didn't even recognize me. It really hurt. Fortunately, most people understood once I explained my story.

On a lighter note, my husband and I gather with the same group of friends every year for our annual Christmas party. We always take a group picture. One year, we decided to organize the pictures from all the previous years. The only way we were able to figure out which year was which was by how puffy my face was!

Changes in your face, as well as in your weight, are some of the most difficult side effects of prednisone. How much your face changes and how much weight you gain depend on many factors, including your own individual reaction to prednisone. However, you can do a few things to help minimize these problems:

- **Don't restrict fluids.** Restricting fluids won't help your situation. In fact, it can make the puffiness worse. If water is scarce, your body will try to hang on to more of it. Drinking more may seem counterintuitive, but it's actually good to drink plenty of water.

- **Restrict sodium (salt).** Restricting your sodium intake—starting the first day you take prednisone—is probably the most important thing you can do to prevent swelling and puffiness. The problem is that most processed foods are laced with it. It's a good idea to check labels and avoid adding salt to your food. Also, consider eating more whole, unprocessed foods—or at least those that are minimally processed—because they rarely have added sodium. If you've had your colon removed, however, it's not recommended that you limit your salt intake. If you have concerns about how much sodium you should consume per day, talk with your gastroenterologist.

- **Eat healthy foods slowly and in small portions.** Processed foods that are high in fat, sodium, or sugar are often tempting when you are constantly hungry. However, consider substituting healthier foods for those that are fattening. Also, try eating small portions of food slowly throughout the day. This way, you're less likely to get so hungry that you'll want to devour large amounts of unhealthy food.

- **Exercise regularly.** If you have difficulty controlling your eating, try to remain as physically active as possible. Both cardiovascular exercise and weight training can help you burn excess calories.

- **Work with your doctor.** It's wise to consult your doctor if you continue to have excessive swelling despite trying the measures just mentioned. Your doctor may have to prescribe a diuretic, a medication that helps eliminate excess fluids.

Clarissa did her best to deal with the weight gain and water retention:

> *Since I'm on a low dose of prednisone now, my face is pretty normal and so is my weight. However, I still have bags under my eyes that I attribute to the prednisone.*
>
> *It was very difficult for me when I was on higher doses. I'd look at myself in the mirror and feel like I was the ugliest person on earth. Not only did the prednisone distort my facial features, but it made me*

gain a lot of weight, too. It also redistributed my body fat so that it was concentrated more in my belly area.

Coping was not easy, but I did my best. A diuretic helped with the water retention, and I also went to Weight Watchers. This helped control my weight, but it didn't do much for the moon face. At times I'd get so upset about my face that I'd cry. I tried to remember that it was only temporary, but it was still hard on my self-esteem.

Emotional side effects

Prednisone affects many parts of the body, including the brain. Hence, it's not uncommon to experience alterations in your mood while on the drug. In the past, some doctors have minimized the emotional impact that prednisone causes. Fortunately, today, most doctors understand the toll the drug can take on one's mental health.

Emotional side effects—if they occur—generally develop in people who take high doses for more than a few weeks. As you taper to moderate and lower levels, the emotional problems may gradually dissipate. The following sections describe some of the most common mental side effects of prednisone.

Anxiety

Prednisone is chemically similar to the natural hormone that your body produces when you are under stress. It's therefore not surprising that feelings of anxiety can occur when taking the drug.

Prednisone tends to magnify feelings of stress or anxiety. If a stressful situation arises, for example, prednisone has a way of making it seem much worse than you'd normally perceive it. You may find yourself overreacting to things that normally never bothered you. Or you may discover you now have trouble dealing with certain people or situations. Once the stressful feelings begin, you may find yourself transferring your worries from one thing to the next. Unfortunately, this can soon lead to a chronic state of anxiety.

The following tips can help prevent anxiety from taking over while you're on prednisone:

- **Minimize your exposure to stressful people, situations, and events.** You can't control everything around you, but you can try your best to temporarily avoid things that trigger your stress response. For example, perhaps you can delay that move to a new apartment for a few months, or postpone that visit to your in-laws till your dose is below 20 milligrams.

- **Schedule time for relaxation.** It may help to incorporate rest periods throughout your day, because it gives your mind a chance to switch gears and relax. Exercise, meditation, listening to music, and watching movies are a few ways to relax.

- **Keep a journal.** Some people find journaling is a good way to release stress and anxiety. Keep a spiral notebook with you and write in it when you feel the need to let off some steam.

- **Remember you're on a mind-altering drug.** If your worries and anxieties are increasing, remind yourself that the drug is making you feel this way. When you taper down, you'll return to your normal self.

- **Seek professional assistance.** It may help to talk with a psychologist or counselor. Try and find someone familiar with the emotional side effects of prednisone.

Depression

High doses of prednisone can cause depression. This mood disorder is not simply feeling sad or temporarily disappointed. Instead, it's marked by a pervasive sense of hopelessness, combined with a loss of interest in things you used to find enjoyable. Furthermore, a diagnosis of depression requires that you have continuous symptoms for at least two weeks. A complete list of signs and symptoms is presented in Chapter 17, *Emotions and Coping*.

Depression is a serious disorder that can be debilitating. Even if you know that prednisone is primarily causing your problems, depression can still be overwhelming. It's therefore very important that you seek professional assistance if you or your doctor suspect you have it.

The good news is that depression is treatable. Your doctor can refer you to an appropriate mental health care professional. Often a combination of both medication and talk therapy is very helpful. Also, consider seeking support from other people with IBD who have also taken high doses of prednisone.

Clarissa used a variety of methods to cope with her depression:

> I've had a variety of emotional side effects from prednisone, including depression. For a while, it was so bad I took an antidepressant drug. Fortunately, I haven't needed the antidepressant for a few years now. But it did help. Faith and prayers helped, too. Other times, just sitting down

and having a good cry made me feel better. It also helped to join a support group where I could talk to others who were going through the same thing. Lastly, over the years, I've gradually developed a different perspective on things. My attitude now is that "This, too, shall pass." And whatever it is, it usually does.

Euphoria

Prednisone makes some people euphoric. You may wonder how a drug that causes some to fall into the depths of depression can also create feelings of elation in others. No one fully understands the intricacies of how corticosteroid hormones affect the brain, and thus mood and emotions. Emotional responses to prednisone can vary widely from person to person, and within the same person at different times.

Stacy describes her ups and downs:

> When I was on high doses of prednisone, I felt like super-woman. I responded to it very quickly and experienced the euphoria. I sometimes felt like I could almost do anything. My mind was always active and it was very hard to sit still.
>
> I was just the opposite coming down on prednisone. I sank into a depression. I was always tired and couldn't keep up with what I had to do. I knew it was temporary, so I held off on any formal treatment. In time, it passed. But when you're on it and then coming down, it's quite an emotional roller coaster.

Insomnia

Sleeplessness is a problem for some people who take prednisone. The drug closely resembles your body's natural adrenaline hormone, so it's not surprising that taking excess amounts keeps some people awake at night. Also, insomnia often accompanies anxiety, depression, or extreme feelings of elation; thus, it also develops from these side effects. So whether you're happy, sad, worried, or depressed, prednisone can interrupt your sleep.

Laura shares her story:

> I had horrible insomnia on prednisone. Sometimes I'd only get two or three hours of sleep. My mind was always racing so it was difficult to rest. And when I did sleep, I'd often wake up drenched in sweat. I tried sleep medications but they didn't work too well for me.

> *What would I do at night then? I always found lots of things to do.*
> *I'd often read or watched television. QVC and MTV were among my*
> *favorites. I was also one of those people who called in to those late*
> *night talk radio shows. And of course, since I was always hungry, I*
> *spent plenty of time eating.*

Different people have success with different methods for helping themselves fall asleep. What works for one person may not work for someone else. However, here are a few suggestions worth trying:

- **Engage in calm activities an hour before going to bed.** Try and reserve the last hour before bedtime for some kind of calming ritual. For example, you might listen to relaxing music, write in a journal, meditate, or take a warm bath. Avoid anything that stimulates you or gets your mind moving quickly.

- **Drink something warm.** Some people find a cup of warm milk or chamomile tea can help. Whatever you drink, try to avoid anything with caffeine.

- **Eat a carbohydrate-rich snack.** Some people find that eating carbohydrates makes them sleepy. You might try snacking on a banana, baked potato, or other carbohydrate-rich food before bedtime to see if this helps.

- **Consult your doctor.** Check with your doctor before taking an over-the-counter sleep aid—whether it's a drug or dietary supplement—to ensure that it's appropriate for you. If your insomnia is severe, he may recommend a prescription sleep medication.

Obsessive thinking and behavior

Some people say they feel preoccupied with certain thoughts and feelings while taking prednisone. This in turn can lead to unusual behavior. For example, someone worried about safety may feel the need to check for locked doors multiple times before going to bed.

Others, like Stacy, may become obsessive about cleanliness:

> *My house was always the cleanest it could be while I was on*
> *prednisone. I'd focus on the minutest details, such as the grout*
> *between the tiles. I'd use a toothbrush and scrub. I'm not sure why*
> *I had a need to do this. I just felt I always needed to be cleaning*
> *something.*

Laura experienced the same thing:

> *I was an obsessive cleaner on prednisone. I was always coming up with new cleaning projects. One time, I decided I needed to wash one of my lampshades. Instead of just dusting it, I took it out in the backyard and hosed it down. Of course, this completely ruined it. But it seemed like such a good idea at the time!*
>
> *I'm glad I can laugh at these things now. In fact, I was even able to laugh when it was happening. I belonged to a great support group and we shared all our crazy stories. We discovered, though, that we really weren't crazy. It was just the side effects, and it was comforting to know that we weren't alone.*

Mood swings and personality changes

Prednisone causes a wide range of reactions. Some may have one predominating emotional side effect lasting weeks or months; others experience many emotional changes within a single day. These mood swings are marked by brief periods of intense feelings. It's not unusual to have a crying spell in the morning and then feel cheery by afternoon. By evening though, you might feel overcome with anger or rage.

It's difficult to cope with wild mood swings. Some, like Gina, have even said they feel as though they're not the same person:

> *Between the changes in my physical appearance as well as my emotions, I really felt like I was a different person. It was kind of scary. I'd look in the mirror and almost not recognize myself. I'd lash out at my husband about something and then wondered what I'd become. I recall one time he didn't take out the garbage and I got so upset. I just blew everything out of proportion.*
>
> *It was a difficult time. Fortunately, most people around me understood. I relied a lot on my faith, family, and inner strength. Support groups helped me, too. It was nice to know that I wasn't the only one experiencing these problems.*

Many people define themselves—at least partially—through their moods, feelings, and reactions to their environment. And unfortunately, prednisone can temporarily change these things. If you feel that prednisone is seriously altering your personality, discuss your concerns with your doctor. Perhaps it's possible to reduce your dosage to a more tolerable level. In the meantime, while waiting for your old self to return, consider seeking support from understanding friends. A good psychotherapist is advisable as well. Above all, remember that you are still you—it's just that you are under the influence of a powerful drug.

Tapering off

You should never stop taking prednisone abruptly. No matter how quickly you want to get off, it's very important to taper the drug gradually. Because prednisone is almost identical to your naturally-produced cortisol, your adrenal glands stop making cortisol while taking the drug. If you suddenly stop your medication, withdrawal symptoms will occur. Signs and symptoms can include extreme fatigue, low blood sugar levels, nausea, and heart rhythm problems. For this reason, everyone who takes prednisone should wear a MedicAlert bracelet. You can call the MedicAlert Foundation at (888) 633-4298, or (209) 668-3333 if you are outside the United States. You can also find it on the Web at *http://www.medicalert.org/*. At the very least, keep a note in your purse or wallet stating that you are currently taking corticosteroids. Also, tell your friends and family to mention to medical personnel that you are taking prednisone if you happen to have an accident or sudden illness.

It takes time for your adrenal glands to return to their normal function after a course of corticosteroids. If you decrease the prednisone bit by bit, however, your adrenals are able to gradually resume their regular production of cortisol. Keep in mind that if you've discontinued prednisone within the last six to twelve months after taking it for years, you may still need a boost of the drug if you experience a major stressful event, such as surgery, a bad accident, or severe illness.

Another reason to avoid coming off too quickly is to prevent your disease from flaring. If you notice a rebound of symptoms when tapering off the drug, let your doctor know. You may need to reduce more slowly. Over time, if you're on prednisone more frequently, you'll learn which tapering method works best for you. Sharing this information with your doctor is helpful so that the two of you can work together to keep your symptoms under control.

There are a number of different ways to taper off prednisone. On higher doses (40 mg or above), you can usually lower by 10 mg every five to seven days. Once you get to 30 mg, it's usually recommended to go down in 5 mg increments. At 15 or 20 mg, some slow the taper to 2.5 mg every week. Once on low doses, such as 5 or 10 mg, some go down 1 mg per week. Along the way, you might need to stay longer at certain doses till your body adjusts.

Another method of tapering involves switching to an every-other-day routine. When down to 15 or 20 mg per day, some people double their dose but then take it every other day.

These methods are just a couple of examples. You may have to go more slowly, or you may find you can reduce a little more quickly. Your doctor can advise you on what tapering method might work best for you.

Clarissa needs to go slowly:

> I've always had to be very careful when tapering. Once I get down to 15 mg, I can't go down more than 1 mg per week. Sometimes I've even lowered it by a half a mg once I've come down this far. It seems minuscule, but I can notice a difference. I don't want to risk a flare. Unfortunately, I can't seem to get below 10 mg without a rebound in symptoms.

Craig, now in his 30s, sums up his thoughts on prednisone and offers hope to those who have been on it long term:

> Prednisone is a drug with which a lot of people have a love–hate relationship. I know this feeling personally, as I was on it twelve and a half years. It's great because sometimes it's the only reliable thing that can get your disease under control. But other times, it can make life so difficult with the changes in physical appearance, as well as the emotional side effects. I know that I and others have at times felt so trapped on it. On the one hand, you feel you can't live with it, but on the other, you feel you can't live without it. It's not a good place to be.
>
> For many years, I was concerned I'd never get off. I knew about all the physical side effects, and was scared what it was doing to me at such a young age. I heard some people say that once people are on it as long as me, they probably won't ever get off. I felt I tried just about everything from both conventional and alternative medicine and yet nothing else worked.
>
> In my case, it turned out that surgery—pretty much the only option left—was my ticket to get off the drug. Within two months

*after my operation, I was completely off prednisone, as well as all
other medications. It felt so liberating. In fact, last year was the
first year I can ever remember that I did not take one single
prescription drug!*

*It's almost been four years now since my surgery and I'm doing
great. Miraculously, I have no damage from all the years on high
doses of prednisone. Surgery is not necessarily the answer for
everyone, but my point is that there is always hope. It didn't look good
for me for a long time, but it turned out there was a way to get off
prednisone and be healthy again. I feel others have hope, too. We're
learning more and more about IBD every year, and I'm convinced that
some day in the not-so-distant future, we'll look back and say,
"Remember when they used to give prednisone for IBD? Thank
goodness that's a thing of the past."*

CHAPTER 13

Personal Relationships

IBD AFFECTS VARIOUS ASPECTS of life, including personal relationships. At times, symptoms are not only difficult to control, but embarrassing to discuss with friends and family. Some people with IBD may avoid people or social situations in an effort to hide the illness. As a result, these people can have difficulty establishing and maintaining relationships with others. On the flip side, others with Crohn's or ulcerative colitis find that their disease has helped deepen their relationships with loved ones. In addition, new relationships are sometimes created through networking with others who have IBD.

This chapter explores how IBD can affect a variety of relationships. Throughout the chapter, people with IBD share their strategies of how they have managed to live with their illness without sacrificing love and friendship.

Family members

IBD can significantly affect family relationships—sometimes for the better and sometimes for the worse. An illness can bring out the best traits in certain family members, while leaving others in a state of stress and helplessness. Predicting how your individual relatives might react to your illness is not always easy. Some may respond with an abundance of love and support. Yet others may become angry, frustrated, anxious, or distant.

The following sections discuss how Crohn's and ulcerative colitis can affect a variety of family members, such as your parents, children, siblings, and other relatives. Suggestions are also offered that may help ease tensions—and possibly enhance the relationship—between you and your loved ones.

Parents

Perhaps one of the most difficult things for a parent is to see her child suffering or in pain. Worse yet is when the parent can't do anything to change the situation. Such is typically the case in IBD. Even if you are an adult with Crohn's or ulcerative colitis, your mother's or father's reaction to it might not be much different from how they would have reacted if you were 5, 10, or 15 years old.

Craig, now in his early 30s, explains how his parents' response to his flare-ups changed little over the years:

> I've had Crohn's disease since I was in junior high school. I'm fortunate that I have great parents who have always provided wonderful support to me when I've been ill. However, it's almost kind of funny how the old parent-child roles tend to resurface during the times I've been sick—even as I was well into adulthood. I can remember times after recovering from a major flare when they'd become very overprotective of me. They'd be concerned about me going out somewhere in the evening. Or they'd express disapproval of my going out on a walk if they thought it was too cold outside. It was like being a kid all over again. I would have to remind them that I'm an adult, capable of making my own decisions, as well as being able to judge whether I'm warm enough! They understood, but still, I know it was difficult for them to let go of the old parental roles. I have to admit though that I'd probably be much the same way if I were in their position.

Most parents want to do everything in their power to help their children. However, what they think of as helpful may not quite fit your definition.

Jamie describes problems with her parents:

> I was diagnosed with Crohn's in my early 30s. My parents have always been there for me and I know their intentions are good. But sometimes they get a little too overly involved. When I get sick, they want to take care of everything for me, such as paying my bills, dealing with the doctors, and making decisions about my care. I would have no problem with this if I were comatose—but I'm not. It sometimes feels diminishing when they take the attitude that I can't handle anything when I'm sick. But I can, and I want to be the one in charge.
>
> One time I even wrote them a letter that expressed my feelings on the subject. We later spoke about it. I'm not sure they totally got what I was talking about, but it certainly helped me to vent my feelings and frustrations. Since having this frank discussion, it's also made it much easier for me to bring the subject up if I feel they're becoming too controlling again.

Following is a list of suggestions to minimize stress between you and your parents when you're having a flare-up:

- **Understand their perspective.** Try to imagine what it would be like to have a son or daughter with IBD. You might feel—and maybe behave—much the same way as your parents. But if you suspect you'd react differently, perhaps you can understand they are probably doing the best they can, given the difficult circumstances.

- **Set boundaries.** Parents often want to do everything they can to help their children. However, there are probably some areas of your life where you don't want or need their assistance. Consider letting them know what they can do to help, while making it clear you can manage other responsibilities on your own.

- **Create open communication.** Both you and your parents probably have a wide range of thoughts, feelings, and emotions about your illness. When they're not clearly expressed, misunderstandings can result. Open discussions with a balance between talking and listening on both sides can do a lot to create an atmosphere of understanding and empathy.

Children

Many parents with IBD fear their disease may have a negative effect on their children. This is understandable, because children often think about illness differently from the way adults do. For example, young children might have trouble understanding what's causing your IBD. It wouldn't be uncommon, for instance, for your 5-year-old to think he is responsible for your being sick. He may believe a negative or angry thought he had about you is causing the disease. This type of magical thinking may also lead him to think your Crohn's or colitis is a punishment for his misbehavior.

Older children sometimes have difficulty accepting the limitations of a sick parent. Your teenager may be embarrassed by your IBD or resentful about the way it affects the family. Children's understanding of the disease and their reaction to it will depend in part on their age and maturity level, as well as their parents' attitude toward the illness.

Some parents with IBD also have concerns about what kind of a role model they are for their children. Because kids—especially younger ones—want to imitate their parents, mothers and fathers may wonder how their illness is influencing their children as they grow and develop.

Susie, who's had Crohn's for fourteen years, explains:

> My kids have definitely felt the effects of my illness over the years.
> For example, I'll never forget what my daughter said to me one time
> when she was 5. She told me that she wanted to have blood in her poop,
> too, so that she could be just like mommy. This scared me considerably.
> It really made me stop and think what effect this disease is having
> on her.
>
> You sometimes forget how young children think. They want to be just
> like mommy or daddy. And although her innocent comment frightened
> me, it was actually a good thing that she had verbalized it since it then
> gave me the opportunity to explain some things to her. I told her that it's
> okay to want to be like mommy, but that there are certain things that
> aren't good to copy. I explained that I have many good traits and that
> I wanted her to have those. However, I emphasized the blood in the
> poop was not one of those and that it's definitely something she'd want
> to avoid.

IBD can interfere with family activities. Unfortunately, diarrhea, pain, and fatigue sometimes make planning time with your family difficult. Children may feel disappointed or upset if plans are suddenly canceled or changed. Or they may feel sad or let down if they have to go out and participate in activities without you. In these circumstances, some mothers and fathers feel guilty if they miss events that are important to their children.

Susie describes her feelings in these situations:

> It is very frustrating when my IBD gets in the way of our family
> activities. It's also kind of sad, too, how I have lost time with my
> children. There have been many things I've missed out on, such as band
> recitals and Christmas parties. I feel bad about it, but there's really not
> much I can do if I'm too sick to go to these events. One time, for a band
> recital, my husband called me on his cell phone so I could at least hear
> the music. It's not like being there but at least it's something. I also talk
> to my kids about the situation as well. On some level, they are used to
> me being like this and they do understand. But it's still not easy.

Having a parent with IBD doesn't necessarily impact a child in a negative way. Although parents would not have chosen to have Crohn's or ulcerative colitis, some mothers and fathers think their illness has shaped positive qualities in their kids.

Clarissa, who was diagnosed with Crohn's disease long before she had her four children, explains:

> I really don't think my illness has had much of a negative impact on my
> kids. They've never known me any other way and have adapted well. In
> fact, I'd say it's possible that the Crohn's has had a side benefit for them.
> All four of my children are very compassionate people. Perhaps they
> would have turned out that way anyway, but I can't help but suspect that
> it had something having a mother with a chronic illness. Also, all of them
> have a very strong sense of commitment in everything they do. Again, I
> think a lot of this comes from how they've seen me carry on and not give
> up despite all I've been through.

Following are some tips on ways to help your children cope:

- **Focus on what you can do.** It's only natural to focus on the things you can't do
  when you are sick. However, this style of thinking usually leads to feelings of
  resentment and frustration. You might consider concentrating on activities in
  which you can participate with your children. For example, instead of focusing
  on how you don't have the energy to coach little league or to go to the local
  amusement park, try reading stories with your kids. Or perhaps you can watch a
  movie on video and then discuss it.

- **Communicate clearly about your illness.** Children sometimes have misconceptions about illness and what causes it. And just because they are not verbalizing
  their thoughts and feelings doesn't mean they're not having them. It's a good idea
  to talk openly about your illness with your kids at an age-appropriate level.
  Explain to young children that it's not their fault. Older children will require
  much more information. Answer all questions honestly. Remember, too, that
  listening is as an important part of communication as talking.

- **Let them help.** Many youngsters are naturally empathic and want to do what
  they can to help. Although it's inappropriate to shift the burden of your care or
  certain household responsibilities onto your children, there are probably some
  things they can do. Older kids can help with chores around the house, such as
  washing dishes and vacuuming. Younger ones can assist with simpler tasks like
  picking up their toys.

Sarah describes her daughter's helpfulness:

> My kids are pre-school age. Even when they are this young, children
> are still capable of helping out. My daughter, for example, is a very

compassionate little girl. Sometimes when I'm having a flare, she'll hold my hand and ask how I am doing. It's her way of helping. It means so much to me how she wants to do what she can to make me more comfortable.

- **Consider therapy.** Having a parent who is chronically ill is sometimes a lot for a child to deal with. Thus, it's a good idea to be attentive to changes in your youngster's behavior. Signs of trouble may include problems in school, changes in friendships, or difficulty in managing emotions, such as anger. If you feel your son's or daughter's difficulties are related to your illness, consider consulting a therapist who is familiar with chronic diseases such as IBD. Your gastroenterologist is a good resource for referrals.

Other relatives

IBD can affect your relationships with a wide variety of other family members, including siblings, grandparents, cousins, or in-laws. Its impact at least partly depends on how much interaction you have with a given relative. Those with whom you are the closest will likely feel the most affected. And as in other relationships, IBD has the potential to create tension as well as strengthen family ties.

Sarah explains how Crohn's disease has affected her and her sisters over the years:

I was diagnosed with Crohn's when I was 12 years old. I'm the second oldest of four daughters and we are all close in age. When we were growing up, there was sort of this ongoing family joke that I was our mother's favorite. It really wasn't true—Mom loves all of us equally— but sometimes it just came across that way since I would get special treatment when I was sick. For example, I'd be given extra money when we'd go out somewhere (a school field trip or grad night at Disneyland) since I might have special dietary needs. Or, if my sisters wanted Mom to make some special kind of food or treat, they'd make me ask her since they knew she would do it for me but not for them.

Fortunately, this special treatment over the years didn't harm my relationships with my sisters. Perhaps if my illness had been more severe, it could have. But we're all adults now and I get along well with each of them. To this day I can still discuss my health problems with them. What's nice is that they are very helpful and supportive, but they don't treat me as a poor, helpless, sick person.

Relatives whom you don't see on a regular basis are probably the least likely among your family to feel the effects of IBD. However, relationships with them can still suffer. If they are not familiar with the illness, they may have difficulty understanding it is a disease that is managed, not cured.

Sarah has had difficulty trying to explain Crohn's disease to her extended family:

> My husband's family and even some of my family just don't seem to understand what I'm going through. Their attitude is that I'm somehow bringing this on myself. They feel that if I just didn't let stress get to me that I would be healthy. One relative even told me that if I just ate enough fresh fruit I'd get better. As insensitive as some of this sounds, I can acknowledge that the people telling me these things probably mean well and are just trying to help. Unfortunately, though, they don't seem to be open to learning about the illness and are content with their preconceived notions, especially the ones about how to better care for acne caused by prednisone. So about the only thing I can do is to thank them for their concern and let it go, because there are only so many times you can tell them it's just a temporary side effect of the meds.

Larry has also had problems with relatives making assumptions about what is wrong with him:

> I've had Crohn's for fourteen years, but it's been especially severe the last several. When I have a flare-up, I can easily lose 30 or 40 pounds in just a month or two. As a result, my appearance can be very startling to those who don't see me on a daily basis. One time, some relatives on my wife's side of the family, when they saw me so thin and emaciated, simply didn't believe that I had Crohn's. Not that they even knew much about Crohn's or what it is. But they just assumed that I must have cancer since I lost so much weight. One person directly confronted me face to face, and we later heard through different relatives about other family members saying the same thing. I tried to explain that the Crohn's caused the extreme weight loss, but I don't think it did much good. Certain people are just going to believe what they want to believe. There's not much I can do about that. It's difficult, but I've learned I need to just let things like that go.

Friends

Good friends are often wonderful resources when you're sidelined by Crohn's or ulcerative colitis. Not only do they provide emotional support, but they can help with some of the basics, such as cooking, cleaning, and child care. For some people with IBD, however, making and maintaining friendships can pose a challenge. Unfortunately, chronic illnesses such as Crohn's and ulcerative colitis are hard for some healthy people to understand. Many people's concept of illness, for example, is something like the following: You get sick; you go to the doctor; he gives you some medication; you get better. It's probably hard for someone who thinks like this to grasp that a health problem can last for months, years, or indefinitely.

Friends may also have difficulty understanding why you are unable to participate in various activities when you seem perfectly healthy to them. Some people with IBD look ill, but others appear just as normal and healthy as the average person walking down the street. The fact that Crohn's disease and ulcerative colitis are frequently invisible illnesses creates challenges, such as having to repeatedly explain why you can't do certain things. Even worse, others may not take your illness seriously and just think you are trying to avoid them or specific activities.

Richard explains his frustrations with friends in college when they couldn't understand his illness:

> My college years were sometimes difficult. I looked completely normal and healthy, but my Crohn's was fairly active during that time of my life. I had limited energy and had to be very careful with what I ate. I remember one time some friends were going on a weekend retreat and wanted me to come. Given my condition at the time, I knew it wasn't a good idea. However, one person was especially putting pressure on me to go. His intentions weren't bad, but he just couldn't understand how I couldn't go away for a weekend when he saw me looking so well and able to go to my classes. Unfortunately, I gave into the peer pressure and went. By the time I got back, I was exhausted and felt awful. I was lucky that it didn't throw me into a major flare, but I still missed the whole following week of school.
>
> It was frustrating how I couldn't make my friend understand. Maybe if the Crohn's had been visible, that would have made a difference. It was almost as if he didn't believe I had a real disease. I didn't like having to defend that there was something wrong with me.

Needless to say, the experience made me realize that I need to listen to my body more than other people who don't know what they are talking about. Also, over time, I learned to surround myself with people who were able to accept me, even if I had certain limitations.

Having a chronic illness such as IBD may also help you realize who your true friends are. Those with severe Crohn's or colitis have especially found some people can't handle having a friend with a serious disease.

Jamie experienced this unfortunate situation after her first hospitalization:

It's interesting what effect your illness can have on those around you. Before I was first diagnosed, I had a friend at work with whom I was very close. When I got sick, it was so bad that I was in the hospital for a month. During this time, I didn't hear from her at all. I thought that it was kind of strange, and didn't know what to make of it.

When I finally returned to work, it was clear our relationship had definitely changed. She really distanced herself from me. Since it was bothering me, I got the nerve to ask her — in a non-confrontational way, of course — what happened to our friendship. She was polite, but just kind of downplayed the whole thing and made some excuse about how she's just been more focused on work lately. I didn't probe. It was clear she didn't want to have much to do with me anymore. I don't know what it was. Perhaps it had more to do with her fear of illness. Or maybe she just didn't know how to respond to it. It hurt, but fortunately her reaction was the exception rather than the rule.

Others with IBD, such as Susie, find having Crohn's and ulcerative colitis brings out the best in their friends:

It's been truly incredible how my friends have rallied around me and my family during this difficult time. I recently had major surgery to remove my colon, and the outpouring of love has been remarkable. In addition to all the cards and flowers, friends were very generous with providing meals for my family. Believe it or not, we received enough food to cover dinner for my family for six weeks! I even had one friend from New York fly all the way across the country to come out and help us on just three days notice. It's just been so wonderful to feel so loved and cared for.

Larry expresses his fears about losing friends because of his illness:

> *I've have a very severe case of Crohn's, especially for the past several years. It's been quite difficult. I have trouble getting out because of the pain, diarrhea, and low energy. I also haven't been able to work as much. Sadly, I've noticed that some people who used to be a part of my life have gradually disappeared. I've made an effort to call and write, but there are some who no longer respond. I'll probably never know the reason, but my theory is that for some people, it brings up issues of their own mortality. In other words, I think on some level they worry that something like this can happen to them. And since it's too uncomfortable of a thought, the easiest option is to just eliminate contact with me. I suppose it's just a coping mechanism.*
>
> *Fortunately, I do have friends who have stood by me. I am very grateful and appreciative of these people and I let them know that. I have to confess though that in the back of my mind, I worry about some of them disappearing since it has happened with others. However, I try not to think about that and instead focus on expressing my gratitude and doing what I can to be a good friend to them.*

Ulcerative colitis and Crohn's disease can impose limitations on your lifestyle. However, it is still possible to maintain existing friendships and cultivate new ones, even if you are living with active disease. Here are a few suggestions that may help:

- **Keep in touch.** Some of your friends may avoid contacting you simply because they don't know what to say or are afraid of saying the wrong thing. Although you may feel as if they should call you, because you are the one who's sick, consider taking the initiative by reaching out first. Calling, writing, and emailing are all good ways of maintaining contact.

- **Share IBD details selectively.** Not everyone wants or needs to hear everything about your illness. It's important to carefully choose with whom you share the details of your disease. Try to keep talk of your bowel problems to a minimum unless you're sure a friend wants to hear about it.

- **Educate friends.** Some friends won't have an interest in learning about IBD, but others may. The Crohn's and Colitis Foundation of America (CCFA) publishes many easy-to-understand brochures on Crohn's disease and ulcerative colitis that are appropriate to give to friends. You might also consider inviting those closest to you to a support group meeting so they can get a better idea of what it is like to live with IBD.

- **Pursue interests.** It's important to make time for activities that do not revolve around your disease. Although having IBD may somewhat limit your choices, there are probably many things you can still do. Participating in these activities also allows you to meet and make friends with others who have similar interests.

- **Meet others with IBD.** You may feel at times that no one in your life understands what you are going through. You might consider contacting other people with Crohn's or ulcerative colitis. Your local CCFA office can give you information on support group meetings in your area. If there are none close to you, they can still give you the names and phone numbers of volunteers with whom you can speak. The CCFA web site also has links to many online message boards, newsgroups, and chat rooms, which are found at *http://www.ccfa.org/links/#ngmb*. The *Resources* appendix lists many resources as well.

Clarissa has made several good friends as a result of attending a support group:

> *I know this might sound strange, but Crohn's has produced a few good things in my life. It's not that I would have ever wished to have the disease. But one good thing about it is that it has led me to some very wonderful people. It has enabled me to establish new friendships with people that I otherwise would have never met. And it's not like my friendships with these people are completely based on the disease. Yes, we can and do talk about IBD, but it's not the foundation of our friendship.*
>
> *I'm so thankful I chose to involve myself in support groups. It's so nice to be in a place where you know everyone understands. Not only have I received an abundance of support, but I have been able to give back to others as well. And that's a good feeling. Strange, but I guess I have Crohn's to thank for that.*

Intimate relationships

Having Crohn's disease or ulcerative colitis can affect your self-image. Symptoms such as pain, fatigue, diarrhea, and excessive weight loss can also contribute to feeling unattractive or undesirable. It's only natural then that some people with IBD have concerns about establishing and maintaining intimacy. Although Crohn's and colitis can interfere with romance, married and single people have found ways to enjoy a good love life despite occasional problems caused by their disease.

Sexual problems

Perhaps one of the greatest concerns of people with IBD is whether they can still have and enjoy a fulfilling sex life. The answer is almost always yes. However, there may be temporary periods—such as during a severe flare-up or in the weeks immediately after surgery—when sexual intercourse isn't possible. This section includes many suggestions from people with IBD on how to minimize or work around these occasional problems. The following situations may temporarily disrupt your desire or ability to have sexual intercourse.

Severe flare-up

One common impediment to sexual relations is a major flare-up. Symptoms such as nausea and pain can certainly dampen both your mood and spirit. Frequent diarrhea can also make you fear an accident during a romantic moment. In addition, the severe fatigue associated with many flares can easily sap the energy necessary for sex. If these or other symptoms are interfering with your love life, consider the following suggestions:

- **Know when you are strongest.** Fatigue can reduce the desire for and ability to have sex. But maybe there are times of the day—such as the morning—when you have more energy. If so, initiate or schedule a romantic interlude at a time of the day when you feel your best.

- **Take steps to control diarrhea.** Several medications are available to control diarrhea. Perhaps taking a dose a few hours before sex can give you confidence you won't have an accident at an inappropriate time. Also, if you know certain foods can cause loose bowel movements, alter your eating accordingly during the hours before lovemaking.

- **Find other ways to express your love.** Many people equate intimacy with sex. However, there are many other ways to share love if intercourse isn't possible. Consider talking openly with your partner on this topic. The two of you can probably come up with ideas for enjoying intimacy that are still satisfying for both of you. The idea is to broaden the goal of lovemaking. Having a goal of giving and receiving pleasure—for example—reduces performance anxiety and increases your potential for enjoyment.

Larry describes how he and his wife had to plan around his illness:

> *During the early years of my illness, the Crohn's sometimes*
> *interfered with our sex life. However, my wife and I found that with a*

bit of planning, we could work around it. For example, I found that if I took an anti-diarrhea medication about an hour before sex, I would reduce my chances of having an accident.

We'd also have to be a bit spontaneous as well. My energy level was never predictable, so we'd just take advantage of the moment when I had enough energy—regardless of what time of the day it was.

There were also times back then when I was so sick that I couldn't have sex for a few months at a time. When this happened, it was frustrating for us. But we found other ways we could be intimate, such as cuddling and caressing. It wasn't quite the same, but it was at least somewhat fulfilling for us.

Recovering from surgery

Having abdominal surgery is a major stress on the body. Although many doctors say you can resume normal activity within six to eight weeks, some people may take longer to recover their energy and rebuild their strength. This is especially true if you were very ill before the surgery or have recently taken corticosteroid drugs. It's not uncommon for people with IBD to have a reduced libido for a few months following surgery.

Larry, now in his late 40s, explains that it took him a while to regain his stamina:

Over ten years ago I had intestinal resection surgery. The Crohn's was out of control and it was not responding well to medication. Not even prednisone was helping. Thus, I was very ill before the surgery. Overall, the operation went well and they were able to remove the diseased segment of my bowel. However, it wasn't like I could just bounce back and resume life as if nothing happened. It took a while to regain my strength. It wasn't until three months after the surgery that I had enough energy to have sex.

Many men have concerns that removing their large intestine may leave them impotent. A small chance of this complication exists, because the nerves that control erection are near where a surgeon cuts when performing this operation. However, the risk is very low for men with IBD who do not have rectal cancer—less than 2 percent.[1] The risk of erectile dysfunction in men with rectal cancer, in contrast, is higher.[2] This is because to remove all of the malignancy, the surgeon may have to cut closer to the nerves that control erection.

It's best to have your surgery done by an expert who has performed at least a hundred colectomies. This way, you'll minimize your chances of impotence following your operation.

David discussed his concerns with his doctor before his surgery:

> *Before having my colon out, I was very concerned that the surgery might leave me impotent. However, my surgeon sat down with me and spent almost a whole hour explaining the procedure. He said he had performed hundreds of these operations and that the chance of impotence in my case was very low. His expertise gave me confidence, so I went into surgery feeling more comfortable than I had been. The surgery was successful and everything worked out fine. My sexual function is completely normal.*

Rectovaginal fistula

A rectovaginal fistula is an abnormal connection between rectum and vagina. It can develop if IBD inflammation tears the lining of the rectum. When this happens, a channel can form between it and the vagina.

Rectovaginal fistulas allow both gas and feces to enter the vagina. This is often very distressing, because a woman can't predict—let alone control—when stool or gas will pass through. Moreover, bacteria from waste products can cause both inflammation and infection.

Having a rectovaginal fistula can make sexual intercourse difficult, if not impossible. Medications, such as 6-MP, azathioprine, or infliximab, can sometimes help resolve fistulas, but most of the time surgery is necessary to fix the problem.

Depression

Living with a chronic illness is as much an emotional challenge as it is a physical one. It's therefore not uncommon for people with severe and persistent IBD to experience feelings of depression.

Depression can cause a loss of interest in activities you previously found enjoyable, including sex. If you suspect your depression is causing a diminished libido, you might consider seeking professional help from a counselor familiar with IBD. For more information on the emotional impact of IBD, including depression, please see Chapter 17, *Emotions and Coping.*

Other effects in couples

Ulcerative colitis and Crohn's disease can have a wide range of effects on couples. Besides sexual problems, people in committed relationships often face nonsexual ones as well. For example, IBD sometimes creates difficulties if the healthy partner has trouble understanding the uncontrollable nature of symptoms.

Larry describes his frustrations with his wife's inability to understand his urgent bouts of diarrhea:

> I've been married for over twenty years, and have had a severe case of Crohn's during much of this time. To this day, I often have problems with urgency and diarrhea. I'm generally good about keeping myself out of situations where I might have an accident, but I'm not perfect. Unfortunately, there have been a few times when my wife and I were out with others and I didn't make it to the bathroom in time. Unfortunately, she's unable to understand that even though I try my hardest, accidents can still happen. She's literally said to me, "Why can't you control yourself? You could if you tried harder and really wanted to." It seems it's embarrassing for her since she's sometimes the one who has to explain it to other people if I have to run off and leave. But then imagine how I must feel!
>
> It hurts me that she can't seem to appreciate my situation. After all, it's not like I want to have accidents just so I can embarrass her. I've tried to educate her that it's not uncommon for people with IBD to have accidents now and then, but it hasn't helped much. We've also been in therapy as well. However, I honestly can't say we ever resolved this particular issue. Sometimes I think the only way she could understand is if she had IBD herself. About the only thing I can do is to continue to adjust my diet and medications before going out so I can avoid problems in public.

Chronic illnesses such as IBD also have a way of bringing subtle problems in a relationship to the surface. Or similarly, some have found their Crohn's or colitis can magnify certain problems that seemed relatively minor before they had the disease.

Larry, who developed Crohn's several years after he got married, explains:

> I was diagnosed with Crohn's about eight years after my wife and I got married. Before I developed my illness, we occasionally had some

> problems communicating clearly with each another. Neither of us saw
> it as too serious, and overall our relationship was going along well.
> However, once I developed IBD—and especially once it became quite
> severe—our communication problem intensified. It became difficult
> to enjoy the things we used to do, such as traveling or even going out
> in the evening. I had trouble relating my frustration and anger about
> this. And likewise, she had difficulty expressing her feelings, too. It
> was significantly affecting both of us, yet neither of us could discuss it.
> We sought help from both a marriage counselor and a minister.
> Unfortunately, this still hasn't been enough to help. Just recently,
> we have decided to separate.

IBD can have a positive effect in couples' relationships. Some people have found the stress of having a chronic illness has ultimately helped bring them closer to their partner. Much like increased resistance on exercise equipment can build stronger muscles, the increased strain on a relationship has the potential to create stronger bonds.

David explains how he and his wife have grown closer over the years:

> My wife and I have been through some pretty tough times. I had a
> really bad case of Crohn's that required many hospitalizations. At one
> point, I came very close to dying. Ultimately, I had surgery to remove
> my colon, but even after that I continued to have problems. I would
> imagine that some marriages would not survive what my wife and I
> experienced. After all, I barely survived it myself physically. But we've
> always had a deep love for each other that's carried us through. In
> fact, I'd say in some ways the Crohn's helped strengthen our love over
> the years. It's made us realize how fortunate we are to have each
> other. We truly appreciate each other more every day. We are
> extremely thankful for what we have and don't take anything for
> granted.

Concerns for singles

Single people with Crohn's and colitis sometimes worry that their illness might affect their chances of finding a life partner. Understandably, having an unpredictable disease such as IBD with its many symptoms can undermine your self-confidence and feelings of attractiveness.

You probably have many questions regarding IBD's potential impact on your future love life. Here are two of the most common:

- Knowing I have this disease, will anyone ever want to be with me?

- How do I tell someone I'm dating about my illness?

The following sections address these two important questions.

Acceptance and lovability

Adjusting to life with a chronic disease such as IBD is often not easy. And if you're having difficulty accepting Crohn's or ulcerative colitis yourself, you may wonder how anyone else can. It's true there are people in the world who may not want to be in a committed relationship with you because of your health condition. But you probably wouldn't want to get involved with such people in the first place—even if you were completely healthy. These are likely the same individuals who avoid others if they think they are too fat, too thin, or have some other perceived imperfection. In all probability, such individuals are not well suited for long-term, committed relationships.

The world, though, is filled with a variety of people who have different needs and preferences. What one person finds unappealing is often attractive to another. It's therefore unfair to take an attitude that you have little or nothing to offer someone in a relationship. You probably have a lot more to give than you realize. It may help to consider the following suggestions:

- **Know that you are more than your illness.** IBD may at times dominate your life, but you still have your personality and identity. No disease can ever take these away from you. You are still you: a unique individual who just happens to also have Crohn's disease or ulcerative colitis.

- **Analyze your assets.** You may consider your IBD a potential liability when trying to find a mate. But instead of focusing on the negative, look at your strong points, such as your sense of humor or ability to listen. Many who've had a chronic illness have also developed traits such as compassion and patience—two highly valued qualities that come in handy in any type of relationship.

- **Find a model.** Many people with IBD in committed relationships developed their illness when they were single. Yet many now enjoy successful marriages. Consider talking to people who've made the transition from single to married life. They can help assure you that it is indeed possible to find a loving partner. CCFA support groups are a great resource for meeting people in all phases of life.

- **Accept and love yourself.** Learning to love and accept yourself with your illness is often a challenge, but it's sometimes the first step needed before others can fully love and accept you. Your attitude sets the tone for how others perceive and interact with you. If you accept and love yourself, others, including potential mates, probably will, too. You might consider psychotherapy if you're having difficulty with this issue.

Vickie explains how her feelings changed over time:

> I was diagnosed with Crohn's when I was 18. It wasn't an easy time since I was already insecure about myself before I had the disease. But now with it, I was even more so. I had difficulty accepting it and did what I could to ignore it. I also worried how I would ever find a boyfriend. I frequently asked myself, "Who would ever love me like this?" After all, I could barely accept myself the way I was.
>
> I can't say I suddenly one day had this revelation that I was totally lovable with my illness. It was more of a gradual thing. After a few years, I began to adapt to it. Even though I still had recurring flares, I noticed that the disease really hadn't changed who I was. I was still the same Vickie with same personality and desirable attributes. I also realized that other people had their own issues, too, and Crohn's just happened to be mine. So gradually, I reached a point where I was much more at peace with myself and the illness.
>
> Interestingly, once I reached this state of peace, I was not even looking for love. But then the man who has now been my boyfriend for the past few years popped up into my life. He's been with me through the ups and downs of Crohn's, and has had no problems being able to love and accept me just as I am—illness and all. It's been such a wonderful experience and I feel so fortunate to have him in my life.

Disclosure when dating

Singles with IBD frequently wonder how and when to tell a potential partner about their illness. Although you can take many different approaches, there's no right or wrong way to inform the person you're dating. Nor is there a correct time to disclose the fact you have Crohn's or ulcerative colitis. The important thing is to choose a method and a time with which you are comfortable. Following are a few examples of how some people handle this situation.

Sandra's approach changed when she fell in love:

> When I was younger, the method I used for telling guys about my Crohn's disease was that I didn't. I felt that no guy could accept me with the disease. I was so afraid of rejection that I would do everything I could to hide the illness. Ultimately, when I would start getting too close to someone, I'd break off the relationship. I felt I couldn't risk anyone finding out.
>
> This went on for many years. However, when I met the man who is now my husband, I really fell in love. At first, my pattern with him was still the same. I'd do everything I could to hide the illness. I didn't want him to see me with all the diarrhea. I would purposely not eat before the times I'd spend with him to reduce my chances of needing to go to the bathroom. If I was at his apartment and needed to go, I would just suddenly leave without explanation. With him, though, I couldn't bring myself to break off the relationship like I did with all the others. It finally reached a point where I just broke down and told him everything. It was scary, but fortunately he really loved me, too. He still accepted me with the Crohn's. We've been married now for many years and have three wonderful children. He's always been very supportive and understanding of me.

Hollie likes to disclose early in a relationship:

> I know some people who wait a long time to tell. But that's not for me. I'm very up-front with my health history right from the start. I have an ileostomy—so I especially want to make sure that someone doesn't have an issue with that.
>
> As for how I tell, it really just depends. It's amazing though how the topic can just naturally come up, even if it's just the first time I'm meeting someone. For example, if we're at a movie, and a guy asks if I want popcorn, I'll mention that I can't have it. When he asks why, it's usually a good segue for me to bring up my health history. Also, sometimes my ostomy will gurgle quite loudly—so that always provides a good opportunity!

Chuck believes in early disclosure, too:

> When I was first dating the woman who's now my wife, it was important for me to mention my illness early on—just to get it out

of the way. It really wasn't a big deal though for either of us. I've always been comfortable with myself. And fortunately, my having an illness like Crohn's didn't bother my wife.

Others, like Vickie, rely on intuition to determine the best time to bring up the subject:

I'm not the type to bring up my illness on a first date. One time, I was on the other side of the fence, so to speak, and a guy told me about a problem he had first thing. It felt inappropriate to me at such an early stage and I have to admit it didn't feel quite right.

So when I began dating my boyfriend, I knew I didn't want to tell him right away. But I was concerned when I should tell him. I decided that there wasn't necessarily a right time—so I waited until it felt appropriate, based on how I thought our relationship was progressing. It turned out that about a month after we started seeing each other, it just naturally came up. We had reached a state where we were both so interested in each other that we wanted to know everything about one another. At that point, I mentioned my chronic condition, how if affects me, and how I have to take medication to control it. It wasn't a problem for him. Our relationship continued to deepen, and we've now been together for two and a half years.

Cathy sums up her philosophy on IBD and relationships:

I've been a support group facilitator for a long time. So I've seen how IBD has impacted many people's lives. There's no doubt that Crohn's and ulcerative colitis can have a significant effect on relationships. But the impact is not all negative. Yes, there will be people who either can't or don't want to understand your illness. And they'll eventually drift away. Sometimes it's just acquaintances, but other times it's people who were previously close to you. Although this is difficult, I sometimes think this works out for the best.

In a way, IBD is like having a built-in screening device. Those who can't handle it probably aren't committed to you in the first place. So in the long run, it's probably good that they left your life. However, you know the ones who stick by you through the bad times are true gems. These are the people who love you, and you know that without a doubt. In my case, for example, I know how hard my illness has been on my husband. But since he loves me, he's stood by and always supported me. My close friends and certain family members have also done the same.

I'm not saying that it's always easy maintaining your relationships when you're sick. But if people truly love and care for you, they're not going to stop loving you just because you have a bowel disease.

CHAPTER 14

Fertility and Pregnancy

IBD OFTEN ARISES during the prime reproductive years. As a result, Crohn's disease and ulcerative colitis can interfere with plans to start a family. Many couples are therefore concerned how IBD may affect their ability to conceive and deliver a healthy baby.

This chapter discusses fertility, pregnancy, nursing, and heredity. The chapter also looks at the major medications used to treat IBD and how they may affect an unborn child. Throughout, those with ulcerative colitis and Crohn's share their stories of how IBD has affected their reproductive capabilities and influenced decisions about having children.

Fertility

Fertility is a man's ability to induce conception or a woman's capacity to conceive. Male fertility depends on making large numbers of healthy, motile sperm, and then the ability to ejaculate them. Female fertility depends on a number of factors, such as having healthy eggs and the ability to release them through hormonal fluctuations, having clear fallopian tubes through which the eggs can travel, and having optimal uterine conditions.

The vast majority of people with IBD do not become infertile from their disease. The most common exceptions include a minority of women with severe Crohn's, a minority of women who've had surgery, and men who are taking the drug sulfasalazine.

Men

Taking sulfasalazine is one of the most common causes of infertility in men with IBD. This drug is made from two components: a sulfa portion (a derivative of sulfur) and a 5-aminosalicylic acid part (also called 5-ASA, an aspirin-like substance). The sulfa component can cause both sperm abnormalities as well as an overall reduced sperm count.[1] The effect is temporary: Sperm quality improves within a few months after stopping the drug. In the early 1990s, a new generation of 5-ASA drugs became available that do not contain sulfa. Although sulfasalazine is still used to treat IBD of the colon, men now have the option of substituting similar medications that do not impair their ability to father a child.

Another medication, methotrexate, can also impair male fertility. Like sulfasalazine, the effect is temporary and should wear off within several months after you stop taking the drug.

Prolonged periods of severe malnutrition can also temporarily impact male fertility, but with excellent medical care this is rare. If it does happen, however, fertility should return once health and nutritional status are restored. Otherwise, there's no evidence to suggest men with IBD have any more problems with fertility than those without a chronic illness.

Women

Women's fertility is sometimes affected by undergoing surgery or by having severe Crohn's disease. Ulcerative colitis, whether active or not, is not usually associated with reduced reproductive ability. A recent study found, however, that having surgery for ulcerative colitis can reduce a woman's chance of conceiving after the operation.[2] Another group of researchers found that among women who had surgery, 12 percent of those with Crohn's disease and 25 percent of those with ulcerative colitis had fertility problems.[3] Of those who did not have surgery, the infertility rate was 5 percent for Crohn's and 7 percent for ulcerative colitis.

Krystal, who had a colectomy because of ulcerative colitis, was unable to get pregnant:

> *During the years I first had ulcerative colitis, my doctor didn't want me to get pregnant since I was too sick. After several years, I finally had a colectomy with a J-pouch construction. I soon returned to good health. At this point my doctor said it was okay to have a baby. But then I found I was unable to conceive. It turned out that that my fallopian tubes were scarred. We don't know whether the scarring was due to the ulcerative colitis, my surgery, or some other reason. However, I participate in an online message board for people with the J-pouch, and I've found that other women have similar problems. My husband and I still wanted to have a baby so I underwent in-vitro fertilization. I became pregnant and now have a healthy baby boy.*

It's generally thought that Crohn's disease, especially if it is active, decreases women's ability to get pregnant. Because Crohn's can cause problems with absorption, malnutrition is perhaps one explanation for this decrease. If a woman is not receiving sufficient nourishment, her menses may cease. In addition, other complications, such as abscesses or fistulas in the vaginal area, can make sexual intercourse difficult or unpleasant. When Crohn's is brought under control, a woman's capacity to conceive usually returns.

Stacy, however, had such a severe case of Crohn's that she was never able to conceive:

> I had a very active case of Crohn's with many complications such as fistulas and abscesses. During the time my husband and I were trying, I was never able to get pregnant. After I had my first surgery, the doctors told me that I probably could never conceive since my female organs were so scarred. They explained that when you have a lot of inflammation in the small intestine, the bowel sometimes adheres to other nearby organs, such as the sex ones, and can cause scarring. They also said that even if I got pregnant, it would be very difficult since my nutritional status was so poor. I could barely support myself with what I could eat, much less a baby.
>
> My husband and I decided that although we didn't want to undergo fertility treatment, we still wanted a family. We decided to adopt. We now have two beautiful daughters, four years apart.

Sandra also had a long history of Crohn's, but was able to conceive very easily:

> I've had Crohn's since I was 3 months old, and had several surgeries as a young child. The doctors told my parents that I'd never be able to have children. My parents told me this as I was growing up—so it was ingrained in me from a very early age. However, they were all wrong. I'm very fertile. In fact, I sometimes joke that my sex organs are just about the only part of my body that work right! Despite the Crohn's, I've never had trouble getting pregnant. I have three wonderful children and they were all born very healthy.

Most IBD medications do not affect female fertility. Prednisone can cause menstrual irregularities, but no studies indicate that it reduces the ability to conceive. Data on how newer drugs such as infliximab affect fertility are still pending. Methotrexate should never be taken if you are trying to get pregnant, because it causes miscarriage and severe birth defects.

Pregnancy

Some women worry that having a baby may worsen their IBD. However, it appears pregnancy has little effect on the course of either Crohn's or ulcerative colitis. A general rule is that about one third of pregnant women improve, one third get worse, and one third remain about the same during pregnancy. These percentages are similar to any group of women with IBD over the course of a year whether they are pregnant or not. Moreover, research indicates that if your illness is inactive at the time of conception, your IBD is likely to stay in remission for the following nine months.[4]

Doctors are most concerned about women who conceive when their disease is active. Unfortunately, under these circumstances IBD has a greater chance of worsening during pregnancy. Furthermore, these women may also experience more problems with their illness postpartum.[5] For this reason, most physicians encourage women whose IBD is out of control to delay pregnancy until the disease calms down.

Amy waited till her illness was under control before trying to conceive:

> *My illness has never been severe. However, a few months before I conceived my first child I was having some problems. I asked my doctor if I should wait a while before trying to get pregnant. He explained that although Crohn's is generally unpredictable, it's probably best to get as healthy as possible before trying to conceive. He said we could always treat it if necessary should anything flare during the pregnancy. So we adjusted my medication. Within a couple of months, I was stable and felt the disease was under control. I conceived within the first month of trying and had a wonderful pregnancy. In fact, I'd say I felt the best ever when I was pregnant— I rarely had any symptoms.*

Other women have also found pregnancy helped their IBD. Sarah, who has Crohn's, explains:

> *I've been pregnant three times. Each time before conceiving I had mild symptoms such as loose bowel movements two to four times a day. Within the first few months, all my symptoms went away with each pregnancy. I also found I could eat just about everything. Normally, I have difficulty with dairy, salads, and fresh fruit, but not when I was expecting. As a result, I was able to gain a good amount of weight, which normally is very difficult for me. I wish I could be pregnant all the time!*

Some women, such as Rhonda, have found that what happens in one pregnancy is not predictive of what will happen in another:

> With my son, I was the healthiest I had ever been. I had no problems with the Crohn's during that pregnancy. My doctor explained that pregnancy produces natural steroids that often help control inflammation. However, she also said that if flares occur, they usually happen within the first three or four months. Sure enough, that's what happened when I was expecting my second child (a girl). I had a flare the first trimester. We were concerned since I was not gaining weight and was fatigued, which made caring for my son a challenge. For a while I was seeing my doctor every two weeks. We also adjusted my medication. Fortunately, we got it under control. By my second trimester I was fine and remained so for the remainder of the pregnancy. It just goes to show though that each pregnancy can affect IBD differently.

IBD sometimes first begins in pregnancy. In this situation, researchers do not know whether pregnancy significantly contributes to the development of IBD or if it is just a coincidence. However, when it happens, the disease—particularly Crohn's—is usually more severe.[6,7]

Laura was diagnosed with ulcerative colitis when she was pregnant with her first child:

> During my pregnancy I began having diarrhea and bleeding. I was very concerned, but unfortunately my doctor at the time didn't take it too seriously. I was told I had hemorrhoids and that they were quite common in pregnant women. I wasn't satisfied with this is as I knew something much more serious was going on. Finally, I got in touch with a gastroenterologist and he was able to diagnose ulcerative colitis when I was seven months along. The rest of the pregnancy was difficult since I was still dealing with the bloody diarrhea. Fortunately, I delivered a healthy baby girl only two weeks before her due date. However, my illness continued to get worse after I had my baby. I suffered for over four years without ever having a remission. It was very difficult during that time, especially when having to care for a young child. When I'd finally had enough of the ulcerative colitis, I had a colectomy. I've been fine now for over fourteen years.

Women who have had surgery often wonder how pregnancy might affect their health. Although previously having an operation or currently having an ostomy doesn't prevent a woman from having a normal pregnancy, it's necessary to work closely with a team of doctors who have experience with other mothers-to-be who have had your particular procedure. One problem to watch for is intestinal obstruction. Scar tissue from your surgery may shift as your baby is growing. It can then push on your intestine, causing it to become blocked. Also, it's important to discuss with your doctor how you will deliver your baby. Many women who've had surgery can deliver their babies vaginally, but a caesarean section may be appropriate, depending on your circumstances.

Julie describes her experience when she was pregnant in the early 1970s:

> I developed ulcerative colitis when I was 9 and had ileostomy surgery when I was 16. In the early 70s, I was pregnant, and unfortunately had a doctor who was not familiar with the possible risks I faced. I don't know what it was, but maybe at that time they just didn't know as much. Or maybe they just took an attitude that everything could still be done as naturally or easily, even with an ileostomy. I was hospitalized twice during my pregnancy for partial intestinal blockages. During labor I had a complete blockage. Unfortunately, they didn't recognize what was going on soon enough and the baby didn't make it.
>
> I'm not in any way saying that women who have ileostomies can't or shouldn't have babies. And I'd like to think what happened to me could never happen again today. But it's not worth taking a chance. I can't emphasize enough how important it is to make sure that you are working with a team of doctors who are very familiar with these types of high-risk pregnancies.

Krystal, who has a J-pouch, worked very closely with her doctors during her pregnancy:

> I wanted to do everything I could to make sure my pregnancy ran as smoothly as possible. I spoke with my doctors, and we decided that I would have a Caesarian section. There was only a very small chance that my J-pouch might burst with a regular delivery. But my gastroenterologist is very conservative and said a C-section is safer in my case. I felt the same way. I didn't even want to take a chance that

my pouch might not make it—so I went with the C-section.
Everything worked out fine.

Women with active IBD, particularly if it's Crohn's, sometimes deliver their babies prematurely. When this happens, the infant is usually smaller than normal for gestational age (the age based on the number of weeks since conception). One study found that among women with Crohn's, 15 percent delivered early and had babies who were small for their gestational age. Women with ulcerative colitis had a rate of 11 percent, whereas those without IBD had a rate of 7 percent.[8] If your disease flares when you are pregnant, therefore, it's a good idea to keep in close contact with both your obstetrician and gastroenterologist. They can recommend treatment that can help get your symptoms under control without harming your unborn child. This way, you'll have the best chance of delivering a normal-sized, full-term baby.

Rhonda describes her flare during pregnancy:

> *I've had Crohn's since age 18. I've had what I would describe as a*
> *moderate case. It's been fairly active, however, causing me cramps,*
> *diarrhea, and fatigue—but at least I've never been hospitalized.*
> *When I was pregnant with my daughter, I flared during the first few*
> *months. It was difficult to eat enough, so I was very worried how this*
> *might affect my baby. I kept in close contact with doctor. We decided*
> *to temporarily increase my medication. Luckily, this helped get the*
> *Crohn's under control. I did well the rest of the pregnancy and had*
> *a healthy baby girl, although she was on the small side—five and*
> *a half pounds.*

Most women with Crohn's disease and ulcerative colitis are able to have healthy babies. One review of several studies on this subject found that women whose IBD was in remission had the same rate of normal pregnancies as those in the general population.[9] The percentages of birth defects, miscarriage, and stillbirths were also very similar. However, this review mentions a couple of studies that show an increased risk of preterm delivery regardless of remission status. So even though chances are good you'll have a normal pregnancy, it's still important for your doctors to follow you closely, especially during your last trimester.

Sandra says IBD had little impact on her when she was pregnant:

> *I feel I was very fortunate that IBD didn't interfere with any of my*
> *pregnancies. Of course, I'm sure a lot of that had to do with the fact*

that my disease was inactive during the times I was expecting. My kids were all on time and had no birth defects. They were normal weight and very healthy. In fact my son weighed nine pounds! I delivered them all vaginally, with no epidural or drugs. I guess one thing IBD taught me was a high tolerance for pain!

Medications during pregnancy

Active disease is generally more of a threat to you and your developing baby than treating your IBD. Although ideally it's preferable to take no medications while pregnant, many drugs commonly used to treat Crohn's and ulcerative colitis can be taken safely when you are expecting. For these reasons, your doctor may prescribe medication if she feels the benefits to you and your unborn child outweigh any risks. Following are a list of drugs frequently used to treat IBD. To learn more about any medication's effect on pregnancy or the health of a baby, talk to your doctor and look up the drug in the *Physician's Desk Reference* (the newest edition will be in your public library's reference section) and read the section called "Contraindications." Another good reference is *Drugs in Pregnancy and Lactation,* which can be found in most medical libraries.

5-aminosalicylic acid (5-ASA) drugs

5-ASA drugs consist of sulfasalazine and relatively newer medications, such as olsalazine (Dipentum), mesalamine (Asacol and Pentasa), and balsalazide (Colazal). They are commonly used to treat mild to moderate IBD, and are also prescribed to help maintain remission. These medications are generally regarded as safe to use during pregnancy. Even though sulfasalazine can cause infertility in men, it doesn't in women. Nor does it appear to cause any harm to a developing, unborn child.[10] However, sulfasalazine can interfere with the absorption of folate, a B-vitamin that prevents certain birth defects. Current recommendations for all expectant mothers, as well as all women contemplating pregnancy, include supplementing with 1 milligram daily of folic acid. This amount is also recommended for women taking sulfasalazine. In addition to your supplement, it's a good idea to include as many dietary sources of folic acid as well, such as green, leafy vegetables, orange juice, and fortified foods.

Olsalazine, mesalamine, and balsalazide are theoretically just as safe—if not safer—than sulfasalazine. They have the same 5-ASA component as does sulfasalazine but lack its sulfa portion. Although the use of these drugs in pregnancy has not been studied as thoroughly as sulfasalazine, research so far has not found any increased risk of birth defects when taking these drugs.[11]

Amy shares her experience of taking 5-ASA medications when pregnant:

> During my first pregnancy, I was a bit nervous taking 5-ASA. However, my doctor said it was safe. He had other patients who were on it while pregnant and none of them had problems.
>
> I asked him why I couldn't just taper off since I was doing relatively well. He explained that if my symptoms came back we'd then have to treat more aggressively. Thankfully, I stayed well and had a normal, healthy girl.
>
> Since I had already been through it before, I was much less worried during my second pregnancy. The only difference was that I took a different 5-ASA medication. Everything worked out fine and now I have two healthy girls.

Corticosteroids

Corticosteroids such as prednisone are one of the most reliable treatments for moderate to severe IBD. Fortunately, their use in pregnancy is generally safe for both mother and unborn child. If your Crohn's or colitis is severe enough that your doctor fears it might complicate your pregnancy, he may recommend a course of prednisone. As when you are not expecting, your physician's goal is to control your IBD on the lowest possible dose. Once you are stable, he'll likely try to taper the amount you're taking as far as he can without risking a relapse.

Trish took prednisone when she was pregnant:

> I've had ulcerative colitis for many years. At times I've needed prednisone to help keep it under control. At first I had some concerns about taking it when pregnant, but my doctor said it wasn't a problem. I was fortunate that during my pregnancy, I only needed to take between 5 and 10 milligrams per day. That's not much, but I was concerned that if I tried to come off, I might risk flaring. So I stayed on the low dose and everything worked out. I now have a healthy six-month-old boy.

6-MP and azathioprine

Azathioprine (Imuran) and 6-MP (Purinethol) are chemically similar medications that suppress your immune system. Although they help maintain remission and allow some people to reduce or eliminate corticosteroids, their use in pregnancy is somewhat controversial. In humans, birth defects have been found in babies born to women taking azathioprine.[12] However, the women did not have IBD and were on dosages higher than those normally prescribed for people with Crohn's or ulcerative colitis. Some evidence indicates azathioprine is also associated with an increased risk of premature birth, as well as impaired immunity and delayed development in the newborn.[13]

Research specifically on 6-MP and azathioprine in pregnant women with IBD, however, demonstrates that the drugs appear safe for expectant mothers.[14,15] Why this contrasts with earlier studies on women with other illnesses on the drugs is not known for sure but may be because the dosage prescribed for IBD is less than for people with other health problems. Although uncertainties remain, many IBD experts currently feel 6-MP and azathioprine can be taken during pregnancy if needed to manage very active IBD. Your gastroenterologist can help you make an educated decision about taking either of these medications based on current data.

Clarissa had a severe case of Crohn's disease. She tells her story of when she unexpectedly became pregnant over twenty years ago:

> My husband and I had been trying for ten years to have a baby. We just assumed it would never happen. Six weeks after having surgery, I had a check-up with my doctor. I wasn't feeling good and thought I might have the flu. My period was late, but that was nothing out of the ordinary with an active case of Crohn's. He ran a pregnancy test and it came back positive. We couldn't believe it.
>
> What should have been one of the happiest moments for me quickly turned quite stressful. I was on 6-MP. At that time, not much was known about the drug's effect during pregnancy, and what was known was fairly negative. My doctor recommended that I have an abortion.
>
> I didn't know what to do. For religious reasons, I didn't believe in abortion. Plus my husband and I wanted a child so much. I just couldn't do it. I decided to proceed with the pregnancy.

A month or so later, I developed some problems. I started bleeding internally. We thought I was miscarrying, but I wasn't. It had to do with the recent surgery and becoming pregnant too soon after the operation. I lost a lot of blood and almost died. At that point, the doctors once again said I really should terminate the pregnancy. Even if the baby somehow managed to live, they said he'd surely be a vegetable. I talked to my clergyman and he even said I had just cause, given the circumstances. However, I still couldn't do it. I decided to keep my baby.

I carried him to full term and he weighed over six pounds. He was fine except that his immune system was suppressed at birth. He developed a fever and he had to be in ICU for one week. However, we then took him home and he gradually built up his immune system. Today he is a six-foot, totally normal, healthy, 22-year-old man. We were truly blessed.

Sarah decided she did not want to take 6-MP while pregnant:

I know that some doctors are now saying that 6-MP is not as risky as they once thought it was. However, I didn't want to take a chance. I was on 6-MP for just a short time, and then decided I wanted to have another baby. I discussed my concerns with my doctor and we agreed that I'd stop the medication. In my opinion, having a baby is already risky enough if you have Crohn's, in terms of passing it on genetically to your child or grandchild. I didn't feel comfortable adding 6-MP to the mix. I'm sure there are others who would have felt differently. But for me, it was the right decision to come off the drug, since I was able to come off it without causing an immediate flare.. Fortunately, my health was excellent during my pregnancy.

The use of 6-MP and azathioprine in men who wish to father children is also somewhat controversial. One recent study suggests that pregnancy-related complications might be higher if fathers have taken 6-MP within three months of inducing conception.[16] More research is needed to clarify if developing babies of fathers who take 6-MP or azathioprine are at a greater risk for problems. Your doctor can help you make an informed choice about taking these medications if you are planning to have a family.

Antibiotics

Antibiotics are prescribed for some people with IBD, particularly for those with Crohn's who have fistulas or abscesses. The most commonly used ones are metronidazole (Flagyl) and ciprofloxacin (Cipro). Because the use of metronidazole in pregnancy is sometimes associated with birth defects, it's generally recommended to avoid the drug if you are pregnant. An exception is made sometimes, however, for women with severe rectal disease during the second or third trimester.[17] Little is known about ciprofloxacin during pregnancy—so it's recommended to not take this medication if you are expecting.

Antidiarrheal drugs

Some people with IBD take either loperamide (Imodium) or diphenoxylate with atropine (Lomotil) to control their diarrhea. Diphenoxylate with atropine is not recommended, because no adequate animal or human studies have been performed during pregnancy.

Animal studies have found loperamide does not cause fetal harm. However, little research has been performed on expectant human mothers. Although one group of researchers recently found the drug is not linked to an increased risk of problems in newborn babies, this is only the first major study that has investigated its use in pregnancy.[18] Some gastroenterologists are comfortable prescribing it to pregnant women if it's really needed, but others are more cautious. Consult with your doctor about the latest recommendations.

Methotrexate

Methotrexate is sometimes used for people with severe Crohn's disease who are unable to stay well when tapering their dose of corticosteroids. Like azathioprine and 6-MP, it suppresses your immune system. If it helps in achieving remission, doctors will often prescribe it for an extended period to maintain health. However, you should never take methotrexate if you are pregnant or planning to have a child in the near future because severe birth defects or miscarriage can result. If you are coming off the drug, wait at least three months before trying to conceive.

Men are advised to avoid fathering a child while on methotrexate. The medication affects sperm structure that can contribute to birth defects. Again, it's best to wait at least three months after stopping the drug before trying to induce conception.

Cyclosporine

Cyclosporine is a potent immune-suppressing drug that is sometimes used as a short-term therapy to treat severe ulcerative colitis. A major review article on cyclosporine and pregnancy (not on women with IBD) suggests the drug may be associated with an increased risk of premature delivery, but not birth defects.[19] However, no well-designed studies have specifically examined cyclosporine's impact on pregnant women with IBD.

Infliximab

Infliximab (Remicade) is prescribed for people with Crohn's who have moderate to severe disease. It's usually reserved for those who do not respond favorably to other IBD medications. Because infliximab is still relatively new and there is insufficient information on its use in expectant mothers, it's recommended to avoid the drug if you are pregnant or trying to conceive.

It's important to remember that all drugs have side effects and potential risks. Some IBD drugs present more risk than others, especially to a developing baby. It's therefore extremely important to work closely with your doctor to evaluate the risks versus benefits for any medications used before or during pregnancy.

Nursing

Women with IBD who wish to breastfeed are usually able to do so successfully. The only things that may affect your choices are the medications you take and your general health. For example, if you are so ill you can barely support yourself nutritionally, it probably doesn't make sense to try and sustain your child as well.

Sarah had some problems breastfeeding her son:

> Breastfeeding was difficult on me. Before I gave birth to my son, I weighed 170 pounds. Within a few months I was already down to 120. It was taking too much out of me. My doctor recommended that I stop nursing, but it was a difficult decision for me to make. I felt guilty because I really wanted him to have the best start in life. But after another month, I knew I couldn't do it anymore. I realized in order to take care of him, I needed to take care of myself first. I've noticed with each of my three children, I've been able to nurse less and less. My

first child I nursed for eight months, the second for four months, and the third for only six weeks. Switching them to formula was the right decision because it prevented me from losing too much weight.

Trish found that she did well breastfeeding:

I had no trouble nursing my son at all. In fact, I really felt that it helped my ulcerative colitis. I was on a small amount of prednisone during my pregnancy, and was able to taper off a month after birth while I was breastfeeding. I don't know what it was, but perhaps the nursing somehow released hormones that helped quiet the disease in my body.

Sandra decided to bottle-feed:

I've had a serious case of Crohn's for most of my life. Although I did quite well during my pregnancies, I knew that nursing would not be a good idea for me. My doctor and I agreed that it was more important to take care of myself in order to avoid malnourishment. After all, what good would I be as a mother if I didn't have any energy to take care of my children?

Some IBD drugs are safe to take when nursing, and some are not. Prednisone is generally safe to use when breastfeeding, because only a small amount makes its way into the milk. If you are on a high dose, however, your doctor may suggest the pediatrician monitor your baby for possible side effects.

Sulfasalazine is also considered safe to use while nursing. A very small amount of this medication transfers to breast milk, but not enough to present any significant risk.[20] Newer 5-ASA drugs are theoretically just as safe but have not undergone adequate testing for use in breastfeeding mothers.

Amy shares how she handled breastfeeding after taking 5-ASA drugs during pregnancy:

I've actually taken two different 5-ASA medications during pregnancy, but at separate times. However, when it came time to nurse, my doctor wasn't comfortable with me breastfeeding while on either of these drugs. He said there wasn't enough information available to know how much comes out in the milk or how it would affect the baby. But it was important for me to nurse.

> *Fortunately, my Crohn's has always been relatively mild. So after I*
> *delivered, my doctor and I agreed that I'd try stopping my medication.*
> *I was able to breastfeed for about nine weeks, after which I felt I*
> *needed to get back on to the 5-ASA. So at that time, I weaned my*
> *baby and then resumed my medicine.*

It's recommended that you do not breastfeed if you are taking azathioprine, 6-MP, cyclosporine, methotrexate, or diphenoxylate with atropine. Doctors also advise against using antibiotics such as metronidazole and ciprofloxacin, because they pass into breast milk. Recommendations on loperamide can vary, so check with your gastroenterologist. Of course, it's always necessary to discuss with your doctor and your baby's pediatrician the latest recommendations about your medications' effects on breast milk, because new information is continually emerging.

Diagnostic procedures during pregnancy

Your doctor will probably prefer to postpone most diagnostic procedures until after you have your baby. If necessary, however, sigmoidoscopies and endoscopies of the upper GI tract can usually be performed safely during pregnancy. Colonoscopies are performed less frequently, as there's little information on their safety in expectant mothers. Most physicians avoid recommending x-ray tests, because radiation can harm the developing baby. Exceptions are only made during emergencies, such as when a complete obstruction is suspected.

Sarah was fortunate she didn't need to have tests when she was pregnant:

> *My doctor and I talked about having a scoping procedure when I*
> *was expecting. But since I was quite healthy, there was really no*
> *justifiable reason why I had to have it. So rather than making me go*
> *through one of those examinations in my condition, we thought it best*
> *to wait till after I had the baby.*

Susie, however, was diagnosed when she was pregnant:

> *Looking back, I realize that I had ulcerative colitis as far back as*
> *college. I just didn't know what it was at the time. But before my*
> *second pregnancy, I was doing great and had no symptoms. However,*
> *during the pregnancy I started having symptoms I couldn't ignore,*
> *such as diarrhea and some bleeding. My doctor recommended a*

flexible sigmoidoscopy. So I had it when I was about three or four months along in the pregnancy, and he was able to diagnose ulcerative colitis. I had no problems during the procedure. There was some talk about doing a colonoscopy, but we were concerned about the sedation needed for that. So we figured we could do that at a later time. Fortunately, my symptoms soon cleared up on their own, and I was healthy for the rest of my pregnancy.

Surgery during pregnancy

Major surgery such as colectomy or intestinal resection is only performed on pregnant women in emergencies. Examples of life-threatening situations that might require surgery include toxic megacolon or complete bowel obstruction. Not much research exists on the outcome of pregnancies in women with IBD when the expectant mother undergoes a major operation. However, what little information is available suggests the chance of losing the unborn child is high.[21] It's therefore very important to keep IBD under control during pregnancy. If you experience a major flare, it's very important to keep in close contact with your doctor. Nonsurgical treatments she prescribes early on may prevent the need for emergency surgery later.

Nutrition

Proper nutrition is essential when you are pregnant. Unfortunately, women with IBD—especially if they have active Crohn's—are at risk of malnourishment even when they are not expecting. The demands of pregnancy further increase this risk, because extra calories are needed for the developing baby. If you are unable to gain enough weight, you may need to supplement your diet with a liquid formula such as Ensure. In more extreme situations, you may temporarily need to go on an elemental diet, which is usually administered through a feeding tube placed in your nose and threaded down to your stomach. In one small study examining the effect of elemental diet during pregnancy, all the women achieved remission and went on to deliver healthy babies.[22]

Intravenous feeding is another option. Total parental nutrition (TPN) can be used in pregnant women with IBD who are unable to eat normally or tolerate an elemental diet. It allows your bowel a chance to rest while you receive all your nourishment through one of your major veins. However, an elemental diet is often strongly preferred over TPN, because there is always a significant risk of infection with intravenous feeding. For more information on elemental diets and TPN, see Chapter 8, *Alternative Forms of Feeding*.

It's a good idea to work closely with your doctor and a dietitian or nutritionist to maintain adequate nutrition during pregnancy. They can help you to:

- Determine how many calories you need per day

- Monitor your nutritional status during pregnancy

- Choose the best foods and supplements to improve or maintain your nutritional status

- Decide whether you can benefit from an elemental diet or TPN

For more information on nutrition and IBD, see Chapter 7, *Diet and Complementary Therapies*.

Laura describes how she managed nutritionally:

> Since I was diagnosed with ulcerative colitis when I was pregnant, I was very concerned about my nutritional status. I wanted to do everything I could to ensure that my baby would grow and develop normally. I worked very closely with my doctor to monitor my weight as well as my lab work. Back in the 80s, they didn't have all the nutritional supplement drinks at the stores like they do today. Fortunately, I was able to manage on regular food, prenatal vitamins, and a lot of extra iron. I never needed tube or intravenous feeding.
>
> It was always a challenge to eat and drink enough. I suffered from nausea, vomiting, and diarrhea. However, I was able to take in enough nourishment by eating small meals. I basically grazed and sipped water throughout the day. I even got up in the middle of the night to eat a snack. I found ginger cookies helped with the nausea, and so did eating crackers in the morning before I got out of bed. I always took my prenatal vitamins with food.
>
> Fortunately, everything worked out okay. I've never been someone who loses weight easily. Of course, this type of metabolism is frustrating now that I'm healthy, but at least it came in handy when I was sick and pregnant. My daughter was born two weeks early, but was normal weight and healthy.

Heredity

Many parents with IBD have concerns about passing their illness on to their children. Crohn's and ulcerative colitis sometimes run in families, but not most of the time. Approximately 5 to 10 percent of people with IBD have a first-degree relative (sibling, parent, or child) who also has the disease.[23] One group of researchers estimates that if a child has one parent with IBD, he has approximately a 9 percent chance of developing the illness during his lifetime.[24]

Little research exists on the rare situation when both parents have either Crohn's or ulcerative colitis. One small study of nineteen couples who both had IBD found that 36 percent of the couples' children developed either ulcerative colitis or Crohn's.[25] The researchers point out, however, that factors other than genetics—such as environmental ones—may play a role in the increased risk. For more information on genetics and IBD, see Chapter 1, *Introduction to IBD*.

Amy wasn't too concerned about passing her IBD on to her kids:

> *I have a mild case of Crohn's. I guess I don't worry too much about handing this down to my children. I'm the only one in my family with it, and it has been very treatable. Besides, there are so many other things that can happen.*

Clarissa's kids are in their teens and twenties now, but she still worries about them:

> *Even though none of my children have IBD, I still worry that someday they will develop it. I've especially been concerned about my 15-year-old son lately, who has been having bad stomach aches. He has no other symptoms, and I know that some people just get stomach aches and they don't have Crohn's. But as a mother, it's difficult not to worry. However, I have absolutely no regrets about having children. It was very important to me to have a family and I didn't want Crohn's to stop me from having kids.*

Sarah shares her philosophy on having children when you have IBD:

> *I've had Crohn's for a long time. I spent some time wondering whether I should have kids. I had many concerns, including whether I could pass the disease on to my children. However, I knew in my heart that I really wanted to have a family. After talking to a genetic*

counselor, and learning the risk of passing it on was low, we decided to go for it. I have never regretted our decision.

Having children has really made me appreciate my life. I'm so glad I didn't let the Crohn's interfere with that. You can always have negative thoughts and think, "What if . . . , What if . . ." But I didn't want to be 60 someday and have regrets. I'm so glad I took the chance—I now have three healthy kids. I have found it essential to try to maintain a calm balance in life, which includes plenty of time for my family and myself.

CHAPTER 15

Children and Teens

RECEIVING THE NEWS that your child has IBD is heart wrenching. Parents don't want to hear their child has a disease, much less one for which there is no cure (although ulcerative colitis can be cured with the complete removal of the colon). Compounding this nightmare is the fact that many mothers and fathers have never heard of Crohn's disease or ulcerative colitis. Fear of the unknown can contribute even more stress. With time and knowledge, however, IBD in children and teens becomes more manageable.

This chapter is a guide for coping with IBD in a son or daughter. It begins with a discussion of symptoms and diagnostic procedures, including methods for helping your child cope with these tests. Parents' emotional reactions are covered next, followed by suggestions of how to tell your child about the disease. The chapter also has sections on treatments, hospitalization, and growth failure. It concludes with how parents and children have coped with IBD's effect on school and family life.

Onset and symptoms

The Crohn's and Colitis Foundation of America (CCFA) estimates that about 1 million people in America have IBD, of whom 100,000 are children under age 18.[1] Although onset and diagnosis are most common during the teen years, they can occur at any age, even in infancy. As with adults, IBD can begin either suddenly or gradually.

Parents whose children are developing IBD may have difficulty figuring out what's wrong with their son or daughter. Several signs and symptoms of IBD, such as stomachaches, diarrhea, bloody stools, fever, growth failure, weight loss, or fatigue, can be caused by many other illnesses. And even though the major features of the disease are similar to those in adults, children—especially younger ones—may express symptoms such as pain or fatigue in different ways. For instance, some children may become irritable, cranky, or moody, whereas others may become quiet, withdrawn, or just different from their normal selves.

Patrick, whose daughter began developing Crohn's when she was 3, explains:

> We started noticing in the fall that Kristy was getting pale and becoming rather sluggish. Her appetite wasn't too good either. On Halloween, for example, we had maybe gone only half way around the block and then she wanted to go home. We knew something just wasn't right. She didn't have stomach pains at first, but mentioned that her back hurt.
>
> The doctors didn't figure out what it was right away. But finally by the following January, they did a colonoscopy and diagnosed her as having IBD.

Diagnostic tests and procedures

The tests and procedures used to diagnose and monitor IBD are often quite scary for children. Unfortunately, these tests sometimes become a regular part of life for many youngsters with Crohn's and ulcerative colitis. It's therefore to your and your child's advantage to develop effective strategies for dealing with blood tests, x-rays, and scoping procedures. Although it isn't always possible to eliminate all of your child's fears, a calm and well-prepared child copes far better during uncomfortable procedures.

Blood tests

Frequent blood draws are common for many children with Crohn's or colitis. Although blood tests alone cannot provide enough information to diagnose IBD, they can help the pediatric gastroenterologist determine what impact the disease is having on your child. They can also help your child's doctor monitor side effects of medications. For example, a complete blood count (CBC) can indicate whether your child has lost significant amounts blood through intestinal bleeding. A CBC can also show if an immune-suppressing drug is lowering your child's white blood cell count too much. For more information on blood tests for IBD, see Chapter 3, *Diagnostic Procedures*.

Blood tests can be traumatic for children, particularly those who fear needles. If blood is taken during every office visit, some children may become terrified of going to the doctor. Fortunately, there are many ways to help your child cope with these tests. Sometimes it takes a bit of trial and error, but you can learn ways to ease your child's fear and anxiety about blood draws. See the section titled, "Coping with tests and procedures," later in this chapter.

Kristy, who is now 9 years old, shares her experience with blood tests:

> When I was little I was so scared of blood tests that I'd start crying and screaming before I got to the hospital. I use to think it hurt super-duper bad but now I don't think so anymore. I don't mind having them now because I've had a lot and I'm used to them.
>
> My right arm has an okay vein, but my left arm has a really good one. When I get a blood test now, I always tell them to take my blood from the big, bulgy vein.

Endoscopic procedures

Endoscopic procedures, such as colonoscopies and sigmoidoscopies, are difficult and unpleasant for anyone. They are necessary, though, because they let the pediatric gastroenterologist directly view the inside of your child's GI tract. The scoping instruments can also take tissue samples of the gut so the gastroenterologist and pathologist can make an accurate diagnosis. For detailed information on the different endoscopic examinations, see Chapter 3.

Scoping procedures are often uncomfortable and scary for many children. As with blood tests, however, adequate education and preparation can make a dramatic difference in your child's response. See the section titled "Coping with tests and procedures," later in the chapter.

Jeremy, who is now 11, had an unexpected sigmoidoscopy during a doctor visit:

> The doctor wanted to take a quick look but it was not quick enough. It was kind of scary, but it was more painful than anything else. It felt like I had a whole bunch of gas but I couldn't let it out. It hurt really bad, but I survived.

X-ray procedures

X-ray procedures are yet another category of tests your child will have to undergo. Barium enema and barium drink tests are prescribed so that your child's physician can see the outline of your child's bowel in great detail. They are especially useful in identifying any narrowed segments of intestine. Computerized tomography (CT or CAT) scans are helpful when trying to diagnose abscesses (areas of infection) or certain types of fistulas (abnormal connections from the intestines to other organs). For more information on these x-ray procedures, Chapter 3 provides detailed explanations.

Like blood and endoscopic tests, x-ray exams can be frightening, uncomfortable, or both. Drinking the barium is also a problem for many children.

Nine-year-old Kristy explains:

> The barium drink is nasty. After about five sips, it makes me feel like I have to throw up. It's not like I have to drink gallons, but it's hard to get through a whole cup of it. And last time, my x-rays didn't show up clearly so then they made me drink even more after I thought I was already done. I'm glad I haven't had to drink it in a long time.

Coping with tests and procedures

Learning how to cope effectively is easiest when parents, children, and healthcare professionals work together as a team. You all have the same goal, and that's to get through procedures quickly and painlessly while learning as much as possible from them (although your son or daughter may not care as much about the latter). Fortunately, parents today have many options and resources available to help. Here are some ideas:

- **Inquire about child life programs.** Child life programs are run by professionals who specialize in helping children and their families cope with medical experiences. Although their focus is generally on hospitalized boys and girls, ask the pediatric gastroenterologist if the medical center offers child life services to outpatient children undergoing medical procedures. A child life specialist may be able to meet with you and your child to explain the procedure in easy-to-understand ways and also help allay any fears surrounding it.

- **Seek out age-appropriate educational materials.** Your hospital library may have books or videos made specifically to help children deal with blood tests or other procedures. Inquire if they have any for the test or examination your child is about to undergo. The STARBRIGHT foundation offers many video and CD-ROM programs for children and teens facing chronic illness. Contact them at (310) 479-1212, or visit the web site at *http://www.starbright.org/*. The Crohn's and Colitis Foundation of America at (800) 932-2423 and the US government's Digestive Disease Clearinghouse at (800) 891-5389 are great resources as well.

- **Reason with your child at an age-appropriate level.** Explain in age-appropriate terms how important it is for the doctor to monitor her blood or view the inside of her intestines. Mention that although the test might be uncomfortable, it's being used to help her get better. If your daughter or son has questions, always answer them honestly so your child is prepared for what will happen.

Terri shares her strategies:

> Kristy, now age 9, has often had a difficult time with procedures. For example, she's unable to drink the laxative solution for the colonoscopy prep. Thus, they have to insert an NG tube to get it down, which is obviously not a pleasant experience for her.
>
> Unfortunately, there's really no good way to prepare her for all this. The best way for us has just been to explain that it has to be done. Both her doctor and I go over with her what will happen and why we need to do it. We emphasize how important it is to see her colon so that we'll know what to do to help make her feel better. She still doesn't like it, but on some level she understands. And she also understands that if she can't drink the solution, she has to have the tube.

- **Take steps to reduce pain.** Many children fear the pain of tests and procedures more than anything else. So it's important to do what you can to keep your child comfortable. For example, you can apply EMLA—an anesthetic cream—to the skin an hour before a blood test to prevent pain. EMLA can constrict veins, so put a hot pad on the site a few minutes before the blood draw. Doctors always use tranquilizing drugs during a colonoscopy but sometimes don't for sigmoid-oscopies or x-ray studies. If you feel your child will need medication to prevent pain or distress, work with the pediatric gastroenterologist so that your child has a pain-free procedure.

Liz tried many things to help reduce pain from needle sticks:

> Although it wasn't diagnosed till he was 2, Ian has had Crohn's since he was born. Needle sticks didn't become a problem for him till he was about 5. Unfortunately, he doesn't have good veins—so it's difficult to draw blood from him. We've used EMLA. It takes away the pain, but sometimes it makes it even harder to draw the blood because it constricts the veins. We've also tried teaching him breathing exercises and even consulted a hypnotherapist. I can't say we had great success with these measures. What's really worked best is finding a phlebotomist with whom he has established a good relationship. And it helps, too, that he can always get Ian's vein the first time.

Terri found her daughter needs more sedation than most other kids her age:

> *Kristy seems to have a high tolerance for the drugs they use for sedation during procedures. Since those medications don't calm her down enough, they gave her other medicines that put her to sleep. This worked much better for her.*

- **Ask if your child wants you present.** Although you may not be able to stay with your child during x-ray procedures, you can during endoscopy examinations and blood draws. Let your child determine whether he wants you with him during these tests. Some children do better with a parent with them, and others prefer to go it alone. Your child may prefer to have the child life person with him for procedures.

Liz's son wants one of his parents to be with him during tests:

> *Ian, who's now 8, has always felt better with either my husband or me with him during procedures. Fortunately, the doctors always let us stay with Ian if we could. Usually, his endoscopic procedures were in a special endoscopy room and we could always be there. Sometimes, however, they did it in an operating room and we couldn't go in with him. It was hard, but it ended up working out okay since they'd give him enough sedation to put him to sleep.*

- **Determine appropriate lead time.** Some children prefer to know well ahead of time what's coming, and some do better knowing closer to the test. You know your child best. So tell her about the upcoming tests at the optimal time beforehand.

Liz explains:

> *Ian has always done better if we let him know well ahead of time what's coming. He doesn't like surprises, so we'd never wait till the last minute to tell him he's having a procedure. I also feel much better doing it this way since it gives us time to prepare.*

- **Provide comfort objects.** Ask your child if he'd like to bring anything with him to feel more comfortable. Sometimes a stuffed animal or other toy can make a difference. Musical tapes or CDs can also be soothing during tests.

- **Reward.** If you feel comfortable with this idea, consider giving your child a reward for his valiant efforts. Remind him of the special treat coming soon to take his mind off the anxiety at hand.

Terri has tried giving Kristy rewards:

> During the time she was having difficulty with blood tests, we tried
> giving her a reward, such as a new doll. Rewards were somewhat
> helpful, but what helped most of all was just time. She eventually just
> got used to it. Time was what desensitized her. She's now 9 and is
> quite the expert when it comes to her veins. She shows the
> phlebotomist where she thinks is the best place to draw her blood.

Reactions to diagnosis

A diagnosis of IBD in a child or teen can create a wide range of emotions. Different
people react differently to stressful situations, and there are no right or wrong emotions
to have. It's therefore just as normal to feel sad or angry as it is to feel fearful or numb.
Here are some of the most common emotional reactions to a diagnosis of IBD:

- **Numbness.** The shock of hearing your child has an incurable and unfamiliar
  disease is often overwhelming. Parents often feel numb for the first few days after
  hearing the diagnosis. This reaction is not only normal but it is often adaptive,
  because you might otherwise experience emotional overload under such stressful circumstances. With time, you'll be able to process all that's happening, and
  the numbness will give way to other emotions.

- **Relief.** Some parents feel relieved once they finally learn their child has IBD. This
  usually happens when their son or daughter has been ill for a long time before
  receiving the diagnosis. If doctors cannot quickly determine what's wrong, some
  parents jump to other conclusions.

Terri didn't know for several months what her daughter had:

> Although we were fortunate that it didn't take years for Kristy to
> get diagnosed, it was very difficult for several months when we were
> left hanging and didn't know what was wrong with her. When she was
> so pale and was so tired all the time, I sometimes feared she had
> leukemia. At times, I also thought she might be dying. It was actually
> somewhat of a relief when she was diagnosed with IBD. At least we
> finally knew what it was and it was something that was treatable. Not
> that I was happy that she had it. But knowing the diagnosis was better
> than not knowing what was wrong with her.

- **Anger**. Anger is a totally normal response to a diagnosis of Crohn's disease or ulcerative colitis in your child. The challenge is in dealing with this anger in a helpful way. Sometimes it's easy to misdirect your anger at the disease toward other people such as medical personnel or family members. When this happens, you may end up alienating the very people who are in the position to help you the most. Thus, it's a good idea to find ways to manage your anger. For example, you might consider talking to a counselor, trusted friend, or other parents who have children with IBD. Writing your thoughts and feelings in a journal is another option. Other people find vigorous physical exercise or punching pillows helps release anger.

- **Fear and helplessness**. Parents often feel fearful or helpless on hearing their child has Crohn's disease or ulcerative colitis. Because many mothers and fathers have never heard of either illness, the prospects of facing the unknown can cause much anxiety. In addition, being suddenly or gradually thrown into the medical system interrupts normal, everyday life. Parents frequently feel helpless because of this disruption and loss of control in their lives.

  Liz describes her experience with fear:

  > *I think it's only natural to feel afraid or helpless when your child is diagnosed with a disease. And when an illness is life-long and chronic, these feelings never really completely go away. At times, the fear or helplessness has felt overwhelming, but most of the time it's not.*
  >
  > *Crohn's is a difficult disease to deal with because it's so unpredictable. But over time, I've lived to learn with the uncertainty. If I look out too far ahead, I can get overwhelmed. Instead, I live with the not knowing one day at a time, and this helps to control the fear and helplessness.*

- **Guilt**. Mothers and fathers may feel guilty, thinking they may have done something to cause the disease or should have been able to do something to prevent it. Some questions that may arise are: Did my son inherit this from me? Did I feed him the wrong food? Have I somehow created a stressful home life for her? Although these kinds of questions are both common and normal, try to remember you are not to blame for your child's illness. You did not cause it, nor could you have prevented it.

  Sylvia has struggled with guilt for a long time:

  > *I think any parent of a child with IBD must have feelings of guilt from time to time. I know it has been a recurring issue for me. My*

*daughter was diagnosed at age 12, and I know for the longest time
I felt I must have done something wrong that caused it. After many
years, I finally reached a point where—intellectually at least—
I understood that I was not to blame. But on an emotional level, it's
been hard to let go of the guilt. Even today, when my daughter is doing
well at the age of 24, I still catch myself. I recall not too long ago I was
reading an article about how the consumption of fast food might be
correlated with IBD. Immediately, my brain started down the old path
thinking, "Sylvia—see, it's your fault. You occasionally took her out
for fast food."*

Terri experienced a different kind of guilt:

*My daughter was diagnosed six years ago at age 3. I don't recall
feeling guilty about causing the disease, but I know I've felt guilt
and uneasiness when deciding what treatments are best for her. My
husband and I receive so much advice from many well-meaning
people, "Take this," or "Don't take that." Whatever we did or didn't
do, I'd feel bad about. For example, I remember our dilemma about
whether to give her an immune suppressing drug. I had a lot of guilt
about giving such a small child this kind of medication.*

Liz didn't have any guilt:

*I'm thankful that guilt was one emotion I didn't have to deal with.
I know it can be a major one for some people when their kids are
diagnosed with something. I really feel strongly that guilt is wasted
energy. My husband and I are clear that we didn't cause it.*

- **Sadness and grief.** Many parents are overcome with grief and sadness on hearing the diagnosis of Crohn's or ulcerative colitis. Even if your doctor assures you that your son's or daughter's prognosis is good, it's hard not to feel grief on hearing that your child will have a chronic illness for life.

Terri didn't feel her sadness till later:

*I can't say I recall feeling overwhelmed with sadness or grief when
Kristy was first diagnosed. So much was going on and we just had to
deal with what was happening. It wasn't until later when I realized
that I was sad, but just didn't notice it at the time. I'd look at a picture
of her when she was puffed up on prednisone, and suddenly become
filled with grief. I felt so sad that my child had to go through that. It's*

a terrible thing for anyone so young to have to go through. I'm so thankful she's doing well now.

- **Hope.** Hope is probably not the first emotion you'll feel after your daughter or son is diagnosed. However, most children with Crohn's disease or ulcerative colitis live normal, productive, and enjoyable lives despite their illness. Time, knowledge, and familiarity with the medical team can lead to hope for your child's future.

Liz has hope:

> *Ian has one of the most severe cases of Crohn's that his doctors have seen. Yet I still have hope. There is always something new around the corner, and one of these days, someone is going to figure it out. I feel that not being hopeful is self-defeating. Yeah, it's not always easy, but you have to believe that there is a better tomorrow.*

Sharing information with your child

Many parents often wonder how much information they should share with their child about Crohn's disease or ulcerative colitis. As you might suspect, there are no hard or fast rules. Over time, you will be able to properly gauge what's appropriate. Although you might feel compelled to hide certain details from your child to protect her, it's usually best not to delay or avoid telling her about the disease. It's also important to be as honest and straightforward as possible, given your child's stage of development.

Children can often sense when their parents are hiding something from them. And if they are going back and forth to the doctor, undergoing various procedures, taking medications, or spending time in the hospital, they already know something is wrong. Your silence about it will probably only make your child more fearful and anxious. Also, because many children have vivid imaginations, trying to cover up things may lead to fantasies that are much worse than reality. Therefore, most experts agree children cope much more effectively if information about their illness is presented to them accurately and honestly in an age-appropriate manner. Encouraging an environment of open communication where questions can be freely asked and answered matter-of-factly is also recommended.

Parents choose different ways to present information to their child. Some mothers and fathers prefer that they be the ones to impart information about IBD to their son or daughter. Another option is to share the responsibility with your child's medical team, including pediatric gastroenterologists, nurses, social workers, and/or child life specialists. If your youngster is a teenager and expresses interest in speaking with his healthcare team in private, respect his wishes.

Whoever discusses IBD with your son or daughter should make a point to emphasize that he or she did nothing to cause the illness. Children—even older ones—may assume they are being punished for misbehaving, doing something wrong, or thinking bad thoughts. Taking the time to clarify this point will help prevent your child from feeling guilty about having Crohn's or colitis.

Charlotte explains how she and her husband share information with their son:

> My son, Jeremy, was diagnosed with ulcerative colitis when he was 8 years old. When he was 9, we went through a very difficult period where he was in the hospital for four and a half months. This isn't typical, but he had complication after complication following his surgery.
>
> From the beginning, my husband and I always told Jeremy everything. We didn't want to keep information from him. I wasn't always completely sure how much he really understood, but we didn't want to hide things. However, during the long hospitalization, the social worker and some of the nurses suggested that we shouldn't talk about it so much with the doctors in front of Jeremy. They even put a note on his door stating this to warn the different hospital personnel coming in and out. Of course, my son immediately picked up on how we weren't discussing his medical situation in front of him. He also read the note on his door. It turned out that this really frightened him. We soon found out that he thought we secretly were planning another surgery. Avoiding discussions in his presence had the exact opposite effect that nurses and social worker intended. We learned we were originally doing the right thing by just being straight with him.

Sylvia also believes in being open with the facts:

> My mother had a philosophy that children will understand what they need to understand, and then the rest will just go over their heads. I used the same philosophy when raising my kids.
>
> When my daughter was diagnosed at age 12, we learned about Crohn's together. I didn't worry about limiting her exposure to information. I figured she'd pick up what she needed to know. I had no problem with her reading the different books and brochures that we

had on IBD. Without sufficient information, you're pretty much just
left with your imagination—which may not work to your advantage.

If you have concerns on how much information is appropriate, consider letting your son or daughter be your guide. Some kids will want to know more, and some less. If you're still unsure, you might simply ask what questions he has about his illness. By reassuring him there's no such thing as an embarrassing or dumb question, you'll foster a safe and comfortable atmosphere where he can air his questions and concerns.

Treatment

Gastroenterologists treat IBD in children very similarly to the way they treat it in adults. However, pediatric gastroenterologists are specifically trained to consider growth and development, as well as potential long-term effects of medication exposure. For instance, there's generally a stronger emphasis on minimizing the use of corticosteroids in children, because they can impede growth and affect bone development. In addition, pediatric gastroenterologists heavily stress the importance of nutritional supplementation to support a child's growth.

Medications

The medications discussed in Chapter 5, *Medications,* are also used to treat children with Crohn's disease or ulcerative colitis. However, your pediatric gastroenterologist will adjust dosages based on your child's height and weight.

Giving medication to young children

Giving medication to young children is sometimes a challenge. However, by taking a cooperative approach with your child, you'll have the best chance of establishing a comfortable routine from the start. A little creativity doesn't hurt either. For example, you can crush pills (check with your doctor or pharmacist first) and mix them in your child's favorite food or drink. Applesauce, puddings, yogurt, or fruit smoothies are a few good suggestions, but let your son or daughter choose the mixing agent.

Liz describes Ian's preferences:

> *Ian is now 8, and he's been able to swallow pills from a very young*
> *age. I realize this probably is not typical. However, he didn't like the*
> *taste of any of his medicines, and especially did not like anything in*
> *liquid form. It's so funny, whenever a doctor is writing him a*

prescription, he says, "You are writing that for pills, aren't you? If not, we'll be back for pills."

Asacol is one IBD drug that must be taken whole. An alternative to it is Pentasa, which is still effective if you open the capsule and mix the little beads in food. The beads are much easier for a child to swallow.

Terri describes what she went through when Asacol was prescribed for her daughter:

> *Trying to give Asacol to a 3-year-old is extremely difficult. The pill has to be taken whole or else it will dissolve in the stomach and not reach the colon. But how can you expect such a young child to swallow this type of pill? My husband and I tried everything. Finally, after much trial and error, we found it would slide right down when we put it in applesauce. Then we followed that with a few sips of milk. This was the only thing that worked.*

Prednisone is easily crushed, but most children—as well as adults—think it tastes bitter and unpleasant. If you're finding it difficult to mask the taste, you might consider breaking the pills and putting them into small gel caps. A 10 mg prednisone can fit into a number 4 size capsule, which is small enough for children as young as 3 or 4 to swallow.

Here are two other tips that may make medication time a bit easier for you and your young son or daughter:

- **Keeping on a regular schedule**. A regular schedule helps you and your child adjust to life on medication. He or she will know what to expect and when.

- **Emphasizing how it helps**. Children are very impressionable and have powerful imaginations. Emphasize how the medication will make him feel better. Also, work with your child to come up with a fun visualization exercise that involves the medicine eliminating inflammation from his body. If you need assistance with this, consult a therapist who specializes in guided imagery. You can call the Academy for Guided Imagery at (415) 389-9324 for a referral.

Older children and medications

Older children present different challenges when it comes to taking medicines. With younger kids, there's no question that you as a parent must manage your child's medication. However, if you have an older child or teenager you'll have to decide how much responsibility you want to give her. It's especially important for teenagers to feel they have some sense of control over their health and bodies. Yet teens are sometimes rebellious, and may decide to express this trait by being lax about taking their medicines. This is potentially dangerous, particularly if your son or daughter is on prednisone. Because prednisone shuts off the body's own natural production of adrenaline hormone (cortisol), it needs to be taken on schedule. Abruptly stopping it can cause serious side effects. Not taking other IBD drugs—such as 5-ASA preparations—is potentially harmful as well, because skipped doses can lead to an increase in symptoms.

You know your son or daughter best. Some teenagers are extremely responsible, others may require some supervision. You might consider negotiating so the two of you can come to an agreement about who is responsible for what.

Ann shares how she handles the situation:

> My son is 14 years old and was diagnosed within the last year. When he was acutely ill, my husband or I would give him his medication. Now that he's doing well and only on maintenance drugs—Imuran and Pentasa—we let him share in the responsibility. I gave him a medication box that has compartments for morning, noon, dinnertime, and bedtime. I let him fill it each week in my presence, referring to a list that I have prepared. It's up to him to take his medicine at the right time, but of course my husband and I are always watching to make sure he is indeed taking it. He wants to get off the drugs, but he also understands that right now it's important to take them.

Mary, whose son is now in his 20s, tells how she eventually let her son be responsible for his medication:

> When my son was first diagnosed at age 13, I was the one responsible for him taking his medication. Although he didn't like the side effects of prednisone, he was always quite willing to take it since it dramatically relieved his symptoms. Fortunately, he was well the last two years in high school and didn't even require any medicine. When he went to college though, he went through some rough times again. Of course, at this point there wasn't anything I could do; nor would it have been appropriate for me to involve myself with his taking his medications. Fortunately, he was good about taking his prednisone and tapering it gradually. The problem was more with

*remission-sustaining drug such as 6-MP. Once he was off prednisone
and feeling fine, he'd question the value of taking the maintenance
drug. Several months later when he was starting to have problems
again, we learned that he had stopped it. But as a parent, there comes
a point where you have to accept that your child is an adult, capable
of making his own decisions.*

Nutritional therapy

Nutritional therapy plays a very important role in the management of pediatric IBD. Children with Crohn's or colitis may not have the ability to consume enough calories to fight their illness and to grow properly. Although it's better to eat a normal, healthy diet, supplement drinks such as Ensure are often helpful, because they provide a concentrated source of calories and nutrients. And they come in a variety of different flavors, so most children can find one they like.

Children with more severe cases of Crohn's are good candidates for elemental or semi-elemental diets. An elemental diet consists of the most simple, basic forms of nutrients. Although you can try finding an elemental formula your child can drink, most are very unpalatable. Peptamen is an exception, but most people still prefer the taste of complete formulas such as Ensure or similar drinks. However, even if your child finds an elemental formula he likes, it's still difficult for a young person to drink nothing but an elemental formula for weeks. For this reason, many doctors suggest tube feeding, where a thin, flexible feeding tube is inserted up your child's nose, threaded down his esophagus, and placed in his stomach or duodenum. A feeding pump is attached to the end of the tube coming out of the nose so that the formula is pumped in. The feeding can often take place at night while your child sleeps.

In the event your child's GI tract is so inflamed it cannot even tolerate an elemental diet, total parental nutrition (TPN) may be recommended. TPN is a complete form of nutrition that is delivered intravenously through a major vein. For more information on elemental diets and TPN, refer to Chapter 8, *Alternative Forms of Feeding.*

Results of research studies comparing an elemental diet to corticosteroids such as prednisone are mixed.[2,3] Usually the pediatric gastroenterologist prescribes one or the other, because their effects are similar. Occasionally, though, both may be recommended for very severe Crohn's, as it was for Mary's son:

*When Carl was 13, he'd been having diarrhea and vomiting for six
weeks. Before this, he was a pretty big guy for his age, but then he lost*

about 30 pounds in this six-week period. He was hospitalized, where they started him on both tube feeding and oral prednisone. He was in the hospital for three weeks, and then was home for three more weeks on the tube feeding. He responded very well to this treatment. It's difficult to say whether the prednisone or elemental diet played the greater role. I think they were both instrumental in his recovery. The tube feeding was, I'm sure, especially useful because it helped him gain weight while we were getting the inflammation under control.

Some children, such as Carl, are put on tube feeding for several weeks. However, other children who can still eat a little bit can benefit from nightly tube feedings. The tube is inserted every night before bedtime, and then taken out every morning before going to school. Although it may initially seem unthinkable to have to insert and take out a feeding tube every day, many children adapt well to this regimen. Often, a thousand calories or more can be infused overnight, which can make a significant difference for a growing child or adolescent.

Nutritional and dietary support can also involve altering your child's diet and taking other supplements. Although scientific studies have not linked specific diet or food sensitivities to Crohn's or ulcerative colitis, some parents have found that specific types of food and supplements can help to control symptoms.

Ann discovered her son had several food sensitivities:

Although my son's current pediatric gastroenterologist doesn't think much of dietary therapy, she knows I've taken my son to see another physician who thinks it can help. We had my son tested for food allergies, and it showed that he is sensitive to wheat, cow dairy, and chicken eggs. So we eliminated these foods from his diet and substituted with spelt instead of wheat, goat and sheep milk products instead of cow, and duck eggs instead of chicken. This dietary change, in combination with supplements such as fish oil, probiotics, quercitin, and L-glutamine have made a remarkable difference. Elimination of all preservatives and chemical additives, along with sugar (honey is acceptable) keeps his digestive tract healthier. He's doing great now. If he has just a little wheat or cow dairy every once in a while, he's okay. But if he strays from his diet for too long or doesn't take his supplements, he starts having symptoms again.

For more information on how diet and supplements can help treat IBD, see Chapter 7, *Diet and Complementary Therapies.*

Surgery

Undergoing surgery is difficult for anyone, but it can be especially scary for a child. However, if your son or daughter has a very severe case of Crohn's disease or ulcerative colitis that is unresponsive to medications, surgery is sometimes the magic bullet that can allow your child to attain a good state of health. In fact, when the diseased section of intestine is removed, a child who was previously physically immature finally has a chance to grow and catch up with her peers.

Surgery really helped Sylvia's daughter:

> When Mindy was a freshman in high school, she still looked like an elementary school student. She had been missing a lot of school, so her doctor decided she should have the barium drink test. The x-rays showed that a six-inch segment of intestine was as narrow as a straw. No wonder she was always in so much pain and not able to eat much. He recommended that she have surgery to remove this constricted area of bowel.
>
> We decided to go for it. It turned out to be a very good choice. Within a few months after the surgery, she grew three inches. She was finally able to mature physically, and she eventually reached a height of five feet, two inches. Maybe if she never had Crohn's she would have been a little taller, but five feet two is still a normal height for a woman.

If you and the pediatric physicians agree that surgery is the best option, it's important to properly prepare your child for his upcoming operation. Here are some steps you can take:

- **Educate yourself.** You may want to take some time to learn as much as you can about the operation your son or daughter will undergo. When your child has questions, you'll feel more comfortable and confident when responding.

- **Educate your child appropriately.** Use your best judgment when explaining the surgery to your child. Some kids want to know everything, and others may prefer not to know every detail. Let your son or daughter guide you and always answer all questions honestly. If you need resources, ask the pediatric doctors if they can recommend any good books or videos for children facing surgery. Child life specialists at your child's medical center can provide age-appropriate instruction. They may also give your family a tour of the operating and recovery rooms.

Liz found child life specialists helpful:

> *Ian needed to have a colectomy when he was 5. The child life people were a wonderful resource. Before and after his surgery, they took the time to explain to him what he'd be going through. They brought in a doll and showed him what it was like having an ostomy on his abdomen. Who knew they had dolls that wore bags? It was nice that he could go into his surgery understanding what was going to happen.*

- **Find another child who's already been through it.** Finding another child of the same sex, the same age, and who has undergone the same surgery is often extremely helpful. If your child can see that another person similar to her has flourished, she will probably feel much more at peace. Call your local Crohn's and Colitis Foundation of America (CCFA) office and ask if they know of another child who might be open to visiting yours. Another resource is your child's doctor. If your son or daughter is undergoing ostomy surgery, call the United Ostomy Association (UOA) at (800) 826-0826. Your hospital's enterostomal (ET) nurse may also know other kids willing to share their experience. Of course, because of confidentiality considerations, you and other children's parents will have to give consent before an introduction can be made.

Pediatric surgeons generally perform the same types of operations on children as general surgeons do on adults. One exception is the Kock pouch. Most pediatric surgeons are reluctant to perform this operation on a child because the child or parents needs to intubate the stoma several times a day after surgery, which may be too complex a procedure or too much responsibility for some children and teens. For more information on the Kock pouch and other operations performed on those with IBD, see Chapter 6, *Surgical Treatments*. For information on living with an ostomy, you can read Chapter 11, *Life with an Ostomy*.

Hospitalization

Having a child in the hospital can be difficult for the whole family. Parents and children often describe hospitals as loud and chaotic places where they experience a significant loss of control. However, there are plenty of things you can do to gain some control over the situation and make your child's stay as pleasant as possible.

- **Prepare your child.** Nothing can fully prepare your child for the hospital if she's never been admitted before. However, if you try to learn as much as possible what it's like, you can share the information in a manner she'll understand. If it's a planned admission, consider seeking help from the child life staff, as they can provide tours and age-appropriate orientations. Most importantly, tell your child that either you or another close relative or friend will stay with her at all times and ensure this happens.

- **Make your child's room festive.** Hospital rooms are often dull and depressing. Fortunately, there's much you can do to liven it up. You can decorate the walls with your child's favorite posters, get-well cards, and art projects made at home and in the hospital. Balloons, plants, and flowers also help bring cheer to the room. You might also consider bringing a few personal pictures, stuffed animals, or other things from home so your child will feel he is in more familiar surroundings.

Liz has helped decorate many hospital rooms:

> Ian has been in the hospital many times. As soon as we get there, artwork from him and his sister starts going up on the walls and so do all of the get-well cards. We also bring stuffed animals, blankets, coloring books, videotapes, and puzzles. We try to make it as much like home as possible.

Jeremy, who's now 11, describes what his hospital room was like:

> I was in the hospital for a long time a few years ago. We decorated it just like my room at home—so that meant lots of stuffed animals and Pokemon cards. By the time I left, it really felt like home.

- **Befriend the staff.** It's to your advantage to befriend as many hospital employees as possible. Try to think of all the nurses, doctors, and other staff members as part of your team. Remember that you all want the same thing: the best care and treatment for your child. Good relationships are formed if everyone is quick to understand and slow to anger. Some parents offer to help with mundane tasks, and are generous with kind words. By working with your child's medical team in this manner, you'll be creating an ideal environment in which your child can best heal and recover.

Liz and her 8-year-old son, Ian, have developed many good relationships with hospital staff:

> We've become quite close with many people around the hospital. Ian has benefited most of all from this since he has a whole network of people who support him—doctors, nurses, phlebotomists, social workers, pharmacists, and even the cleaning staff. When Ian is hospitalized, everyone is there rallying and supporting him. They do

special things for him. For example, the pharmacist will come and give a tour of the pharmacy. Other staff will come in on their breaks to visit or play with him. Some people have even come in on their days off to see him. They all know and love him. Sometimes, I'm not sure if he really wants to leave the hospital and come home after all the attention he receives there.

- **Be an advocate for your child.** Hospitals are staffed by human beings. Thus, mistakes can happen, and not everyone is always treated in the most respectful manner. It's important to watch out for your child when she's hospitalized. Become familiar with all her treatments and speak out diplomatically if you see something you don't think it correct or right. You can enlist a few other friends and family members as advocates, too, so you're not the only one carrying the burden.

Liz explains:

I think most parents instinctually know what's right for their child. It's just that in the hospital, it's easy to be intimidated or think that the medical staff knows better than you. I always recommend though that if a parents isn't comfortable with something, she should speak up. I know I've had to do this on many occasions. For example, it's not easy to draw blood from Ian. If the phlebotomist that can do him isn't around, I make it clear to other phlebotomists that they have two chances. After that, I call in the anesthesiologist.

- **Encourage play and recreation.** Children's hospitals usually have a wide variety of things to keep children entertained in the hospital, including play rooms, arts and crafts rooms, and plenty of books and videos. Your hospital's child life department may also put on special activities for the kids. By participating in these activities, your child will not only have fun, but he'll have the opportunity to interact with other children in similar situations.

Jeremy describes all the things there were to do at his hospital:

There was a computer room that I used a lot when I had the energy to walk over there. I mainly used it to play games. They also had something where you could have a video chat with kids in other hospitals, but I didn't do that. Also, every once and a while, the child life people brought pets in—mostly dogs. My favorite though was when they had a giant lizard—I think it was an iguana.

- **Encourage exercise.** If your son or daughter is up to it, encourage as much physical activity as possible. Walks around the hospital can be an adventure. If weather permits, try to include some outdoor time as well. Fresh air and sunshine can do wonders for anyone in the hospital.

- **Stay overnight.** Teenagers may not want you stay overnight, but younger children often do. Most children's hospitals provide special sleeping chairs or roll-a-way beds so parents can stay overnight in their child's room. If you can't stay, try to find another trusted friend or family member who can. And in the rare case that the hospital has a policy forbidding you to remain overnight, talk to the nursing supervisor on duty and insist that you must stay with your child.

Charlotte highly recommends that one parent should remain with a child, if possible:

> I'm a big advocate of parents staying with their children in the hospital. I can't imagine doing it any other way. My son was 9 years old when he had to remain in the hospital for an extended period. He really needed me, and I was very thankful I could be there. I felt so bad for other children whose parents couldn't stay. It was sad to see them alone.
>
> Many of the hospital staff recommended that I should take some time off, but I just couldn't do it. For me, it was the right thing to stay with him every night. Of course, I'd take short breaks during the day when I'd go walking or out to dinner with some friends in the area. I also had the opportunity to socialize with other mothers who were staying with their children. This kind of support really helped during such a stressful time.

Liz also makes sure that either she or her husband stays with Ian:

> Ian is still young and I cannot imagine leaving him alone overnight. I assume one day when he's older he'll tell my husband or me that he doesn't want us there anymore. But until then, one of us will always stay overnight with him.

For further information on hospitalization, see Chapter 10, *Going to the Hospital.*

Growth failure

Some children with IBD fail to grow normally. Having active IBD often reduces appetite, preventing your child from consuming enough calories for normal growth. In fact, kids with IBD frequently have a higher-than-normal caloric requirement from chronic inflammation. So just when your child actually needs to eat more to battle the disease, he can't because symptoms—such as pain, cramping, and reduced appetite—make it difficult to consume enough food. In addition, if Crohn's disease is present in the small intestine, he may not absorb nutrients properly despite eating well. This might partially explain why a higher percentage of children with Crohn's fail to grow normally than those with ulcerative colitis. Of course, loss of blood and nutrients from inflamed intestinal tissue can affect growth in all children with IBD. Medications such as prednisone can also do the same.

Delayed puberty is possible for some youngsters with IBD, especially if they are ill during their preteen years. Like growth failure, this delayed development is usually a result of malnourishment.

The best way to treat growth failure and delayed puberty is by treating the IBD. Once symptoms are brought under control and your child achieves remission, he will likely catch up with his peers. Nutritional therapy is often very helpful. If prednisone is needed, efforts should be made to reduce the dosage to the lowest amount possible. If medications and nutritional therapy fail, surgery may be recommended.

Experiencing a delay in physical growth and development is often very stressful for children with Crohn's or ulcerative colitis. Children usually don't like being different from their peers, especially when it's something so noticeable.

Sylvia describes what happened to her daughter:

> Although Mindy wasn't diagnosed with Crohn's till she was 12, she fell off the growth chart when she was five. For the next several years, the doctors said nothing was wrong with her, other than she was short.
>
> Being small was difficult for her. By the time she was 12, she still looked like a third or fourth grader. And when she first started high school, many of the kids at her new school would come up to her and ask if she was lost and needed directions to the nearby elementary school. And they weren't teasing her—that's what they really thought. It was very embarrassing and humiliating for her.

Fortunately, Charlotte's son, Jeremy, didn't have this problem:

> Jeremy has always been a big guy. When the ulcerative colitis
> started at age 8, he was already 90 to 95 pounds. He certainly lost
> some weight during the time he was very sick and in the hospital for
> several months, but it didn't delay his growth. He's 11 now and is the
> biggest kid in his class at five feet five inches and 140 pounds.

Liz's son, Ian, is small for his age:

> Because Ian has been very sick since he was a baby, Crohn's has
> significantly affected his growth. He's 8, but looks more like four.
> He's on Remicade now and has finally gotten off prednisone. We
> also have him on growth hormone shots, which have begun to help.
> We're hoping that a combination of him staying well, staying off the
> prednisone, and getting the shots will give him the growth spurt
> he needs.
>
> We're fortunate that he's been at the same school with the same
> group of kids since he was age 3. The kids accept him the way he is
> and he has some really good buddies. On the rare occasion that he is
> teased, his buddies stand up for him.
>
> When we're at the mall or grocery store, people assume he is a
> 4-year-old. However, Ian seems to handle this in stride, often using
> humor. If someone asks how old he is, he sometimes jokes and says,
> "I'm 3, but a smart 3."

Some people experience delays in growth, but later catch up with their peers:

> I was fortunate that my IBD didn't interfere too much with my
> physical growth and development. Prior to developing it, I was
> always one of the tallest boys in my class. For about one year in
> junior high, it seemed like others were passing me up, but I eventually
> caught up again in height once I had some remission time. However,
> even though my height was within the normal range, people would
> still think I was a couple of years younger than I was. I recall the
> summer before I went off to college, some thought I was only 15 or 16.
> I eventually grew to six feet tall and full, physical maturity by the
> time I was 21.

School

Mothers and fathers often have concerns about how IBD can affect their youngster's schooling. Some children miss days or weeks of school and may need tutoring in the hospital or at home to keep up. Children who are able to go to school have to learn how to manage their IBD while there.

Missing school

Children and teens with severe IBD are sometimes away from school for lengthy periods. It's important for parents to notify school administrators, teachers, and the school nurse about the child's situation. A child who is out of school longer than two weeks for any medical reason is entitled by law to instruction at home or in the hospital. The ideal time to request this service is as soon as you find out your child may remain in the hospital longer than two weeks. A letter is required from the physician stating the reason and expected length of time for this service.

If the child is in the hospital, the school district in which the hospital is located must provide the teacher. If the child is at home, the home school district provides the teacher. The teacher is responsible for gathering materials from the school and judging how much the child is capable of handling.

If your child is intermittently able to attend school, you should work with your school district to come up with a plan that works for her.

Sylvia explains how she negotiated with her daughter's high school:

> Mindy was missing a lot of school days during her freshman year. At first, the counselor had suggested that Mindy go to one of their special schools. However, this place was really geared for drop-outs and other kids with behavioral problems. When the man who headed it saw my daughter, he immediately said, "No way, this wouldn't be the place for her. She's not a teenager who doesn't want to be in school."
>
> It was then suggested that she try another school that was designed for teenagers who need to work. They meet with a teacher once a week and then do the assignments on their own at home. We negotiated so that my daughter could take half her classes through this school, but then the other half through the regular high school. She had difficulty with morning classes since she was often up much of the night with diarrhea. But she was usually fine in the afternoon. So she took a half-load of classes at her

regular school in the afternoon, and took her other classes through the special school. They don't normally let kids do that. But all we had to do was ask and then negotiate. We got what we needed.

Educating teachers

Most teachers want to do what they can to help their students, including those with special needs. Although some youngsters might prefer that their parents don't discuss IBD with their instructors, it's usually important for teachers to be educated on the topic. For example, if your son or daughter needs special bathroom privileges, the teacher needs to understand why. Also, if your child is having difficulty keeping up with coursework, most school instructors are generally much more understanding and flexible if they know a student is having serious health problems.

Sadly, some teachers are either insensitive or just don't understand, as Sylvia explains:

> *My daughter faced a very embarrassing situation once in PE. One day, she arrived late to class because she had to go to the bathroom. In front of all the other students, the teacher demanded to know where my daughter was and why she was late. It was so humiliating for her. Fortunately, the school nurse went to bat for us and pulled her out of that class.*
>
> *We tried to do a variety of things to educate her teachers, including meeting with them. We also gave them the pamphlet from the CCFA that is specifically written to give to teachers. Some teachers were helpful and understanding, but others just didn't seem to get it.*

Mary also spoke to her son's teachers:

> *Carl's Crohn's involved a lot of arthritis. Sometimes he could barely walk and get around. This part of it was often much more debilitating than any of the bowel problems.*
>
> *Carl would have been extremely upset if I had tried to get him any special bathroom privileges—so I didn't. Fortunately, prednisone always controlled the bowel inflammation, and he never ended up needing special permission to use the restroom.*
>
> *He was not open about telling people he had Crohn's, but he was okay with people knowing he had arthritis. When the arthritis was really bad, he could not carry all his books around. Although he didn't want to have to ask for special help, he was relieved when we arranged with his*

teachers for him to have two sets of books—one for the classroom and one at home. He wouldn't have been able to get by without this extra help.

Bathroom privileges have really helped Charlotte's son:

We've made an arrangement so that Jeremy has access to the staff bathroom near the nurse's office. Boys' bathrooms can be nasty. At my son's school, they are never clean and the toilets are frequently plugged. When Jeremy needs to go, he needs to go—so having access to a clean, private bathroom is essential. We also keep a backpack in the nurse's office with extra underwear. He still has some occasional, minor leakage with his J-pouch—so this comes in handy, too.

Terri's daughter has always had supportive teachers:

We've never had any problems with school or teachers. We've made a point to set up appointments with Kristy's teachers to let them know about her illness. We of course always come armed with the CCFA teacher brochure. Fortunately, all of her teachers have always responded supportively. In fact, many of them have made a point to personally show her where the bathroom is and have said she can use it any time.

If you are having problems with your child's school or teachers, consider discussing options with your youngster's healthcare team. Physicians, nurses, or social workers may have suggestions for assistance or can go to bat for you if problems arise.

Children with IBD who are undergoing medical treatment may be eligible for services and accommodations under the federal Rehabilitation Act (Section 504). Section 504 applies when the child does not meet the eligibility requirements for specially designed instruction, but still needs accommodations to perform successfully in school. For example, a child with IBD may need some special accommodations, such as full-time access to a bathroom, different behavior management while on high doses of prednisone, a water bottle on his desk, different medication administration policies, reduced homework during periods of frequent illness, a waiver for regular attendance/tardy policies and procedures, two sets of books, or more time to get from classroom to classroom. Check with the school's special education department to learn about your legal rights to accommodations for your child.

Peers

Crohn's disease and ulcerative colitis have the potential to affect your child's relationship with his peers. Of course, this impact will depend on how severe your son's or daughter's IBD is. Mild cases will probably have little effect, whereas severe ulcerative colitis or Crohn's has a greater chance of causing problems.

Battling a chronic illness is not a typical experience for most children and teenagers. As a result, your child may feel like he is different from or can't quite relate to other kids his age.

Sylvia describes how it was for her daughter:

> I felt so bad for Mindy at times. She was in the hospital four different times during her teen years. When other girls her age were learning how to deal with boys, she was learning how to deal with hospitals and doctors. It didn't seem fair, and I know it was hard on her.
>
> Another problem was her physical maturity. During her freshman year, she could still pass for a 9-year-old. Of course, her peers all looked their age. The problem is, many 14-year-old girls don't want to be hanging out with someone who looks like 9. It's not cool. It was also difficult for her to do normal teenage girl stuff with her friends. If they went to the mall, for example, her friends could find things in the teen section, but Mindy could only find clothes that fit her in the children's department.
>
> Fortunately, although there were some girls who ditched her, she always had a few friends who understood and stood by her. This really helped her get through the hard times.

Terri knows it has been difficult sometimes for Kristy:

> I know Kristy sometimes feels lonely. Intellectually, she's ahead for her age, but socially, I think she's a little behind. She just knows way too much because of her Crohn's, and most other kids haven't had to deal with anything like this.
>
> I'm glad to hear though that her teacher says she gets along well at school. However, I know she still has some anxieties and insecurities. For example, she never tells people about her Crohn's. I remember once I said something about it to someone, and she reacted quite strongly, "Mom, don't do that!"

*My husband and I have been worried about her anxieties and social
development so we have her in counseling. I think this is very
important for a child like her who has been through so much at such a
young age.*

If you have concerns about your child's peer relationships, here are a few suggestions
that might help:

- **Consider psychotherapy.** IBD is often as emotionally draining as it is physically.
  Psychotherapy often provides the tools your child needs to adjust to his illness,
  which can include helping him get along better with his peers.

- **Respect your child's wishes about disclosing information to friends.** Some children are okay with friends knowing about their illness, and some are not. In
  general, older children and teens will have stronger feelings on whether to tell
  their peers. It's probably best to not interfere with this, and to let your youngster
  be the judge.

- **Encourage your child to keep in touch with friends.** If you notice your son or
  daughter is withdrawing from social situations, do what you can to help him or
  her maintain contact with friends. For younger children, you might consider
  initiating play dates. Older kids may pose a greater challenge, but you can be
  creative. Inviting other families to your home (that have kids your child's age) for
  a dinner or barbecue is one idea.

- **Take your child to a CCFA support group for children and teens.** The CCFA
  has support groups for children and teens all across the United States. Although
  these groups are usually in metropolitan areas, call your local CCFA office for
  information. Even if there isn't a group in your area, perhaps another child of
  similar age lives not too far away, whom your son or daughter can meet.

- **Encourage your child to attend a CCFA summer camp.** The CCFA also has
  summer camps for kids with IBD. Like the support groups, they can be found all
  over the United States. Call CCFA at (800) 932-2423 for details. In addition, the
  United Ostomy Association (UOA) has an annual youth rally. It's a summer camp
  for kids with ostomies and is usually held on a university campus.

Charlotte is very thankful for IBD camp:

*Jeremy went to IBD camp for the first time this last summer. He
had a fabulous time. I'm so glad he can go to a camp where there are
other kids his age who have experienced so many similar problems.*

> *I am so thankful that CCFA has put these camps together. Jeremy can't wait to go back next summer!*

Jeremy sums it up succinctly:

> *IBD camp is the most fun thing that this illness has entitled me to do.*

IBD's impact on the family

Having a child with Crohn's disease or ulcerative colitis affects the whole family. Parents often find themselves under tremendous stress, and siblings may feel neglected when so much attention is focused on the sick child. Although not easy, it's very important to make time for yourself, as well as to address the needs of your other children.

Parents

Having a sick child is very time and energy consuming. As a human being, you only have a limited amount of resources. If you overdo, you run the risk of a massive burnout, in which case you won't even be able to take care of yourself or your ill son or daughter. Here are a few tips:

- **Ask for help.** Most friends and family members usually want to feel useful but they just don't know what to do. Often, if you ask, they will be happy to help. A handful of people giving just a few hours a week can make a surprising difference.

- **Don't skimp on good food, exercise, or sleep.** Although it may seem advantageous to skimp on these basics in the short run, you'll be hurting yourself long term if you do. The last thing you or your child needs is for you to be sick, too.

- **Occasionally treat yourself.** It helps to occasionally treat yourself to something special, even if just for a few hours a week. Try and think about what you really enjoy and go for it. Going to see a movie or having a massage are just a couple of ideas that may help renew or rejuvenate your spirit.

Liz shares what she does to help herself:

> *You have to make at least some time for yourself. I spend time with a couple of my girlfriends every week or two. We go out to dinner, have a glass of wine, and just hang out. We make these get-togethers a priority or else they won't happen.*

- Seek support from other parents. Contact your local CCFA chapter and ask to be put you in touch with other parents who have been through what you are experiencing now. Perhaps there is a support group in your area for parents and children.

Charlotte tells how she copes:

> I'm the type of mother who totally involved myself with every aspect of my son's care. Some might say that it's a bit unhealthy. However, I know I'm the type of person who would worry and stress more if I didn't. So I truly feel I'm doing the right thing for both him and me. I realize my style doesn't work for everyone, but it works for me.
>
> This being said, during the really stressful times, I did make sure to take care of myself. I made time to exercise, sleep, and even socialize when I could. A wonderful resource, too, was actually my computer. When my son was undergoing his J-pouch surgery, I received a lot of help from the discussion boards on the jpouch.org web site. I could remember times when I was so stressed out, and I would literally get responses to my posting within hours. I even got to meet some of these people at a retreat not too long ago. I can't emphasize enough how important it is to seek support from others who have been there, done that.

Husbands and wives frequently have concerns about how having an ill child might impact their relationship. Although many couples find they have little time left for each other, it's very important to do what you can to nurture your relationship with your spouse.

Patrick explains:

> My oldest daughter, who is now 9, has had Crohn's since she was 3. My wife and I also have two younger kids.
>
> When Kristy was extremely ill, it really took its toll on my wife and me. We forgot all about ourselves because we had to focus our energy on her. And what little energy we had left went to taking care of our other two children. Not surprisingly, we started having some problems in our relationship. We didn't want to let it get out of hand so we saw a counselor. This really helped us get through the stressful time. Today, I'm happy to say that my wife and I are getting along really well.

Sylvia recounts how she and her husband managed during the years their daughter was ill:

> My husband and I have our own business; so one of us had to take care of Mindy and the other, our company. We mutually agreed that I would be the one to help Mindy and he would run the business. Although at times I know he needed me, he also understood that Mindy needed me even more. It ended up working out, because he knew he could trust me to be her best advocate, while I knew I could trust him to manage the business.
>
> All this said, it was still not easy at times. There was a lot of stress in our family, particularly between my husband and me. Of course, we had other issues, too, besides just having a child with Crohn's. But somehow we managed. We never went to counseling, but we both came to a point where we could really empathize with the other. By taking the time to see and understand what was going on with each other, we were able to get through this difficult time and maintain our relationship.

Siblings

Siblings of an ill child often have a difficult time. Understandably, if one of your kids is sick, you need to temporarily give him more time and attention. However, because IBD is chronic, this extra time and attention may extend for weeks, months, or longer. Your other children may begin to feel angry, sad, or resentful. These emotions may be directed at you, the sick brother or sister, friends at school, or everyone.

Patrick describes how his 7-year-old son has been affected by his sister's IBD:

> All and all, my son has handled his older sister's IBD fairly well. We're careful to make sure that everyone receives enough attention, and it doesn't seem like he feels jealous or resentful. However, every once and a while something comes out that makes us wonder. I'm in the military, so we have to make sure that wherever we live, there is a pediatric gastroenterologist available to us. There's actually only handful of places where they can station me. No too long ago, my wife had taken the kids to visit her parents. My son loved it there so much that he wanted to move to their area. But then he said, "We can't live there though because of Kristy."

IBD has occasionally caused tension among Ann's children:

> I have a 16-year-old daughter and a 14-year-old son. My son is the one with Crohn's. My son and I have a lot of food sensitivities, so I generally make a lot of our food from scratch. It's a lot of work for me to do all the cooking, and I can't always please everyone.
>
> Occasionally, my daughter will make a comment about why she has to go along eating all this different kind of food, or not eating food that my son is allergic to in his presence, when she's not even sick. So I occasionally make something more "normal" for her. But then when I do that, my son sometimes gets upset and says, "How come she can eat that, and I can't? Of course, he does understand why. It's just that it's frustrating for him that he has to follow an unusual diet to minimize symptoms. My daughter has now come to enjoy spelt and goat milk products.
>
> Overall though, my daughter has been very supportive of her brother. She really feels for him and understands his plight. Occasionally, she has felt left out when all the attention is on him. But my husband and I handle this by talking about it with her. We don't let things go silent. That's when trouble can arise. By being conscious of the situation and actively dealing with it, I feel we have prevented many potential problems between our children.

Liz feels for her daughter:

> Callie, who is 12, is four years older than Ian. Ian's IBD has been difficult for her. On one hand, she's afraid of losing him. On the other, she often feels second in line. At times, she's even said things like, "You love him more than me." Of course, my husband and I tell her that's not true. But it takes more than words.
>
> We always make sure that when one of us is staying with Ian, the other is with her. We also are very open and encourage discussions with her about how she's feeling. She's also been seeing a counselor recently. I think the therapy is helping, as she seems better adjusted lately.

Some siblings respond with a lot of compassion. Sylvia's son was deeply affected by his sister's IBD:

> My son is six years older than his sister. When Mindy was diagnosed at age 12, Chris was already away from home at college. However, he has

always had a close relationship with his sister and was significantly impacted by her illness. He'd tell me of his recurring nightmares about how Mindy disappeared and no one could find her. But somehow he felt he was the one responsible for locating her and bringing he back. I think these dreams symbolized the sense of helplessness he had. He was always her protector, and there was nothing he could do to protect her from Crohn's.

Your relationship with your child

Many parents are concerned about how IBD might impact their relationship with their child who has the illness. As children grow and develop, it's only natural for them to try and separate from their parents as they try to establish their own identities and independence. Crohn's disease and ulcerative colitis, however, can sometimes interfere with this process. If your child is so sick he can barely take care of himself, he'll have to be more dependent on you—at least temporarily. This is often very frustrating for a young person. It's therefore not surprising adolescents sometimes react with anger or resentment toward their parents.

IBD's impact on your relationship with your son or daughter can also be positive. With the help of open communication, a willingness to work out conflicts, an empathetic attitude, and sometimes a good family therapist, the parent–child relationship can improve. Despite potential problems, your son or daughter having a chronic illness can ultimately lead to both of you having a deeper understanding and appreciation for each other.

Mary describes her experience with her son:

> *Carl had a difficult time accepting his illness. I think he was often in denial about a lot of it. If he was having problems with his arthritis, he'd blame his mattress or his shoes. If his belly ached, it was something he had eaten. He always blamed something external. I think it was just too upsetting for him to accept the fact that he had a chronic illness. Rather than face his anger about his disease, I think it was just easier to deny it.*
>
> *Some of this anger was occasionally transferred to me. If I knew he wasn't feeling well, I'd sometimes come to his room and ask him how he was doing. He'd angrily reply with questions directed at me, like, "Well, how's your belly?"*

I know, too, that he resented it when I was trying to research the disease and provide information to him. I'd leave reading material around—even in the bathroom. I'm not sure if he ever bothered reading any of it, but I'm sure he didn't appreciate it.

Despite being dysfunctional at times, we've managed to maintain a good relationship over the years. Although at times he needed our help, he grew up and has become a self-sufficient man. He went to college and he's had a great job now for many years.

He's in his twenties now, and thankfully he has come a long way in terms of accepting his Crohn's. There was no magic formula. I think it just took time. He's married now, too, and I know his wife has helped him a lot as well.

Ann believes in the importance of open communication:

My husband and I have been very concerned how IBD might affect Scott, who is 14. I know some people don't like to talk about a bowel disease, but my husband and I decided early on that we'd be open with it. We discuss the illness with Scott, including the fears that he or we may have about it. One time I asked him if he had concerns about his future, and he said he didn't. But then a while after that, he came to me and asked, "Are you afraid for me?" I explained that at first I was, but now that we're learning so much about it, I'm not as much anymore. I was really glad that he felt comfortable enough to ask me. I think it was a direct result of the openness we have.

Sylvia describes her process of learning to let go as her daughter has grown up:

My daughter and I have been through a lot together. During the years she should have been pulling away from me, we had—what I would call—an "over-closeness" that was a direct result of her disease. There really wasn't much other choice when she was so sick. I therefore totally understood her desire to go to college 3,000 miles away. She needed to assert her independence. Fortunately, we've always maintained a good relationship, regardless of physical distance.

Today, at age 24, she still lives on the opposite side of the country. As a mother, I still worry. I think all parents do. But I think parents of those with IBD or similar illnesses probably worry more. It's hard to let go. But at some point, you have to do it and trust that your son or daughter will be okay.

CHAPTER 16

Record-keeping, Insurance, Employment, and Disability

LIVING WITH THE MEDICAL AND emotional aspects of IBD isn't always easy. And as if this weren't enough, there's also a business side to managing a chronic illness. Handling this part of IBD frequently involves dealing with insurance and workplace problems that may arise because of your disease. Fortunately, there is much you can do to effectively deal with this side of having Crohn's or colitis. In fact, you may become more of an expert on insurance and employment law than you ever imagined.

This chapter begins by discussing the importance of record-keeping. It then provides a brief guide to insurance and how to cope with problems commonly associated with it. The next section focuses on employment and how others with IBD have dealt with challenges in the workplace. Last, the chapter covers how to apply for disability if you've become too sick to work.

Record-keeping

Many people think they don't really need to keep track of all their medical and insurance records. They assume it's the doctor's, hospital's, or insurance company's job. In a perfect world, such an arrangement would be ideal. You could focus on healing, and you could let someone else take care of organizing the mounds of paperwork. However, because errors are commonplace in the insurance and healthcare industries, it's definitely to your advantage to take as much responsibility for your records as you can. Comprehensive records are invaluable if you ever feel you have not been receiving the proper standard of care from your medical team. In addition, it's frequently helpful to keep up with all your records, because you can use the information to make educated decisions regarding your health care.

Jamie explains:

> I found it very helpful to get my medical records and read over
> them. It was an empowering experience because it helped me gain
> a better understanding of my condition.

> When I was first diagnosed and in the hospital, it was just so overwhelming. I was certainly getting information from the doctors, but it was difficult to process at the time since I was so sick. Plus, having Crohn's was all so new. So I waited till I got out of the hospital to request the records. I'm the kind of person who needed to learn all I can about my case. I realize not everyone is like this, but reading my records gave me a sense of control over what I was going through. I pored over every inch of them many times, and used my medical dictionary when there were terms I didn't understand.

Cathy has also found that keeping records is useful:

> I make sure to get copies of my various records—not just the Crohn's stuff but other things like bone density tests and mammograms, too. It's nice because I can look back and see what I did and when. And I can keep track of what needs to be done as well. I also like to know where I stand on my blood work and how it changes over time.
>
> I can honestly say that I have needed to find things in my records. One HMO I was with many years ago lost my parts of my records on several occasions. My doctor and I needed to know when I had certain tests, such as my last colonoscopy or barium x-ray. It was a good thing I had the information! So I'm quite thankful I've taken the time to maintain and organize my records.

Keeping your financial medical records is also essential, because it can be used to justify deductions from your income tax. You can deduct medical expenses if they are over 7.5 percent of your adjusted gross income. This is a low threshold for many people. In addition, many medical insurance premiums can be included as part of your medical expenses. For detailed information on what can count toward medical expenses, see the IRS Publication 502 at *http://www.irs.gov/pub/irs-pdf/p502.pdf* or consult your tax adviser for the latest information.

Accessing your medical records

Some Americans have difficulty obtaining copies of their medical records. Surprisingly, only about half of US states have laws that specifically grant individuals the right to see their own records. Although your information is confidential, it's actually considered the property of your doctor or hospital. And even though your signature is required to release the information to other parties (like insurance companies), it is sometimes difficult to get copies of your own records. Be aware, too, that some hospitals or medical centers may charge a hefty fee—sometimes hundreds of dollars—for copies of everything in your file. In this case, look through the records to only request copies of records relevant to your continuing care.

If you wish to obtain your medical records but are having trouble doing so, here are a few suggestions:

- **Know the law where you live.** It's important to educate yourself on local laws regarding medical records. Contact your state senator's or assemblyperson's office and ask them to send you information on this topic. Most state legislators have staffs that are well equipped to respond quickly to this type of constituent request. You can find their numbers and addresses in your phone book government pages. You can also call the Health Privacy Project at (202) 687-0880. Summaries of each state's medical privacy laws are available on the HPP web site, *http://www.healthprivacy.org/* (click on "State Law.")

- **Ask your hospital or doctor.** Just because your state has no specific law stating that your doctor or hospital has to give you access to your medical records doesn't mean they won't. If you ask them, they may say yes. If they have a formal process or procedure, follow it precisely.

- **Find a new doctor who will share information.** If your hospital or current doctor won't give you access and the law is on their side, find a new doctor who will. Because you do have the power to release the information to another physician, your hospital or old doctor has no choice but to comply. You can then see your records once your new doctor receives them.

- **Make copies of anything you're transferring.** If you are personally transferring records from one physician or medical center to another, make photocopies of everything given to you. If, for example, you are moving to a state that makes it difficult to access your records, you'll be glad you made copies before handing them over.

- **Get involved.** If you live in an area where it's difficult for consumers to access their own medical records—and you strongly feel consumers have the right to have full access—consider taking steps to change the law. For instance, you can to write to your state legislators, representatives, or governor.

- **Educate yourself.** Public Citizen, a consumer rights organization founded by Ralph Nader, publishes a book called, *Medical Records: Getting Yours.* The book discusses various topics, including the importance of medical record-keeping, how to access your medical records, and how to understand and interpret them.

Stacy describes how she got her records:

> I was fortunate that I didn't have much difficulty getting my medical records. We were moving to a different state and I didn't yet know who my doctor would be. I simply put in a request to my old doctor. The only minor problem I had was that the administrative people didn't want to photocopy everything for me since there was so much. They called and asked me what part I wanted. Of course, I wanted it all. My doctor actually had to call them a couple of times to insist that they photocopy everything. I guess they just didn't want to take the time. I also drove 40 miles to pick them up—I didn't want to take a chance that they'd get lost and then I'd have to request another copy. Once I got them, I made photocopies of everything for myself before I handed them over to my new doctor. However, I haven't had any problems getting records from my new doctor either.

Jamie tells her story:

> Before putting in my request, I learned that my state allows patients access to their records. I braced myself for a problem before asking but it turned out I had no difficulties. However, they did charge me for photocopying my records.
>
> I think it's ludicrous that some states deny people access to their own records. It makes absolutely no sense. It's like saying other people have more of a right to your personal information than you do. What are people who made the law afraid of? Thankfully, I live in a state that has respect for patients' rights.

Deciding what records to keep

You may have questions regarding what records you should keep. Opinions vary, but it's usually a good idea to keep as much documentation as you have room to store. Here are some suggested items:

- Dates of medical appointments and the name of the healthcare professional seen.

- All written reports of your doctor appointments.

- Dates and written reports of all hospitalizations.

- Dates and written reports of all surgeries.

- Dates and written reports of other procedures such as colonoscopies, barium x-rays, and so forth.

- Dates of lab work and test results.

- Medication history for all drugs taken, including dates, doses, as well as positive and negative reactions.

- Complementary therapy history, including what you tried and when, as well as positive or negative reactions.

- A log where you keep track of any other pertinent information, including number and quality of bowel movements, pain level, energy level, and so on.

- All medical bills, including those for doctors, hospitals, or prescription drugs.

Jamie keeps a variety of material:

> I keep files on most of my medical records, including hospitalizations, surgeries, procedures, lab work, pathology reports, and notes from my doctors. Since I have an HMO, I don't have to worry about keeping files on bills and claims, other than my monthly payments.
>
> When I flare up, I often look back to see how my current reports compare with past ones. This is helpful—so good record-keeping does come in handy. I have to admit though I'm not as vigilant and organized about my record-keeping as I was the first few years I was sick. Since I feel I have more of a handle on things now, it's not quite as organized as it once was. But still, I keep my records and would recommend that others do the same.

Managing and organizing your records

Figuring out the best way to store and organize your records can be easy or difficult. Most people with IBD accumulate a lot of paperwork, and you'll have to figure out a system that works best for you. Most importantly, you'll need to organize your records in a way that enables you to locate specific information when you need it. Here are some ideas you might consider:

- **Keep financial and insurance records separate from your doctor and hospital records.** It makes sense to keep these types of files in different folders. Even when keeping everything in chronological order, it often takes longer to find specific information if you combine everything.

- **Organize financial and insurance records by year.** You might consider having a separate hanging file for each year's financial and insurance records. The flat-bottom hanging files are a good choice if you have multiple manila folders full of material. Another option is an accordion-style monthly file with twelve pockets.

- **Organize medical records in a way that's logical for you.** People have different preferences for organizing their doctor and hospital records. For example, you may want to keep a separate file for each hospitalization, another file just for blood tests, another for procedures, and possibly separate files for each different doctor you see as an outpatient. Whatever you do, try to keep the material in each file in chronological order.

- **Request copies of records as they happen.** It's a good idea to get copies of all your records as they are generated. When you go the doctor, for example, ask for a copy of your latest lab results before you leave. Do the same thing before you are discharged from the hospital.

Jamie's doctor provides copies of reports:

> *I've generally asked for my records as things have occurred.*
> *In fact, my gastroenterologist actually gives them to me now at my*
> *appointments without my asking. I suspect he probably doesn't do this*
> *for everyone. He just knows me really well and knows what I want.*
> *It's kind of nice.*

- **File things immediately.** As soon as you receive anything—whether directly from your doctor or through the mail—file it right away. If you leave it lying around, it may get misplaced. When you need something immediately, it's frustrating to spend hours trying to find it. The two minutes it takes to file something properly is well worth the investment of your time.

- **Keep a journal.** Keeping a written log of your medical history is an excellent idea. It can help you track the different therapies you've tried and how you responded to them. Sometimes it's easy to forget the details of what helped and what didn't. If you have a journal, you'll always have written documentation. A bound journal is a great option, because it keeps pages together and you can take it anywhere.

Keeping a journal worked for Larry:

> *I make an effort to keep a journal. It's nice having everything in*
> *writing because and I can go back and read things that I wouldn't*
> *normally recall as clearly. Sometimes I can forget how helpful*

something was—even something as simple as how keeping busy with my hobbies can do a lot to take my mind of my illness when I'm going through a bad bout. When I re-read my journal, it reminds me of all different things that work and don't work for me. I also use it to keep track of my medicines, pain levels, and dates of treatments. In addition, my journal came in handy when I was applying for social security because it provided other details that my medical records lacked.

- **Use your calendar.** Some people find using their calendar is a good way for them to track information. Obviously, you can use it to record significant dates, but you can also write other notes on it as well. For many people, their calendar also functions as a personal journal.

Stacy explains:

At times I have used my calendar for record-keeping purposes. I tracked a variety of things on it, including my physical state, my diet, and even the number of bowel movements I had per day. This worked better for me than keeping a separate journal.

- **Use your computer.** If you are computer savvy, you may decide to use your computer to help manage your records. Spreadsheets are often valuable tools because you can enter your data and make all sorts of nifty charts and graphs. For instance, a weekly/monthly bar chart of your hemoglobin or sed rate can help you and your doctor analyze certain trends. You can even create reports on the average number of bowel movements you have per day during different times of the year. Yes, you can really have fun with this, and the possibilities are endless.

- **Get a friend or family member to help you.** If you are too sick to manage your own records, enlist a trusted friend or family member to help. The people who love you may feel helpless, and this could be one area where they can assist you.

Insurance

Obtaining insurance is sometimes difficult for people with IBD. Because Crohn's disease and ulcerative colitis often require expensive medical treatment, insurance companies generally don't welcome people with these illnesses with open arms. Although some people with IBD are able to secure good plans, others face high premiums, less than ideal coverage, or no insurance at all. The following sections review life and health insurance.

Life insurance

Insurance companies usually offer two types of life insurance: term and whole life. Term insurance is cheaper—although prices rise with your age—and only insures you for a given time period or designated term. Whole life is more expensive. However, the whole-life premium will never go up, and if you continue making your payments the insurance company cannot cancel the policy. Part of your premium goes toward insuring your life, and another portion is deposited into an investment account from which can take a loan should you have unexpected expenses.

People with IBD may have problems obtaining either kind of life insurance policy. Although many people with Crohn's or ulcerative colitis live as long as the average person, insurance companies are still wary, because the diseases can contribute toward other life-threatening situations, such as peritonitis, toxic megacolon, or colorectal cancer. However, if you've been in remission for a significant length of time and require little or no medication, you'll probably have a good chance of acquiring a policy. But even if you're not in remission, don't lose hope. Here are a few tips that may help:

- **Take advantage of your employer's life insurance plan.** This is probably the best option, assuming you have an employer who offers this benefit. In many cases, you can get at least some life insurance coverage regardless of your health status, such as one to two times your annual salary. You then usually have an option to buy more without having to provide evidence of insurability. With some flexible plans, you can cover other family members as well.

  If you have questions about your company's life insurance plan, ask for a summary plan description (SPD), which explains in detail how the life insurance plan works. Under the federal Employee Retirement Income Security Act (ERISA) of 1974 (a law that sets minimum standards and provides protection for people participating in private industry voluntary pension or health plans), companies must provide you with an SPD. If you are interested in learning more about ERISA, go to the US Department of Labor's web site: *http://www.dol.gov/dol/topic/health-plans/erisa.htm*.

- **Consult an insurance specialist who has experience helping people with chronic illnesses acquire life insurance.** If you cannot obtain life insurance through your job, consulting an insurance specialist can probably help. If you don't know where to find one, call your local CCFA office or other chronic illness organization and ask if they can recommend an agent who has experience working with people who have diseases such as IBD. Make sure you are working with an agent who can be a good advocate for you instead of someone who is just an intermediary charging a substantial commission.

- **Apply to many different companies.** Another option is to apply to many different places. Probably some company out there will offer you a policy. However, you may have to pay more for less coverage than the average person.

- **Consider obtaining whole life insurance in small amounts.** Although whole life insurance is generally more expensive, a small policy, such as $25,000, may be more easily obtainable. It presents relatively little risk to the insurance company. Also, insurance carriers may look more favorably on someone who's interested in whole life, because the decision to purchase it implies you think you're going to be around for a while.

Brenda had difficulty obtaining life insurance:

> *I've found that it's not easy for someone with Crohn's to get life insurance. Even though my doctor said that I was basically fine, I discovered that insurance companies generally don't view Crohn's disease favorably. One person even told me I that I'm a "walking uninsurable."*
>
> *My solution was to just keep shopping and hope that some company would offer me a policy. Fortunately, I finally found one. It's certainly not as much coverage as my husband has, but at least it's something.*

Health insurance

Health insurance is frequently a major concern for people with IBD. Although federal laws have been passed to help people maintain or acquire health insurance if they change or lose their job, the current situation is still far from ideal. People with chronic illnesses—or pre-existing conditions, as they are often called in the trade— can still face obstacles when trying to secure adequate coverage.

The following is a brief overview of information on health insurance for people with IBD. For more information, see the *Resources* appendix. The CCFA web site also has information on health insurance: *http://www.ccfa.org/medcentral/library/legal/.*

Obtaining health insurance

Many people with IBD are healthy enough to work. As a result, these individuals with Crohn's or ulcerative colitis obtain health insurance through their jobs. Most large companies offer a variety of plans. The three most common types are as follows:

- **Health maintenance organizations (HMOs).** An HMO is a company that provides health care to subscribers for a prepaid monthly premium. They may hire doctors to work for the HMO or contract with independent doctors or groups of doctors. Most HMOs are for-profit companies that generally take a preventive approach to health care. HMOs cover a wide range of services, including diagnostic tests, doctor visits, emergency room services, hospitalization, and sometimes prescription drugs. Their main advantage is that they are usually the most affordable option: premiums are often low, co-payments for services are quite reasonable (generally $5 to $20), and there are often no deductibles (the amount you have to pay before coverage kicks in). In fact, many HMO members never even see a bill or have to deal with claims. The main disadvantages stem from the tightly managed policies to contain costs. For example, you cannot make an appointment with a gastroenterologist unless your primary care physician refers you to one. In addition, subscribers only have access to healthcare professionals in the network and almost always have to pay out-of-pocket if they wish to see someone outside the organization.

Jamie discusses her feelings on her HMO and health insurance in general:

> *My feeling is that my HMO is as good or as bad as any other type of health plan out there. I've found a great gastroenterologist in it so that is a big incentive for me to stay with it. I also like the convenience of having everything all in one place. On top of this, I never have to worry about paperwork, bills, claims, or whether something is going to be authorized.*
>
> *The downside with my HMO—that's probably also true with any insurance plan—is that you need to learn the system and use it to your advantage. I've been fortunate that I've been able to do this, but I feel bad for others who—for whatever reason—are unable to do so. It's too bad, because people really need the system most when they are sick and down. But this is when they are least able to stand up for themselves and be their own advocate. It's sad, but it almost seems like insurance companies count on a certain percentage of people not demanding benefits they should rightfully have under their policy.*

- **Preferred provider organizations (PPOs).** A PPO is a managed care organization that contracts with healthcare professionals and hospitals to provide medical care for subscribers. Physicians agree to accept lower payments and restrictions on how they can treat their patients in exchange for referrals from the insurance company. One advantage of a PPO is that people have more flexibility to choose their physicians. For example, you don't need a referral from a primary care physician to see a specialist, such as a gastroenterologist or surgeon. You can also see professionals outside the network, although your plan will pay a smaller percentage of the bill. The main disadvantage is that PPOs are more expensive than HMOs. Co-payments are usually higher, and plans usually cover only a percentage of costs (75 to 85 percent is common). Annual deductibles can range from a few hundred dollars to a few thousand dollars.

- **Traditional health insurance plans.** HMOs and PPOs are products of the managed care movement, which was implemented to help contain soaring healthcare costs. Before HMOs and PPOs became so prevalent, most people had traditional health insurance plans called fee-for-service. This system has no networks or pre-arranged agreements for set fees. People can go to any doctor or hospital they choose, and the insurance company is not involved with healthcare decisions. Thus, physicians can spend as much time as they want with patients and are free to prescribe whatever treatments and tests they think are necessary. Plans usually cover a percentage of costs and include deductibles. Once your costs exceed a certain amount in a given year—which can easily be surpassed by someone with an active case of IBD—the insurance covers the rest. Traditional health insurance plans can be expensive but they generally offer the most freedom and flexibility for your health care.

Not every employed person has medical benefits. These people—as well as those who are unemployed or too sick to work—must find alternatives. Here are some other options:

- **High-risk insurance pools.** Some states specifically offer health insurance to people likely to have high medical costs, such as those with chronic illnesses like IBD. To find out if your state provides such a plan, call the National Association for Insurance Commissioners at (817) 842-3600 or your state department of insurance. The CCFA web site at *http://www.ccfa.org/medcentral/library/legal/highrisk.htm* also lists phone numbers for the states that have high-risk insurance pools.

- **Individual plans.** Some insurance companies, such as Blue Cross/Blue Shield, have open enrollment periods when you can apply for an individual health insurance plan. Contact local offices of various insurance companies to see what's available in your area. You'll likely have to pay more for an individual plan, but you might find one that can fit your budget.

- **Medicaid.** Medicaid is a health insurance program funded jointly by the states and the federal government. It provides coverage to 36 million low-income individuals in the United States, including many elderly or disabled people, children, and those in certain government assistance programs. For more detailed information, call The Centers for Medicare and Medicaid Services toll free at (877) 267-2323 or see the web site at *http://cms.hhs.gov/medicaid/consumer.asp*.

- **Medicare.** Medicare is a national health insurance program. It covers approximately 40 million Americans, including people age 65 and older, some disabled individuals under age 65, and those with end-stage kidney disease. For detailed information on Medicare, call The Centers for Medicare and Medicaid Services toll free at the number just listed, or visit the Medicare web site at: *http://www.medicare.gov/*.

- **Professional associations or trade groups.** Self-employed individuals should check to see whether any trade or professional organizations they belong to—or could belong to—offer a health plan. College alumni associations are another place to look. Chambers of commerce may also offer health insurance to their small business members. These plans may have limited coverage and/or cost more than average, but most are probably better than no coverage.

- **Short-term insurance.** Short-term health insurance policies provide coverage for brief periods—typically from one month to one year. These policies are often marketed to high school or college graduates who are dropped from their parents' insurance and have not yet found a benefit-providing job. Premiums are extremely low, but deductibles are very high. The downside to these plans is that they almost never cover pre-existing conditions. The definition of a pre-existing condition can vary, but these policies often deny coverage for any illness diagnosed or treated within the previous five years.

- **Financial assistance.** If you are unable to pay your hospital or doctor bills, consider asking for financial assistance. Some doctors accept reduced fees from people who have no insurance. However, to get it you generally have to ask. Many hospitals sometimes write off a percentage of your bill if you can't pay. Ask to speak to a financial counselor at your hospital to learn about your options.

- **Free medicine programs.** Many pharmaceutical companies have free medicine programs for people who are uninsured and can't afford their prescription drugs.

For more information, contact the Pharmaceutical Research and Manufacturers of America (PhRMA) at (202) 835-3400. The web site also has information on patient assistance programs: *http://www.phrma.org/pap*. Another web site to check is *http://www.needymeds.com*. You might also consider calling the drug company whose medicine you need and asking whether they have this kind of a program.

Stacy comments on the difficulty people with chronic illness have when trying to get health insurance:

> *I personally know how difficult it can be to get health insurance when you have a pre-existing condition. When my family and I moved in 1993, my husband no longer worked for a large company. He and my two daughters had no problem getting insured, but I was declined everywhere I applied. It was very scary. For one year I had no health insurance. Thankfully, nothing major happened to me, but I felt like I was holding my breath the whole time. Finally, my husband had to take a part-time job at a major company so I could be covered. He works four hours, five days a week starting at 3:30 A.M. Then he has the rest of day to dedicate to his business. It's a sacrifice, but it's the only way I could get adequate coverage at a reasonable rate.*
>
> *It's kind of sad that people with chronic illnesses have so much trouble getting insured, especially since they are the ones who need it the most. I know someone with Crohn's who's self-employed who pays half his salary just for medical insurance. It's unfortunate, too, that young people with IBD have to think about insurance when deciding on a career. I'm not saying that young people have to give up their dreams. But sometimes the reality is that they feel influenced to pick a career that enables them to work for the government or a large company in order to get good benefits at an affordable price.*

Laws that can help

People with chronic illnesses such as Crohn's disease and ulcerative colitis often fear losing their health insurance if they change or lose their job. Although the current situation in the United States is still not ideal, two major amendments to ERISA have been passed to help protect individuals if they leave their job or if their employment is terminated.

- **The Comprehensive Omnibus Budget Reconciliation Act (COBRA)** is a federal law that requires public and private companies employing more than twenty workers to provide continuation of group coverage to employees if they quit, are fired, or work reduced hours. Coverage must extend to surviving, divorced, or separated spouses, and to dependent children. You must pay for your continued coverage, but it must not exceed more than 2 percent the rate set for your former coworkers. By being allowed to purchase continued coverage, you have time to seek other long-term coverage. Because you are paying out of pocket, COBRA premiums can be significant. However, they are generally worth the peace of mind you'll have until you find new coverage. The US Department of Labor provides a COBRA fact sheet at *http://www.dol.gov/dol/pwba/public/pubs/cobrafs.htm.*

Jamie expresses her gratitude for COBRA:

> *I'm very thankful for COBRA. About a year after I was diagnosed with Crohn's, I lost my job. It was scary being unemployed and having a new disease that I was just beginning to learn about. At least I had the reassurance that for the next 18 months I wouldn't have to worry about finding new health insurance. In fact, I negotiated with my former employer to pay for the first six months of it. With all the other things I was panicked over, at least I had some peace with my COBRA coverage. Fortunately, I found a new job relatively quickly, but the new employer didn't offer the HMO I was on. So I decided to stay on the COBRA for the full 18 months and then converted to an individual plan with my HMO.*

- **The Health Insurance Portability and Accountability Act (HIPAA).** This act— sometimes called the Kennedy-Kassebaum bill—was passed in 1996 and took effect in July 1997. As its name implies, the law makes health insurance more portable, meaning that people who lose or switch jobs have a much greater chance of remaining insurable, even if they have a pre-existing condition. For example, if you previously had group health insurance for at least twelve months (eighteen months in certain cases) with no significant breaks in coverage (defined as 63 days or more) and then leave your job (voluntarily or involuntarily), you not only can't be denied a new plan, but the new insurance company has to cover your pre-existing condition. If you were previously insured for less time, the new company can delay coverage for your condition for up to—but generally never more than—a year. This denial period is based on a predetermined formula: twelve months minus the number of months you were previously insured. Thus, if you had coverage under your old plan for three months, the new company can lawfully exclude coverage of your IBD for your first nine months on the new policy.

If you need evidence of your previous coverage, your former plan administrator is obligated to provide this documentation. Keep in mind, too, that time spent on COBRA counts toward your previous coverage. There are some loopholes in HIPAA, however; you might consider consulting a health insurance specialist if you have questions. You can also contact the Centers for Medicare and Medicaid Services at (877) 267-2323 or visit the HIPAA section on their web site at *http://cms.hhs.gov/hipaa/hipaa1/default.asp*. The US Department of Labor (DOL) has two web pages that describe HIPAA: *http://www.dol.gov/pwba/faqs/faq_consumer_hipaa.html* and *http://www.dol.gov/pwba/pubs/hipaafs.htm*.

Understanding your policy

Insurance policies are sometimes difficult to understand. However, it's important that you make a point to learn the details of your policy so there are no unexpected or stressful surprises. Here are a few suggestions:

- When the new insurance manual is sent to you each year, review your entire policy and pay attention to changes

- Know what all your co-payments and deductibles are

- Learn what percentage of your healthcare bills the insurance company pays

- Find out at what point—if any—coverage becomes 100 percent

- Determine if there is a yearly limit on coverage, either for total expenses or specific expenses such as prescription drugs

- Find out if there is a lifetime limit for coverage

- Determine whether you need to prenotify the insurance company before hospitalization or before diagnostic tests such as a colonoscopy

- Ask your company's benefits specialist or call the insurance company directly if you have any other questions about your policy or what it covers

Carla emphasizes the importance of knowing your policy:

> It's very important to know and understand the details of your policy. I know in my case it gave me peace of mind knowing what was covered and the procedures I needed to follow so that I could get maximum reimbursement. An example of this is when I needed to get pre-approval for anything. When I knew I was heading to the hospital, I got everything pre-approved before I left. This way, by

the time I got there, I didn't have to worry about how much the insurance was going cover. It made my hospital stay much less stressful. I strongly recommend that people take the time to understand their insurance policy as soon as they can. When an emergency comes up, you know exactly what to do. It saves a lot of worry.

Managing claims

Some people have no problems with their insurance, but for others it's a nightmare. The lucky ones may never even see a bill or have to battle their company regarding a claim. Others, however, may have to routinely fight. Here are some tips that may help prevent problems, or may help if problems develop:

- Keep meticulous records of all your medical bills, claims, and all documentation your insurance company sends to you.

- Photocopy and keep all correspondence with your insurance company.

- Pay all your insurance and medical bills by check and request that your bank send you your canceled checks so you have proof of payments.

- Keep a logbook of all conversations you have over the telephone with your insurance company, including dates, times, topics discussed, and the names of the people you spoke to.

- Try to talk to the same person each time you call your insurance company, so you have someone familiar with your case.

If your insurance company denies a claim you think it should accept, you have a right to appeal the decision. Here are a few suggestions:

- **Review your policy and follow the guidelines and procedures for challenging a denied claim.** Usually you'll have to submit something in writing, outlining the reasons why you think your claim is valid.

- **Enlist the help of your healthcare provider.** Your doctor probably will want to help, because that's how he's most likely going to receive payment for his services. Sometimes all it takes is a letter from your physician explaining why something was necessary. Other times, it's just a matter of re-submitting the claim with the correct coding.

- **Try negotiating with the insurance company.** It's possible they may make exceptions to their rules if you present a good case and appeal to their sense of fairness. You certainly have nothing to lose by trying.

- **Contact your elected government officials.** Senators or members of the House of Representatives are paid to represent their constituents. They represent you, so consider giving their local office a call. Their staff is equipped to handle all sorts of problems. State government officials, such as your state senator, assemblyman, or insurance commissioner, may also be able to assist you. Their numbers are listed in your phone book government pages.

- **Exhaust all your administrative remedies.** It's required that you do this before retaining an attorney and going to court. The best way to exhaust all your administrative remedies is to request your insurance plan's summary plan description (SPD), because it outlines in detail how you can appeal a denied claim. Follow the process as described in the SPD.

- **Take the matter to court.** If all the preceding suggestions fail, your last resort is to sue the insurance company. People have done this and won. However, it can be a lengthy and stressful process, which is often difficult on someone with a chronic illness like IBD. And of course, there are no guarantees you will win. If you decide to pursue a lawsuit, make sure you have indeed exhausted all your administrative remedies as just described, and find a lawyer who has expertise in healthcare and insurance law.

Carla frequently had to challenge denied claims:

> When I was in school, I had a student insurance policy that was not too good. They frequently denied my claims. However, I'm the kind of person who doesn't take no for an answer. I fought them on a lot of claims and frequently won. Some of it had to do with the doctor coding the claims improperly. So I worked with him and his staff and they were happy to re-submit the claims with the correct coding. I also made a point to always deal with the same person at this company so that someone was familiar with my case.
>
> It's hard when you are sick to fight the insurance company. But it's so important to be reimbursed for what's rightfully yours. If people can't do it themselves, they should get someone to help them. You can fight and win, but you have to make the effort.

Employment

Having IBD can affect your work life. Although people with milder cases may not have apprehensions regarding work, others with Crohn's disease and ulcerative colitis have a variety of concerns about their employment. Some worry about whether they may face discrimination when applying for jobs; others may fear discrimination in jobs they already have. People with severe cases might worry about whether they can work at all. Even if you're well enough to work, active Crohn's disease and ulcerative colitis have the potential to interfere with your job performance.

Applying for a job

It's important to know your rights before you fill out job applications and go to interviews. Unless your IBD physically prevents you from performing the job you are applying for, having Crohn's or colitis should not make a difference on whether you are hired (see the section on the Americans with Disabilities Act later in this chapter). Here are a few suggestions that may help you avoid discrimination if you are searching for work:

- **Don't volunteer information about your IBD.** During a job interview, employers don't have the right to ask whether you have a chronic illness. However, they can ask questions about your abilities to perform specific job functions mentioned in the job description. If you are capable of performing the job, there is no need to mention Crohn's disease or ulcerative colitis.

- **Never lie.** Don't lie on an application or during an interview. If the employer later discovers your dishonesty, you can be fired. Answer questions accurately and honestly without going out of your way to mention that you have IBD.

- **Don't agree to a medical exam before you're hired.** Employers can only require a medical exam after they've made a job offer, not before. Moreover, the exam can't be used against you unless it proves you are physically unable to perform the job.

- **Consider not asking about health insurance options until you are offered a position.** Opinions on this topic vary. It's possible the employer may wonder why you are concerned. If you wait till the employer makes an offer, you can then inquire about health insurance (for example, ask for the plan's SPD) before accepting the job. However, a lot of healthy people are concerned about benefits, too; therefore, inquiring about them may be okay.

Disclosure

It's often difficult for people with IBD to decide how much they should share about their illness with their coworkers and boss. Some fear by mentioning the illness they may later face subtle or outright discrimination when it comes to advancements or promotions. Yet other people with Crohn's or colitis feel it's important to let their supervisor know what's going on so she knows there is a valid reason for missed days or for projects not getting done on time.

There's really no cookie-cutter formula for disclosing your illness. People who have a supportive boss and coworkers will generally have few problems if they disclose, whereas those who are not working with understanding people may have many problems regardless of whether they say anything. Use your best judgment.

Carla describes her approach:

> First of all, I never mention anything about my ulcerative colitis in an interview. It only gives someone an excuse to deny you and there's really no way to prove that someone didn't hire you because of it.
>
> I don't mention anything about my ulcerative colitis until I've had a chance to prove I'm a very capable employee. Fortunately, I've never needed to mention it sooner. I've been lucky that I can keep my symptoms under control when I'm having a flare. My supervisors and coworkers over the years have ranged from at least tolerant to supportive.

Jamie tends to wait a long time:

> Disclosure of my Crohn's in the workplace is a touchy subject for me. I know it's against the law to discriminate based on illness, but I felt that my disease probably played some role in my termination at a job many years ago when I was first diagnosed. In my following job, I waited three years before I fully disclosed my Crohn's, simply because there was no choice when I had a major flare and had to take time off. I have another job now—that I've had for a year and a half—and I still have not mentioned it to anyone except for one co-worker. And the only reason I told her is that I noticed one day that she was taking Asacol. It turned out she had ulcerative colitis. However, she's left the company, and now, no one there knows.
>
> I would never lie if someone directly asked me if I had a chronic illness, but I never go out of my way to tell. I just don't want to take a chance

that it might somehow affect how I'm perceived. In a perfect world, I'd prefer to be open with it. But in reality, I'm not comfortable sharing information about my IBD at work. I feel bad because it feels like I'm being kind of secretive. Crohn's is part of who I am, and thus I can't fully share myself with those at work. But right now, I feel the cost of disclosing is still higher than the cost of not sharing.

Working well with IBD

Maintaining a good work record is sometimes a challenge, particularly if you have an active case of ulcerative colitis or Crohn's disease. However, it is possible and many people have done it. Following are some workplace suggestions:

- **Give a little extra when you are feeling well.** Establishing a great work record is always a good idea. If there are times when you know you won't be performing as well, you may need to compensate by giving a bit more when your health allows it. This strategy, however, may or may not work, depending on the type of job you have.

- **Never use sick days for vacation.** People with a chronic illness like IBD should definitely avoid this practice. Besides the fact that it's not the right thing to do, if you have repeated flares you may need to take all your allotted sick time. Because of people who abuse the system, some employers now just combine vacation and sick days and give their employees a specific number of days off (for any reason) per year.

Jamie comments:

> *I never use sick days for vacation. I have to say, though, that it really annoys me when I see other people calling in sick when they are not actually sick. I suppose it's none of my business. And I realize these people probably have no concept of what it's like to be chronically ill. But it's especially frustrating for someone like me to see someone taking advantage of the system in this manner. If someone wants to take a day of vacation, they should just use one of their vacation days.*

- **Be conscientious and responsible.** Do your best to demonstrate these traits. For example, if you start getting behind on tasks, keep your supervisor and others posted on your progress. Most people would rather be kept abreast on what's going on, than hear nothing.

- **Try to get an office or cubicle near the bathroom.** Not only will you be less conspicuous, but over the long run you'll save on travel time to and from the bathroom. If asked why you are requesting this, at the very least explain that you generally need to go frequently and that walking a shorter distance is more productive for you and the company.

- **Ask for help.** If you feel this is appropriate, it might not hurt to ask for some assistance. Perhaps a coworker can pick up a little of your slack if you're having a difficult time keeping up. Or maybe your boss might consider hiring some temporary help until you are feeling better.

Michael shares how he asked for a special accommodation at work:

> At my workplace, they have code boxes on all the bathroom doors. So to get in, you have to take the time to press several buttons. If you are in a hurry to go, it's easy to accidentally enter the wrong code. Of course, then the door won't open and you have to wait a few seconds until you can try again. Needless to say, this is not an ideal situation for someone with IBD! Although I don't have urgent diarrhea that frequently, there are still times when I need to get to the restroom quickly. So I spoke to our disability coordinator to see if I could get a master key to all the bathrooms I use. She said it was possible, but that she needed me to have my doctor send her a letter to verify my condition. It took a while, but I was finally able to get my key. Now I can get into the bathrooms more quickly and easily. But I still wish that the boxes were gone.

- **Communicate clearly and honestly if you are away for a significant period of time.** If you have to take a lot of time off for a major flare, hospitalization, or surgery, it's best to honestly explain your situation to your boss. Try as well to give an estimate of when you'll return.

Laws to protect you in the workplace

Some people with IBD don't realize that federal laws exist to protect them in the workplace. Your state may also have other laws that provide further protection. It's definitely to your advantage to know the law and to keep up with any changes, because most are continually undergoing reinterpretation or are frequently amended.

The Americans with Disabilities Act (ADA)

The ADA was signed into law in the early 1990s to prevent employers from discriminating against those with disabilities. This law covers companies with fifteen or more workers. Under the act, a person is considered disabled if she has a physical or mental impairment that prevents or substantially restricts her participation in at least one major life activity, or is perceived to be disabled. Since its passage, the law has undergone many revisions and interpretations. Currently, it's still not totally clear how the most recent interpretations might affect those with IBD.

Recent federal court rulings suggest that mitigating measures, such as medications, may prevent some people from being classified as disabled, because these measures substantially reduce symptoms and allow for normal functioning. It's still possible, however, that your IBD is a disability if medications do not adequately control your symptoms. But what happens if you are one of those people who finds that medications work at times but not at others? Unfortunately, there are no clear answers at this time.

Several US states have enacted their own versions of the ADA. Many of these states have defined disability much more broadly than the federal government, which means it's easier for someone to be considered disabled. It's therefore very important that you contact your state legislators to find out what disability laws are in place where you live.

Assuming your IBD is classified as a disability, here are some major protections provided by the federal act:

- If you are otherwise qualified and capable of performing a job, a potential employer cannot decide to not hire you because of your IBD.

- Unless doing so constitutes an undue hardship, an employer must provide reasonable accommodations. An example is giving you extra break time for going to the bathroom.

- An employer cannot discriminate against you because of a family illness.

- You are not only entitled to lost wages but also compensation for emotional distress if your employer is found liable for discriminating against you because of your IBD. They may also have to pay your attorney fees.

The Equal Employment Opportunity Commission (EEOC) enforces Title I (employment) of the ADA. Call (800) 669-3362 for enforcement publications. Other sections are enforced or have their enforcement coordinated by the US Department of Justice (Civil Rights Division, Public Access Section). The Justice Department's ADA web site is at *http://www.usdoj.gov/crt/ada.html*.

The Job Accommodation Network (JAN) is an international consulting service that provides free information about how employers can accommodate people with disabilities. The service also provides information about the Americans with Disabilities Act (ADA). JAN can be reached by calling (800) 526-7234.

If you think an employer has treated you in a way that violates the ADA, you might consider taking action to remedy the situation. Here are a few ideas:

- **Keep a journal.** It's smart to maintain a bound notebook to record all relevant events. Be sure to include dates and specific details.

- **Get a note from your doctor.** Sometimes all an employer needs is a letter from your physician stating you must have certain accommodations.

- **Review your employee handbook.** This booklet should outline the steps you need to take if you feel you are experiencing discrimination in the workplace. If necessary, speak to someone in your employer's human resources department who can explain the procedure you need to follow if you want to file a grievance.

- **Clearly identify your grievances and put them in writing.** When writing out your grievances, suggest potential solutions that create a win–win situation for you and the company. Then submit your letter to your employer.

- **Enlist the help of your union, if you belong to one.** Unions typically offer many resources and have experience fighting for people's rights.

- **Contact the Equal Employment Opportunity Commission (EEOC).** The EEOC is a federal agency where you can file complaints about discrimination or harassment in the workplace. You can call the EEOC toll free at (800) 669-4000. Or check out the website at *http://www.eeoc.gov/*. Most states also have their own Equal Employment Opportunity (EEO) agencies. For a list, see *http://equalopportunity. monster.com/agencies/*. If you feel you have been discriminated against because of your disability or a relative's disability, contact the EEOC. In the United States, a charge of discrimination generally must be filed within 180 days of the notice of the discriminatory act.

- **Exhaust all your administrative remedies.** As with insurance claims, it's required that you do this before retaining an attorney and going to court. Much of this process has already been described earlier. For example, if your company has a department that handles discrimination claims or has a handbook outlining a grievance process, follow these guidelines precisely. If you are in a union, file a grievance through its process. You must then register a complaint with EEOC and your state's EEO agency, although in some situations one or the other is sufficient. Remember that some state governments provide more protection than the federal one.

- **Go to court.** This is a last resort and one that many people—especially those who have a chronic illness—would prefer to avoid. Discrimination cases are sometimes difficult to prove, and the whole process of filing a lawsuit is often lengthy and stressful. If you choose to follow this course, make sure you have exhausted all your administrative remedies as described, and then find a lawyer who is an expert in employment law.

Stacy describes what she went through in the 1980s:

> I had recently started a new job at a major company when I started getting very ill. I barely got a few months in before I had to take some time off. My boss was not at all pleased. In fact, he literally said straight to my face that he'd never hire anyone again with Crohn's disease. Of course, I was in no condition to put up a fight. I went out on disability, and there was very strong pressure on me to leave the company. After six months they terminated me. This was before the ADA, but I'm sure what happened must have been illegal. However, I knew I wasn't going to be able to return to work. And I would not have been welcomed back by my boss. So I just let this one go. But it was a terrible experience to go through.

Not everyone has had such a difficult experience at work, as Cathy explains:

> I worked in accounting for many years. When I developed Crohn's, I kept working for a while, but it got harder and harder. Fortunately, I faced absolutely no discrimination at work. In fact, my supervisor was very concerned and understood about my need to go to the bathroom frequently. However, all the accommodations in the world weren't going to make a difference because it just became too difficult to get to work and function normally when there. However, I was very thankful I had a supportive work atmosphere during this difficult time. At least there was one less thing to worry about.

Family and Medical Leave Act (FMLA)

The FMLA was signed into law in 1993. It gives employees the option of taking twelve weeks of unpaid leave every year to attend to their own healthcare needs or to those of a child, spouse, or parent. To qualify, you need to

- Work for a company with at least 50 or more employees within a 75-mile radius

- Work for your company for at least one year

- Work at least 1,250 hours within the last year, which is a little more than half time

You don't have to take the twelve weeks all at once. You can spread your time away throughout the year, if necessary. However, the law requires that you give a 30-day notice to your employer if your need to take time off is foreseeable. You may have to pay for your own health insurance benefits during your time away, but this depends on your employer's policy. What is certain is that your benefits do not cease and your coverage is identical to that of when you are working. Your employer cannot penalize you for taking leave and also must guarantee to save your job or provide an equivalent one on your return. For more detailed information on this act, contact the US Department of Labor at (866) 487-9243 or see the web site at *http://www.dol.gov/esa/whd/fmla/*.

If you think your employer has violated this law, follow the steps outlined in the ADA section. The only difference is that you'd file a complaint with the US Department of Labor instead of the EEOC. Again, also file a complaint with your state's agency if it has one. Some states provide more rights and even paid leave under their own family leave laws. For a comparison between federal and state family leave laws, see the US Department of Labor's web site at *http://www.dol.gov/esa/programs/whd/state/fmla/index.htm*.

Disability

Most people with IBD are able to work. However, some with severe Crohn's or ulcerative colitis can reach a point where they can no longer work. This is often a scary prospect for people, but fortunately disability income is available for those who qualify.

Types of disability income

There are three main sources of disability income for people who are unable to work for extended periods: long-term disability insurance, Social Security Disability Insurance (SSDI), and Supplemental Security Income (SSI).

Long-term disability insurance

Many employers offer long-term disability insurance free or very reasonably to their employees. If your company offers such a plan, definitely sign up for it. If you get sick and have to take significant time off work, your insurance will pay a certain percentage—often 40 to 60 percent—of your salary. Most companies either require or strongly encourage you to also apply for SSDI so that this government-funded insurance will either completely take over or cover most of your monthly benefits. If

SSDI doesn't pay all you're entitled to, your long-term disability insurance will pay the difference. Some policies are renewable even if you leave the company, and some are not. If you have a choice, pick one that's not dependent on whether you stay with the company.

Cathy describes the process she went through:

> After my doctor recommended that I stop working, I first went on my company's short-term disability. When that ran out, my company's long-term disability plan kicked in. Under this, I was able to receive 60 percent of my original salary. I also had to apply for Social Security Disability Insurance, which was quite difficult for me to get. However, I finally did after about a year. However, once SSDI kicked in, it and the long-term disability insurance could still only equal 60 percent of my original salary. It's not the same as making what I was used to making, but I was very thankful for being able to get the benefits I did.

Social Security Disability Insurance (SSDI)

SSDI is available to disabled people who have worked long enough to acquire sufficient social security credits for their age. For you to qualify, your IBD must prevent you from doing the work you previously did as well as any other work you could do to earn a living. Your incapacity to work must last—or be expected to last—for at least one year. This definition of a disability is rigid, but both Crohn's disease and ulcerative colitis are included as illnesses that can qualify. However, your case must be severe enough to meet this disability definition as well as other criteria specific to these diseases. Monthly payments depend on your age and past earnings, but typically people can receive amounts equal to 40 to 60 percent of their original salary. For more information, call the Social Security Administration (SSA) at (800) 772-1213 or go to the web site at *http://www.ssa.gov/dibplan/index.htm*.

Supplemental Security Income (SSI)

SSI is available to the blind, disabled, or those over age 65 who have limited income and resources. Disabled people with IBD may decide to apply for it if they have never worked or have either worked too long ago or not long enough to qualify for SSDI. SSI is not funded through social security taxes, but instead through the federal General Revenue fund. As a result, eligibility is not based on whether you or other family members have worked or contributed a minimum amount into social security.

SSI is administered by the Social Security Administration (SSA). The criteria for having a disability are the same those for SSDI, but there are very strict limits on what other resources you can have. As of 2003, individuals who are eligible for SSI can receive up to $552 per month. Some states supplement this amount. To see if you qualify, call the SSA at (800) 772-1213 or go to *http://www.ssa.gov/notices/supplemental-security-income/*.

It's possible you can get both SSI and SSDI if your SSDI benefit is lower than the SSI income level for your state.

Getting disability

Receiving approval for SSDI or SSI is not always easy. Some people with IBD have no problems getting accepted; others experience a bitter, uphill battle before finally receiving benefits.

The SSA reports that 60 percent of people in 2001 were denied disability benefits the first time they applied.[1] Of the people who appealed for reconsideration in 2001, 84 percent were denied. However, those who persisted to the third level where they attended a hearing (before a judge) were accepted over 63 percent of time. If you are still denied after your hearing, you have another chance to appeal through an Appeals Council Review. In 2001, 20 percent of people who appealed through this council were granted approval. Thus, you generally have the best chance of acquiring benefits if you persist long enough to appeal before a judge. Keep in mind, too, that even if it takes months until you are approved, SSDI benefits are retroactive up to twelve months from the date of your application. In addition, SSDI claimants must wait five months from the onset date of their disability before receiving benefits. SSI benefits are retroactive to the date of your application or when you first contacted the SSA to apply for SSI.

Sandra had success at her hearing:

> *I had a wonderful job and great boss at a financial institution. I really wanted to keep working, but my illness was just too severe. I had tried applying for disability but was rejected. I appealed, and it eventually came to the point when I was to appear in court before a judge. I didn't really feel I needed a lawyer, but I hired one anyway since I thought he might be somewhat helpful. If anything, I think it makes you look like you are really serious. My lawyer didn't think I had a very good chance of getting disability because I looked too*

healthy. But I knew if I could explain my situation to a fair judge, I'd
be accepted.

At the hearing, the lawyer didn't have to do much. The judge wasn't
interested in hearing much from him but instead wanted to hear from
me. I explained from my heart everything I've been through with the
Crohn's. It's not an easy disease to discuss, but I told him all about in
a way that was clear, accurate, and personal, but not in anyway
crude. Usually, after a hearing, you have to wait 30 to 60 days before
receiving an answer. But right after my testimony the judge said he'd
accept my appeal. My lawyer said in the fifteen years he's been doing
this he'd never seen anyone get an answer right on the spot. But I did.
It just shows you can work within the system and win.

The following tips may also help increase your chances of getting on disability:

- **Work with your doctor.** Your gastroenterologist will play a major role in the process, because the SSA will partially rely on reports from him. Make sure you inform your physician about all the details of your symptoms and explain clearly what you can and can't do. Provide him with any written documentation you have. Your physician must write a very thorough report and state his opinion based on objective tests and findings. This is where organized, detailed, and comprehensive medical records come in handy.

- **Contact your congressperson.** If you are denied disability, you might try asking your elected officials for help. As mentioned earlier in this chapter, your representatives are there to help you. Their staff is equipped to handle all kinds of problems, including those regarding disability.

David had difficulty with the SSA, but found his congressman's staff very helpful:

I found the whole experience of applying for disability very
unpleasant. Although I came across a few caring people, some of them
were not too nice and treated me rather disrespectfully. For some
reason, they could not understand why I wasn't out interviewing for
jobs, when I had recently dropped to 134 pounds and had one of the
most severe cases of Crohn's that my doctor had ever seen. The
interviewers I had were condescending and didn't treat me kindly.
They also made me fill out forms that I had already filled out. I tried
to explain they already had them, but they insisted I fill out the same
forms again.

It's hard enough when you're already so sick, but then to be treated this way was just terrible. I'm not saying it's like this at all social security offices, but this was my experience. And after going through all this, my application was denied.

I visited my US representative's office and related my story to a woman there. She told me to write a letter, explaining my situation and why I needed their help. She simply gave me a notepad and I wrote it right then and there in the office. They must have acted fast, because within a month, I heard from the SSA and they accepted my application.

- **Hire a lawyer.** You might also consider hiring an attorney who specializes in helping people get disability benefits. Having a lawyer is often helpful for some people, especially if they are preparing for the hearing before a judge. Fees can vary, but commonly the attorney will only receive payment if you win. Most lawyers who specialize in disability law will also supplement your own doctor's reports with those of another physician who has experience writing reports for SSA.

Not everyone has problems getting disability; Stacy didn't have any:

My application was accepted the first time. I was never rejected. I'm not sure why I never had any problems. Perhaps it had something to do with my doctor and his ability to clearly state why I had to be on disability or why I couldn't work. I guess I can really never know. But I'm glad I didn't have to suffer through the stress that so many others have had to go through.

Getting off disability

Coming off disability is sometimes frightening for those who have been ill for a long time. People with IBD are often especially worried, because of the capricious nature of their disease. Crohn's and ulcerative colitis are often unpredictable, remitting and re-flaring for unknown reasons. Consequently, someone with IBD may fear going back to work after several months of good health. He wouldn't want to risk losing his disability benefits, because the disease may return with a vengeance only a few months later. Fortunately, the SSA has a process that gives people a trial period for going back to work. During this time, you don't lose your disability benefits. They are only discontinued if you are able to earn—on average over the trail period—an amount greater than what the SSA has determined to be a substantial income.

The SSA has a special voluntary program that can help people return to work. It's called Ticket to Work. This program:

- Gives people more choices for rehabilitation and vocational services to help them reach their employment goals

- Helps remove barriers so that people don't have to choose between work and healthcare coverage

- Allows people with disabilities to participate in the workforce and reduces their dependence on the public welfare system

For more information on Ticket to Work, go to *http://www.ssa.gov/work/*.

The SSA will review your case periodically to see if you still qualify for benefits. Time between reviews varies and is based on whether your health is expected to improve. If there is a strong likelihood of this happening, your reviews may occur as frequently as every six to eighteen months. If significant improvement is moderately possible, your reviews will occur every three years or so. If your medical condition is not expected to get better, the SSA may wait seven or more years.

Two things determine whether your benefits will stop:

- **If the SSA determines your health has significantly improved, and you are therefore no longer considered disabled.** This can happen if you inform them of a change in your health or if the SSA determines this based on one of your periodic medical reviews.

- **If you are able to earn what the SSA considers a substantial income.** In 2003, substantial income for people on SSDI is $800 per month. If you are on SSI, your benefits change based on your earned income. After your first $65 earned, they subtract $1 from your benefits for every $2 you make.

Stacy was able to get off SSDI:

> *I was on SSDI for almost twelve years. I was reviewed periodically and they kept renewing it for many years. Several times along the way I tried to work, but I was still too sick to earn a sustainable income. However, after I had my ileostomy surgery, my health improved. They determined that within a certain amount of time I should be able to earn a sufficient income.*
>
> *I was nervous about whether I could earn enough while maintaining my health, but I definitely wanted to give it a try. I*

decided to go into real estate since I felt I could have more flexibility with my schedule. Fortunately, my new career worked out—I was able to consistently earn a good amount of money per month. After about a year, I stopped receiving the benefits. I've been off over three years now and continue to work.

I wouldn't be able to work a regular eight to five job. Fortunately, I found something that allows me to regulate my schedule. Some days I can work; others I can't or have to work a short day. Since my husband and I work together, he can cover for me if I can't make it. I average about thirty hours a week.

It was scary when I first tried to go off because I really didn't know what my body would be able to handle. However, I tried and found something that worked. So it is possible to get off disability, even if you've been on it for as long as I was.

The stigma of disability

Some people have mixed feelings about receiving disability benefits. On the one hand, they may feel it's a lifesaver because it provides crucially needed money at a time when they are too sick to work. On the other, some people sometimes feel guilty about receiving it even though they qualify for and are totally deserving of it. For example, they may think others are more needy, or that they themselves should be contributing to the social security system instead of drawing on it. Or they may worry that other people are thinking they are taking advantage of the system.

Having these kinds of feelings is normal, especially if you are used to working and supporting yourself. If you are too ill to work, however, consider that SSDI and SSI were created to help people in just your situation. So instead of losing energy to guilt, try to accept the help you are receiving and focus on living the best life you can live, regardless of your health status.

Stacy shares her feelings:

I've always been open to talking about my Crohn's or my ostomy. However, it was difficult for me to talk about being on disability. It's not something I've shared with many people. I guess in some ways I felt guilty about it. I thought about others who were less fortunate than me financially. Or I thought how there were probably others out there who were even sicker than I was. My feelings were probably rooted in my strong work ethic, and how I felt I needed to earn my way. Sometimes I also felt like being on disability represented how I must have somehow failed or let the disease get me. I wanted to present a positive image that I could still keep doing everything despite the illness—and being on disability wasn't congruent with that image.

How did I learn to accept it? Well, it wasn't easy and it took a lot of time. I started with acknowledging that I was always honest with the SSA about my condition. Nothing was ever falsified and my medical records spoke for themselves. I realized, too, that I was very sick. I made sincere efforts to work on various occasions, but for twelve years my body couldn't handle it. I also had paid into the social security system—so I was eligible for benefits based on my condition and work history. My case was reviewed many times over the years, and the answer was always that I qualified to receive benefits. It wasn't till I had my ileostomy that they suggested I could work—and it turned out they were right. So really, the system worked the way it was intended.

Of course, for a long time, all the facts still didn't convince me that it was okay to be on disability. I'm not sure at what point I accepted it and let go of the guilt. I'd say it was just a gradual process that happened naturally over time. But even now—after three years of working again—it's one detail I don't go out of my way to mention when I discuss my experience with Crohn's.

Cathy shares her thoughts:

Yeah, at first I had some mixed feelings being on disability. It's hard to describe, but it just felt kind of strange going on it after working for seventeen years. But what can you do when life throws a severe case of Crohn's at you? I couldn't work anymore in my condition. So I had to go on it in order to take care of myself financially. I'm comfortable with it because it was designed for people in my situation. I'm thankful our society provides this safety net.

CHAPTER 17

Emotions and Coping

A CHRONIC ILLNESS such as IBD is often an emotional burden as well as a physical one. Although people with mild cases of Crohn's disease or ulcerative colitis may not experience much psychological impact, those with more serious or complicated illnesses frequently do.

This chapter focuses on the psychological aspects of living with ulcerative colitis or Crohn's. It covers the gamut of emotions people with these diseases often experience and offers practical ideas for coping with IBD and its associated symptoms. The chapter also discusses many different ways people with IBD seek emotional support.

Emotions

People with Crohn's disease and ulcerative colitis experience a wide range of emotional reactions to their illness. Different people have different responses, which is totally normal. Some may develop anxiety or depression; others may feel guilty, angry, fearful, or lonely. You may even feel a bit of all these at one time or another. Whatever feelings emerge, however, it's important to recognize them and realize they are a natural reaction to your situation. You'll then want to figure out the best way to deal with these feelings and take appropriate action.

The following sections review some common emotions people with IBD encounter as a result of their disease.

Anger

Some people with Crohn's or ulcerative colitis go through periods where they feel a lot of anger. Understandably, having a chronic illness that is often unpredictable and can interfere with your life plans is quite upsetting. It's therefore not unusual for people with IBD to feel angry at times.

Anger is a natural, human emotion. Many people get angry at the unfairness of having to live with a chronic illness. Others feel angry when symptoms interfere with their relationships, jobs, or hobbies. Problems with anger arise if it gets misdirected. Although people with IBD are usually angry at their disease, they sometimes direct this anger toward themselves or others. Anger at yourself usually solves nothing and often limits your ability to move forward and find solutions. Anger at others can alienate the people around you who might otherwise be able to help and support you.

Many people don't have effective ways to manage their anger. If you think you fall into this category, consider seeking support from a counselor who specializes in working with people who have chronic illnesses.

Susie had difficulty expressing her anger:

> *I never learned how to properly express anger when I was growing up. I guess it was just thought of as something bad. So when I got sick, I didn't know what to do with my feelings. I was actually quite angered by the injustice of it all. I feel I missed out on so much, like activities with my kids or holiday parties. But I either just kept the anger in or displaced it onto someone else.*
>
> *Over the years though, I've gradually learned how to manage my anger. I've worked with a therapist on and off for a long time. Also, I think I have slowly learned to just let go and move on. As a result, not only do I handle anger better but I have also learned to be more patient.*
>
> *My advice to anyone dealing with anger is that they indeed have a right to feel this way. Having IBD is lousy and it's 100 percent normal to feel angry about it. Acknowledging and expressing it are very important because you can then let it go and focus on dealing effectively with the disease.*

Mary discusses the anger her son experienced:

> *My son went through some significant anger and denial with his illness. Occasionally, some of the anger was directed at me, which was frustrating. But he was dealing with it the best way he knew how at the time.*
>
> *Working through the anger was not easy for him. It took a lot of time. Ultimately, he found he needed to work with his illness rather than continue with the anger against it.*
>
> *Another person I was speaking to probably explained it best. He described how a disease is like a river. You can't hold it back, because*

*there is too much force. If you try, it can sweep you away and you'll
drown. But if you can find a way to go with it, you'll find your way.
It was hard for my son to hear and accept this concept. But within the
last few years, I think he's been catching on to this idea. Instead of
fighting, resisting, and being angry with it, he's now more accepting
and working with the illness in order to get through it. It's not an easy
thing to do, especially when you are used to handling it with anger
and denial. But in long run, I think the anger and resistance make
things a lot more difficult.*

Anxiety and fear

The unpredictable and sometimes severe nature of Crohn's disease and ulcerative
colitis can provoke fear and anxiety in some individuals. This is completely normal.
When people experience a loss of health, they are also experiencing a major loss of
control in their lives. This can lead to feelings of fear and helplessness as they face the
unknown. If steps are not taken to help alleviate the situation, a constant state of
anxiety can sometimes set in.

Jamie explains how fear drained her energy:

*I've spent a lot of time worrying about my Crohn's. And I can't say
one moment of it has done anything to help. But for some reason, the
fear is hard to let go of. I think of so many different "what ifs," like
what if I don't get better, what if I lose my job, what if I don't make
it to the bathroom in time, or what if such and such happens. The
problem is that this type of thinking drains me of so much energy.
And in my case, I can't afford to waste any energy. It's too precious a
resource.*

*To help solve my problem, I've come up with a mantra: No fear.
Whenever my mind starts down the "what if" path, I just keep
repeating "no fear." It's not 100 percent effective, but it really has
helped calm me. I then focus on letting go of the things I can't control,
and then that frees me to focus on the things I can. This way, I make
the best use of my energy.*

Susie has had different fears and anxieties over the years:

*IBD has been difficult to deal with, and it certainly causes a variety
of fear and anxiety. You name it, and I've probably feared it at least at*

some point: colon cancer, being sick all time, my future, and also
pooping in my pants if I don't get to the bathroom in time.

What's really helped me is having such tremendous support from
my family, friends, and a supportive therapist. But after a while, I
reached a point, too, when I asked myself, "What's the worst that can
happen now?" I've been through so much. Although it's been very
difficult at times, I've always managed to get through. So whatever
happens in the future, I know I'll have the resources to get through
that as well.

Corticosteroid drugs such as prednisone can also contribute to anxiety in people taking high doses. For information on prednisone and its emotional side effects, see Chapter 12, *Coping with Prednisone*. For additional ideas on how to manage anxiety and other emotions, see the section on seeking support later in this chapter.

Depression

Depression is a serious disorder that sometimes arises in people with IBD. Contrary to what some people think, depression is not the same thing as being sad or dejected about a particular situation. Instead, it involves a pervasive sense of hopelessness that is often very overwhelming and paralyzing. Although most people with IBD do not develop depression, it does occur, especially in those who have been severely ill for a long time.

The good news is that depression is treatable. However, before you can treat it, you must first determine whether you have it. Here are some of the major symptoms of depression:

- Depressed mood for two or more weeks
- Loss of interest in pleasurable activities for more than two weeks
- Changes in appetite or weight
- Changes in sleeping patterns (either insomnia or excessive sleep)
- Noticeable agitation or a slowing-down of speech and movement
- Excessive fatigue
- Inappropriate feelings of guilt
- Poor concentration, indecisiveness, or hopelessness
- Recurring thoughts of death or feeling suicidal

If you believe you have depression, contact your doctor immediately and ask for a referral to a mental health professional. There's no use suffering when help is so readily available. Talk therapy is often very useful, and antidepressant drugs are also an option. Most experts think a combination of talk and drug therapy is the most effective way to treat depression. If your depression is mild and you want to avoid medications, ask your doctor or mental health care professional if they'd recommend any nondrug therapies. For example, many studies have found aerobic exercise reduces depressive symptoms as well as anxiety.[1]

Fish oil, which is sometimes used to treat IBD (see Chapter 7, *Diet and Complementary Therapies*), may also help depression. People in countries that consume large amounts of fatty fish—such as salmon or herring—have lower rates of this mood disorder.[2] If you opt for any herbal or other nonpharmaceutical supplements, check with your doctor and pharmacist to make sure they will not interfere with your other medications.

Larry has been battling depression for many years:

> *I've been under treatment for depression for about seven years.*
> *I've had a difficult time dealing with my Crohn's since it has involved*
> *many complications, including arthritis, kidney stones, and chronic pain.*
>
> *I've had the best success with a combination of both talk and drug*
> *therapy. Unfortunately, my HMO doesn't have a very good mental health*
> *program, so I've had to seek counseling from a psychotherapist in private*
> *practice. It's expensive, but it has been worth it. Fortunately, my*
> *depression is under control, but sometimes it's still a struggle. I'm very*
> *grateful though that there are now so many different treatment options*
> *available for people with depression.*

Corticosteroids, such as prednisone, can cause many changes in your mood, including depressive symptoms. Please see Chapter 12 for more details on the emotional impact of taking prednisone.

Frustration

Frustration is commonly experienced by people with IBD. Although not as serious as something like depression, probably almost everyone with Crohn's or ulcerative colitis has felt frustrated from time to time. This is likely due to IBD's chronic and unpredictable nature. Others may get frustrated because there are usually no simple answers when dealing with IBD.

Jamie comments:

> *I've experienced a lot of emotions with my Crohn's. Frustration is certainly a major one. The problem with Crohn's is that it's not a simple illness and often manifests itself in different ways. I can recall times when my doctor ordered tests and all they lead to were more questions and more tests. It gets exhausting and exasperating. It's not like you have something like strep throat and you can just take an antibiotic and be done with it. It's a lot more complicated. And that's what makes it so frustrating.*

Gina was very frustrated during the years she was sick:

> *When I was very sick it was extremely trying for me. I was doing everything right, but it didn't always help. It seemed so unfair. I was taking my medication, working closely with my doctor, and taking really good care of myself. Yet I could be doing all of this and still remain sick. And then you look around and see others not taking care of themselves and they are totally healthy. It was very frustrating.*

Guilt

Some people with IBD feel guilty about their illness. For example, some believe that if they only ate healthier when they were younger, or hadn't been so stressed recently, they could have prevented the disease. Others feel they did something to deserve this terrible illness, or think they are being punished for past deeds.

Larry discovered he had some guilt initially:

> *When I was first diagnosed, I found myself thinking that I must somehow have caused my illness. Sometimes I'd feel like God must be punishing me for something I did wrong. I was blaming myself for it.*
>
> *Fortunately, I managed to let go of this kind of thinking. It's not something that suddenly stopped one day. It just gradually happened over time. I took the time to learn about the illness and spoke to many other people about it, including others who had IBD. In combination with simply living with Crohn's for a while, this was enough to eventually make me realize that I really had done nothing wrong. I still don't know why I have it, but I have to trust that there must be a reason. In the meantime, I no longer blame myself or feel guilty that I caused it.*

Blaming yourself for your illness or feeling guilty that you somehow caused it serves no useful purpose. First of all, you did not cause your IBD; no scientific evidence suggests that people cause their Crohn's or ulcerative colitis. Second, guilt and blame are not going to do anything to help you get better. In fact, by blaming yourself, you are only making yourself a victim who—by most definitions—is powerless to improve his situation. Guilt and blame are therefore only going to immobilize you and interfere with your ability to take steps to improve your condition. If you have difficulty letting go of guilt or blame, it might help to talk with a therapist who specializes in adaptation to chronic illness.

An alternative to blaming yourself is simply to take responsibility in the present. Blame binds you to the past, where you are powerless and have no control. Taking responsibility for your situation in the present, however, is empowering. Regardless of why you have IBD, you can still take action and make choices that can positively influence your future. For example, by learning all you can about IBD and working proactively with your doctor, you can help make educated decisions regarding your treatment.

Carla has at times blamed her parents for her IBD:

> I was diagnosed with ulcerative colitis when I was 14 years old. Occasionally, I'll go through periods when I find myself blaming my parents for my IBD. When this happens, my strategy is to first let myself vent—not to my parents, of course, but just to myself. I'll give myself a half-hour or so on the "pity-pot," and then I tell myself that this is enough. Regardless of how I got ulcerative colitis, I know my parents were doing the best they could with what they knew at the time. I then tell myself that I have to accept what has already happened and take personal responsibility to deal with it. After all, it's my life and no one else's. I realize that there is much I can do, such as to take good care of myself, make an effort to work well with my doctor, and engage my mind in other thoughts and activities. This way, I divert my attention away from the illness. It's not always easy to do this, but I've been working with a therapist and have made considerable progress.

Guilt was never an issue for Jamie:

> I've never really taken a "why me" attitude or felt guilty about my illness. I mean, why anyone? I know I didn't cause it. As for having

IBD, I've never taken it personally or felt I was singled out. Sometimes things just happen and we can't fully understand why.

What does annoy me, however, is when other people—especially those who have never been seriously ill a day in their lives—imply that I somehow caused my illness. Or that if I just thought the right thoughts it would go away. It's really unfair to put that on someone. I think that kind of talk does much more harm than good. I'm not saying that there isn't any mind–body connection or anything like that, but I think it's really unfair to just go around saying people have caused their own illness. After all, how would they account for infants, from loving families, who develop life-threatening illnesses? It doesn't make sense.

Loneliness

People who have severe IBD may sometimes feel isolated or lonely. Unfortunately, if Crohn's or colitis is extremely active, symptoms such as severe fatigue and diarrhea can keep people temporarily homebound. If this goes on for too long, people can start feeling as if they are missing out on life or are not as much a part of it as before. Although symptoms may be difficult to control, there's still much that people with IBD can do to help alleviate feelings of isolation. The sections "Practical coping" and "Seeking support" in this chapter offer some ideas to help you feel less isolated.

Practical coping

People with IBD face many day-to-day challenges. Consequentially, they need various plans or strategies if they want to effectively get through a rough flare—or even a typical day. Many obstacles they face are directly related to various symptoms of their Crohn's or colitis. The following sections review how people with IBD have capably dealt with symptoms such as fatigue, pain, and urgency to minimize the illness's impact on their lives.

Fatigue

The fatigue associated with IBD can range from mild to severe. For some, it can be incapacitating. Many people, however, find themselves somewhere in the middle, where they can engage in some activities but have to limit others. If you're in this category, it's essential that you develop some kind of energy management plan. This way, you'll have the energy to accomplish the things that are most important to you.

Jamie explains how she manages with limited energy:

> I've had a lot of problems with fatigue over the years. My best advice is to just trust yourself since you know your body and energy level best. Listen to what it says and know your limitations.
>
> Even if I'm feeling well, I still think it's a good idea to pace myself. I'm relatively healthy now, but I still have to plan my days carefully. For example, if I have to put in a little more at work than I normally do, I'm careful to balance that with more downtime afterward. If friends want to do something after work, I'll often have to say no because I know I'll need to go home and rest. Likewise, if I'm going to be out late at night, I always make sure I'll have plenty of time to take it easy the next day. I know myself and what I can and can't do. Occasionally a few people can't seem to understand my limitations, but most do.

Susie shares an important lesson:

> I've had to deal with a lot of fatigue and exhaustion. If there's one thing I've learned from it, it's that you really have to honor your body. Before, I would always keep pushing myself to get everything done. And of course, my body would pay the price. Now that I've learned the lesson, I'm a different person. If I'm tired, I'll take a nap or go to sleep. If the kids need rides to places, I'll arrange for them to carpool with their friends' parents.
>
> There's only one of me and I only have one body. So if I need to rest, I need to rest. If there are errands or tasks that need to get done, I've learned to either ask for help or accept that it's okay to do them later.

Pain

Pain is a warning that some part of the body is injured or under distress. Nerves in the affected tissue send electrical impulses to your brain, causing you to have a very unpleasant sensation. Pain is very difficult to measure, because different people have different thresholds for it and various ways to describe it. Similar damage to tissue can cause unbearable pain in one person and only moderate discomfort in someone else. Not surprisingly, various people with IBD-associated pain experience a range of severities. Some have little or no pain, and others have severe pain quite often.

People with Crohn's disease and ulcerative colitis also report different types of pain. Certain individuals may have a crampy kind of discomfort that's at least partially relieved by passing gas or stool. Others may experience sharp, localized, abdominal pains, or just a dull, generalized stomachache. People with IBD-associated arthritis have pain in their joints.

Fortunately, not all people with IBD experience chronic pain. But for those who do, it's one of the worst aspects of the disease. When you're in pain, nothing else seems to matter.

If your pain suddenly worsens, it's important to contact your doctor immediately or head to the nearest emergency room. If, however, you live with a certain level of pain on a daily basis, or experience it from time to time, you'll have to find some way of dealing with it.

Jamie explains her strategies for dealing with pain:

> Although I avoid pain medication when I can, I will take a Vicodin if I really need it. However, if the pain is bearable, I'll first try and handle it on my own. I try to use a variety of mind–body techniques, such as meditation, visualization, or simply some deep breathing exercise to induce relaxation. I try to relax into the pain as much as possible. This is a lot easier said than done. Sometimes it works, but sometimes it doesn't. Other times it just works partially. Like I said, if it starts getting too bad, I will take a pain pill. Otherwise, it becomes what I call a "pain drain," depleting my energy.
>
> Another thing that I do is keep a heating pad hanging on my bed's headboard. I keep it turned off, but I leave it plugged in. This way, if I'm having pain in the middle of the night, I barely have to move to put the heating pad on my belly. I simply grab it and flip the switch.

Larry has suffered from chronic pain for many years:

> My case is unusual in that I have pain from four different sources: abdominal pain from Crohn's, joint pain from my IBD-related arthritis, acute pain from recurring kidney stones, and back pain from a damaged disc. It's not a good combination, to say the least. I'm fortunate, however, that my hospital has a very good pain program for people in my situation. I've been in it for three years now and it's a godsend. The people are not only willing to listen, but they actually understand what I'm going through. I have access to different pain medications when I need them, and they never treat me as if I'm some kind of drug addict. They treat me like a regular person who just happens to have some severe medical

problems. I'd recommend to anyone with chronic pain to get into some kind of pain program. I can't imagine how my life would be without it.

Susie shares her advice:

> I think it's really important to find a pain specialist if you're dealing with chronic pain. I know it made a big difference for me. It was reassuring that I was working with an expert who knew how to properly prescribe the various medications. I was extremely afraid of getting addicted. But my doctors explained to me that it would be very difficult for me to heal if all my energy and calories were going towards fighting the pain. They also assessed me and said that not only did I not have an addictive personality, but that I would be under very close medical supervision. This made me feel better, so I tried the medicines. I was on high amounts for a while. But sure enough, the doctors were right. The medications helped me to manage my pain and I didn't become addicted.

Urgency and diarrhea

Urgency and diarrhea are two of IBD's most dreaded symptoms. Not only can they cause much embarrassment, but they can significantly interfere with people's lives. If you're constantly worried about where the nearest bathroom is and whether you can make it there in time, your quality of life is sure to suffer. Some people may become so worried about having an accident that they even fear leaving their homes. If this describes you, please know that many others with IBD have faced similar circumstances and have found creative ways to work around their urgency and diarrhea.

Cathy shares her strategies:

> Diarrhea and urgency have always been a problem for me. There were times I was scared to leave the house because I didn't want to have an accident. I was especially concerned, too, when I was driving around in my car. One solution that worked for me was to become very familiar with areas I traveled through. I'd then make a point to know where all the good bathrooms were. Certain fast food restaurants and gas stations were always convenient. But you really need to scope each one out because some places have terrible restrooms. It also helps to have a handicap sign in your car. This way, you always have a close parking place to stores and won't have to run across large parking lots to make it to the bathroom in time. The handicap parking spots also come in handy when fatigue is a factor.

Unfortunately, all of this was still not enough for me. Sometimes when I have to go, there's no time to reach a good restroom. I solved this problem by buying a minivan. In the back, I have my own porto-potty. If I'm in unfamiliar territory, or there's just no time to make it anywhere, I can pull over and go in the comfort of my own van. I don't need to do this very often, but the security it gives me is priceless.

Larry shares his tips:

Wherever I go, I always bring an extra pair of clothes, including underwear, of course. Along with that, I keep roll of paper towels and roll of toilet paper. These go with me in my car everywhere I go. If on a given day I know that there is a greater chance of having an accident, I'll take some anti-diarrhea medication and limit what I eat. Sometimes I'll also wear one of those Depend undergarments. I call it my extra layer of hope!

Diarrhea and urgency never got the best of Stacy:

I strongly believe in not letting my illness interfere with my life. There's too much to do and too much to live for. When I still had my colon, I wouldn't hesitate to wear a big diaper if I needed to go somewhere. If I felt insecure driving in rural areas where there were no restrooms, I'd bring a big coffee can and toilet paper, pull over on the side of the road, and go behind the trees. I would then just snap the lid back on and then dispose of it when I get to my destination. I wasn't going to let IBD stop me from going anywhere.

Seeking support

People with IBD have access to many sources of help. Some find great strength from their faith; others use humor to cope. Face-to-face support groups and online support communities are relatively new resources many people are taking advantage of today.

The most common methods of support are reviewed next. Different people have different preferences for what provides comfort and support. The important thing is to choose something—or several somethings—that can help restore a sense of peace, balance, and control in your life.

Faith

Faith, religion, and spirituality are integral parts of many people's lives. They are often a source of strength and sustenance for those with IBD, especially when Crohn's or colitis is creating chaos and uncertainty in their lives. Having a regular spiritual practice can help you feel calm, secure, and at ease, even if your physical body is out of whack. In fact, research has shown that people who pray frequently—even if they have more physical health problems—have better mental health than those who pray less often.[3]

Facing a chronic illness can cause a wide range of effects on people's spirituality. Some may experience a deepening of their faith, whereas others may start questioning long-held beliefs.

Brenda experienced both:

> *I think having a chronic illness like IBD makes you really take a look at what you believe. I know in my case—at first—it made me seriously question my faith. So many different "why" questions came up, such as "why would God let this happen to me?" I wrestled with these questions for years. Along the way, I'd try to bargain with God, but over time I realized the disease didn't have anything to do with what I did or didn't do. Over time, I learned to trust and have faith that all would work out. And really, it has, and I've learned so much along the way. Ultimately, my whole experience with Crohn's has truly deepened my faith.*

Attending religious services and/or being a part of a spiritual community is often very helpful for people with chronic illnesses and their families. The social and spiritual support from such groups is priceless. Other members of the community are usually more than happy to provide an abundance of whatever is needed, including prayers, hospital visits, home-cooked meals, and baby-sitting.

Ann is very thankful for her church community:

> *Our church community has been a wonderful source of support for our family since the time my son was diagnosed with Crohn's disease. At first, my husband and I wondered if we were being too open about the illness. But we didn't want to hide what was going on since hiding things only inspires fear. Plus, my son was okay with us sharing the information. In fact, I know he has really appreciated how the whole*

church community has been rallying around him and praying for him.
I know it's made a positive difference for him, as well as our whole
family.

Humor

People with various chronic diseases often use humor as a means of coping with their illness. Humor can distract your attention away from your problems, while at the same time lightening your mood. Laughter initiates the release of endorphins, which are naturally produced, mind-altering chemicals that make you feel good. Although controlled research is needed to determine its true efficacy, laughter may help people with various health problems, especially if they deal with a lot of pain.

Everyone has a slightly different concept of humor. What's funny to one person is sometimes offensive to another. Hence, it's important that you be the one to choose what comic material you want. Some may prefer the old sitcom classics, whereas others may get more laughs out of modern-day movies or people doing stand-up comedy routines. Consider taking advantage of all that's around you. Cable companies now offer viewers hundreds of channels and some video stores can locate just about any video available. Experiment and see if you can find something that can make you laugh, or at least lighten your mood.

Humor helped Larry:

> *I've read Norman Cousin's book,* Anatomy of an Illness, *which describes how Norman helped heal himself of his illness—not IBD— by incorporating laughter therapy with his other treatments.*
>
> *I believe humor is a powerful therapy. I prefer comedy movies and watch them on video. I also listen to audiotapes of stand-up comedians. They are a good distraction and help me take my mind off my illness. Laughter though is not only a distraction, but it creates a physiological change in my body. I have chronic pain and I've noticed it helps lessen it a little.*

Jamie discusses how humor has helped her:

> *I think humor is a great coping mechanism. Sometimes it's easier to make a joke about something rather than talk seriously about what's going on. I use it around everyone, including friends, family, and even*

hospital staff. IBD is of course a serious illness, but sometimes it helps to joke about it, especially since it's such a crappy disease.

Mary shares a story about her son:

> *My son has been undergoing Remicade treatments. I was talking to him recently after an infusion and asked him how he was feeling. He said, "I'm fine, Mom. But I had to stop at the store on the way home and pick up some cheese. I'm nibbling on it now." He was trying to be funny, since Remicade is partially made from mouse proteins!*

Richard shares some of his IBD humor:

> *Crohn's and ulcerative colitis are serious diseases. However, I've found over the years that people with these illnesses appreciate a good IBD joke now and then. Several years ago, CCFA used to have an annual bowl-a-thon to raise money for research. I'd sometimes ask my IBD buddies and other friends if they wanted to sponsor me for the bowel-a-thon. Another joke goes as follows: What did the IBD patient say to Vanna White when he was on Wheel of Fortune? The answer: Vanna, I'd like to buy a bowel. I know, these are corny. But sometimes corny can help put a smile on your face.*

Mind–body therapies

Researchers are just beginning to understand the intricacies of how the mind and body are connected. The good news is, you don't have to wait till they figure everything out to take advantage of potential benefits. Many different mind–body therapies are available to help ease symptoms and restore some balance and harmony in your life. The following therapies are some of the most common ones used today.

Biofeedback

Biofeedback is a method that teaches people how to consciously control certain bodily processes by using signals from their own bodies. People can learn to control heart rate, blood pressure, muscle tension, or other physiological indicators that are normally regulated involuntarily. Although scientific evidence for biofeedback's use in IBD is lacking, biofeedback can potentially benefit people with Crohn's or ulcerative colitis, especially for those with pain, diarrhea or urgency. Biofeedback can possibly help people slow their peristaltic contractions so that bowel contents do not move through so quickly.

Guided imagery

Guided imagery is a technique that uses your imagination to invoke a relaxation response. Once in this peaceful state, you can continue to use imagery to visualize anything you want for yourself, such as a healthy, un-ulcerated colon, a balanced immune system, a better relationship with a loved one, or normal bowel movements. The possibilities are endless; the only limit is your own imagination.

Guided imagery uses all your senses, including smell, sight, sound, touch, and even taste. The idea is to create imagery exercises that incorporate the types of images you enjoy. There are many good books and tapes on this topic, which are listed in the *Resources* appendix at the end of this book. You might also consider working with a therapist who specializes in guided imagery. The Academy for Guided Imagery can help locate a specialist near you. The phone number is (415) 389-9324, and the web site is at *http://www.interactiveimagery.com/*.

Cheryl has used guided imagery:

> Guided imagery has helped me, especially when I've been in a lot of pain. One exercise I do is to visualize my bowel in my mind. I begin by seeing the redness and inflammation and then watch as the sores heal over. I also picture myself breathing out the "darkness" of the disease and breathing in a nourishing, golden light. As this golden energy permeates my body, I see the inflammation subsiding. This exercise certainly didn't cure me, but I really do believe it helped with the pain and made some of my flares less severe.

Guided imagery has helped Larry:

> My guided imagery exercises provide me a sanctuary where I can go when I need to get away. My special place is one where I went as a kid. There's a creek as well as a pond with a little waterfall. It's definitely an aquatic environment, with plenty of frogs and fish. There are also lots of trees. I've found that coming here during my visualization exercises really helps with my pain and can even slow down my bowels. It's definitely a wonderful adjunct to my other treatments.

Meditation

Meditation is a technique people use to calm and center themselves. It usually involves focusing your attention on a single object, word, or thought. It's generally suggested that you pick a quiet spot and sit in a comfortable position. Then you might close your eyes repeat the word "love" or "health" to yourself over and over. Others try to concentrate on their breathing. It's natural at first to become distracted. You'll find your mind wants to wander to other thoughts or worries. Calmly let these other concerns pass through, and gently bring your attention back to your chosen thought. In time, you'll get better and better at staying focused. The idea is to clear your mind of all distracting thoughts and achieve an inner state of calm, peacefulness, and heightened awareness.

Cheryl has found meditation very beneficial:

> I'm the kind of person whose mind is always going and going. I grew up in an environment that always emphasized productivity and doing as many activities as possible. Meditation has been great since it helps me clear my mind and slow down. I've been doing it a year and a half now, and I still set aside twenty minutes a day for it. I have to say for the first six months it was very difficult for me to focus and let all my other thoughts go. But then I finally got the hang of it. On one hand, you have an almost "out of body" experience while doing it. Yet when I'm through meditating I feel more connected and in touch with my body. I realize that sounds paradoxical, but it's been my experience.
>
> Like guided imagery, meditation did not cure my Crohn's, But I now function much more productively and cope with things much better with a clearer, more calm—as well as more relaxed—mind.

Online support

It's hard to believe that as recently as the mid-1990s, the average person had not even heard of the Internet. Yet by 2002, it was estimated that nearly two-thirds of Americans have access to it.[4] One out of five Americans even state that the Internet is the most essential communication medium in their lives.[5] As computers reach into more and more households across the United States and the world, having Internet access is destined to become as commonplace as having a telephone or television.

The Internet has become an important resource for people with various chronic illnesses. Those with IBD who are very sick and temporarily homebound often consider it a godsend. Regardless of the severity of your disease, the Internet offers benefits for just about anyone who is interested. Internet chat rooms, discussion boards, and listservs make the world a much smaller place. They enable people from almost any place on earth to network, share ideas, and offer support—all from the comfort of their own home and at any time of the day. The CCFA web site at *http://www.ccfa.org/* offers links to many of these resources (click on "Links.")

The Internet has been valuable to Susie:

> *The Internet has been a wonderful resource for me. I've used the CCFA web site a lot for general information. I've also made use of a couple other web sites that have chat or discussion rooms. My favorite is the jpouch.org site. I can't say enough good things about it. I've gotten everything from this community: medical tips, practical tips, empathy— it's really been an uplifting experience. I've made many good friends, too, that I've talked to on the phone and even met in person.*

Pets

Pets are often very therapeutic for people with chronic illnesses. Dogs, cats, and other animals can provide their owners with much love, affection, comfort, and companionship. They can also ease some of the loneliness and isolation that some people with severe IBD face.

Larry has derived many benefits from his dog:

> *I'm a big advocate of pet therapy for those with chronic illness. I know in my case, it's made a tremendous difference. First of all, having to take care of an animal helps me take my mind off myself. My dog is also very loyal and affectionate and is always there when I need him. When I'm having an acute episode of pain, for instance, he curls up with me and just stays with me till it passes. I'd say pet therapy is at least equivalent to a few pain pills a day!*

Researchers have studied the therapeutic benefits of having pets, and many have found them helpful to people facing illness. Although no studies have specifically looked at pet therapy for IBD, researchers have found that pet ownership helps reduce blood pressure response to mental stress in people with hypertension.[6] Although it hasn't been formally studied, conceivably this kind of stress-reducing effect might improve the quality of life in those with Crohn's or colitis.

Psychotherapy

Psychotherapy—whether individual, couples, or family—is often helpful for people facing chronic illness. After all, developing a disease such as IBD can be a major blow. You may experience the gamut of emotions, including many of the ones discussed earlier in this chapter. Remember, it's not a sign of weakness to seek professional support if you need help managing your feelings or assistance in adapting to the Crohn's or colitis. In fact, it takes a strong person to realize he needs help—and an even a stronger one to go out and get that support.

Types of mental healthcare professionals

There are many different kinds of mental health professionals. In making your decision, it helps to understand the different levels of training and education for the various types of mental health care. You will be able to choose from professionals trained (see the academic degrees noted in parentheses) in one of these five related fields:

- **Psychology (EdD, MA, PhD, PsyD).** Marriage and family psychotherapists have a master's degree; clinical and research psychologists have a doctorate. (Some states may also allow those with a master's degree to use the title "psychologist.")

- **Social work (MSW, DSW, PhD).** Clinical social workers have either a master's degree or a doctorate in a clinically emphasized program.

- **Pastoral care (MA, MDiv, DMin, PhD, DDiv).** Laymen or members of the clergy who receive specialized training in counseling.

- **Medicine (MD, RN).** Psychiatrists are MDs, medical doctors (and only medical doctors are permitted to prescribe medications). In addition, some nurses obtain postgraduate training in psychotherapy.

- **Counseling (MA).** In most states, school and agency counselors must have a master's degree and a year of internship before they can be hired as a counselor. To be a licensed professional counselor (LPC) requires a master's degree, additional coursework, hundreds or thousands of hours of supervised counseling experience, and passage of a state licensing exam.

The designations LCSW (Licensed Clinical Social Worker), LSW (Licensed Social Worker), LMFCC (Licensed Marriage and Family Child Counselor), LPC (Licensed Professional Counselor), LMFT (Licensed Marriage and Family Therapist) refer to licensure by state professional boards, not academic degrees. These initials usually follow others that indicate an academic degree. If they don't, inquire about the therapist's academic training.

You may hear all these professionals referred to as "counselors" or "therapists." Most states require licensure or certification in order for professionals to practice independently; unlicensed professionals are allowed to practice only under the supervision of a licensed professional (typically as an "intern" or "assistant" in a clinic or licensed professional's private practice).

Choosing a psychotherapist

Choosing a psychotherapist is similar to choosing a doctor. Here is a brief list of items you might consider when trying to find the right therapist:

- **Identify what you are looking for.** What kind of therapist do you want? For instance, you probably want someone who has experience working with people who have a chronic illness. Would the gender of your therapist make a difference? Would you prefer someone who uses a psychodynamic approach or one who specializes in cognitive-behavioral therapy? To learn more about different types of therapy, go to *http://www.strisik.com/therapy/approaches.htm*. The *Resources* appendix also lists resources on psychotherapy.

- **Get referrals.** You may not know where to begin looking for a suitable therapist. However, you probably already have many resources to assist you. Gastroenterologist, nurses, hospital social workers, other people with IBD, and the CCFA are all good places to start. The American Association for Marriage and Family Therapy (AAMFT), the American Psychological Association (APA), the National Association of Social Workers (NASW), and the American Psychiatric Association (also abbreviated APA) can provide referrals as well. Please see the *Resources* appendix for the phone numbers and web sites of these organizations.

- **Interview.** Once you have a handful of referrals, it's time to start calling therapists. When calling, be candid and explain you are in the process of searching for a therapist. You can choose to interview candidates over the phone or in person. Some therapists provide fifteen or twenty minutes free of charge to meet; others charge for their time.

- **Check credentials.** It's a good idea to check your therapist's credentials to ensure you are seeing someone who is professionally qualified. Depending on what type of therapist you choose, you'll need to contact one of the professional organizations just mentioned. Because psychiatrists are physicians (MDs), you can also refer to the information contained in Chapter 9, *Working with Your Doctor,* when checking their credentials.

- **Go with the one who feels right.** After talking with several therapists and evaluating their credentials, it's time to make a decision. It's important to choose someone with whom you feel comfortable.

Richard explains the process he went through:

> When I was trying to find a therapist, I started by asking a few
> people in the psychology field whom I already knew. I especially

wanted someone who was familiar with working with people with chronic illness. I assembled a list of about five people or so and just started calling. A couple of them weren't taking new clients, but then they referred me to another colleague who they thought might be appropriate. I spoke to several on the phone, and then narrowed my choices down to two—one PhD and one LCSW—who I wanted to meet. I asked if I could visit with each for just ten or fifteen minutes free of charge so I could get a better feel for them. I had in mind that I really wanted to see someone with a PhD, but after meeting with them, it was clear that I felt much better about the therapist with the LCSW. So I chose her and it worked out really well.

Getting the most out of psychotherapy

Some people are not clear on what psychotherapy can offer, especially if they have never experienced it. People with IBD can derive a variety of benefits from seeing a mental health professional. For instance, psychotherapy can help you:

- Learn to accept your illness

- Learn to use specific coping skills for disease-related problems

- Deal with emotions that arise

- Gain insight into how your mind and body are connected

- Get along better with friends and family if IBD is contributing to disharmony

- Live more productively and meaningfully with your illness

Psychotherapy was very helpful to Susie:

> *I've been in therapy on and off since 1995. I go in spurts. I have to say it's nice to have a long-term relationship with a therapist for so many years. The support she has provided has been invaluable. She listens with a non-threatening ear, and helps me focus on where I am, whether it's with basic survival or higher-level things. For example, when I was extremely ill and in a lot of pain, she suggested I focus on living breath-to-breath—not even day-to-day or hour-to-hour. She has also given me many ideas for coping over the years and has really helped me to accept the limitations that come with my illness. I've always been able to count on her.*

Cheryl has derived a lot of benefits from seeing a psychotherapist:

> *I'm a big proponent of psychotherapy. I realize it's not for everyone, but I think it can help a lot of people. Crohn's and ulcerative colitis — especially if they are severe — can be so emotionally debilitating. It's important to get professional support when you need it.*
>
> *Psychotherapy has helped me deal with so many different issues surrounding my illness, such as learning to accept it and learning to let go of things I can't control about it. The invisibleness of the disease was also difficult for me. When I was sick I felt so misunderstood by others since I looked healthy. My therapist helped give me a new perspective. I learned to give up trying to control other people's reactions, and instead have learned methods to cope with whatever situations arise. Overall, my therapist has helped me to drastically reduce the level of stress in my life — and this makes life so much more enjoyable.*

Support groups

Attending a support group where you can meet and interact with others who have IBD is often an empowering experience. No matter how loving and supportive everyone else in your life is, no one can understand or empathize quite like another person who has Crohn's or ulcerative colitis. These meetings are a place where ideas and information are exchanged, feelings are shared, and support and empathy abound.

There are hundreds of IBD support groups across the United States. Go to the web site at *http://www.ccfa.org/chaptevents/* or call (800) 932-2423 to find out if there is one near you. If not, you might consider trying to start your own. Your local CCFA chapter can list your name and phone number in their local newsletter as someone interested in forming a group in or near your hometown. Others living near you may also be interested.

Stacy found a demand for such support groups in her local area:

> *After having a serious bowel perforation, I decided it was finally time to go to a support group. Although I lived in a metropolitan area that had other meetings within a half-hour's drive, there wasn't one in my local area. I called the CCFA and they put me in touch with another woman who was also interested in setting up a group. We worked together to form the support group, and we became the co-facilitators.*

Support groups are also found in other countries besides the United States. The Resources appendix has contact information for IBD organizations in other countries, as does the CCFA web site: *http://www.ccfa.org/overseas/overseas.htm*.

Support groups are not for everyone, however. Some people prefer not to attend the meetings and find other ways of coping that work better for them. If you have a mild case of IBD, for example, it may be too overwhelming to hear about others having so many different problems or complications. You might go to a meeting once or twice to see what it is like and continue to go for years, or you might decide that it's just not the right thing for you.

Susie went to a meeting once:

> I went to a support group meeting one time. I found it somewhat helpful, but I decided it really wasn't what I needed. I have my own self-made support system that consists of a core group of friends and family. Along with my therapist and the support I get online, I have what I need.

Many people, like Stacy, have found support group very beneficial:

> Support group was such a wonderful experience. There wasn't anything negative about it, except for an occasional difficult person coming to the meetings. I've always found that the best way to take control of a situation is to educate myself about it. And support groups were a major way for me to stay informed of everything. As a facilitator, I worked closely with my local CCFA chapter, and they always provided me with all the latest information. I also learned so much interacting with so many different people. It was a good feeling, too, knowing that I was doing what I could to help others with IBD. But as much as I gave, I also received. It was such a relief for me to know that others were going through the same thing as I was. And I certainly received a lot of emotional support from the group, too. I highly recommend the meetings for anyone facing Crohn's or ulcerative colitis.

Susie sums up her feelings on all the resources available to her:

> It's really amazing what's out there. We're fortunate that we live in a day and age where we have so many different resources available. However, it's not going to make much difference what's out there if you

are not open to receiving it. I know at first this was a big issue for me. I didn't know how to accept help. I was always used to being self-sufficient. But IBD taught me that accepting and receiving is as important as giving. It's been an extremely valuable lesson. I'm glad I didn't miss out on the outpouring of love and support that I have received the last few years.

CHAPTER 18

Living Well with IBD

LIVING WITH IBD is frequently a challenge for newly diagnosed individuals and long-time veterans alike. However, as horrible as Crohn's disease and ulcerative colitis are at times, people with these illnesses can lead enjoyable, productive, and meaningful lives. It may be more difficult for some than others, but most people with IBD find creative and effective ways of doing so.

The major goal of this final chapter is to give you ideas on how to make the most of life despite having IBD. Even if you continually struggle with your illness, it's still possible to experience a sense of healing in your life despite a lack of healing in your intestines. Throughout the chapter, people with ulcerative colitis and Crohn's share how they have used the negative experience of having a life-altering disease to create a renewed sense of meaning and purpose in their lives.

Finding positive in the negative

It may seem strange to think anything positive could ever result from having IBD. Crohn's disease and ulcerative colitis are potentially life-threatening illnesses that can cause many different problems, including much grief. The physical and emotional toll is significant, and no one should try to minimize the negative impact of either disease. However, some people with IBD have managed to find positive things—not in the disease itself, but in the different life experiences generated by having the disease. Although they probably wouldn't have chosen this path for themselves, some people with Crohn's disease and ulcerative colitis have found their illness has guided them directly or indirectly to different but more meaningful careers, new relationships, or new perspectives on what's really important in life.

Work and volunteerism

Most people with IBD are able to work and excel in their chosen fields. However, Crohn's disease and ulcerative colitis can sometimes interfere with employment and professional goals. But instead of giving up hope, many with IBD have taken the opportunity to create more meaningful vocations for themselves. And many have realized what a difference they can make through volunteering.

Crohn's disease prompted Karen to carve out a new career:

> Before I was diagnosed with Crohn's disease I was working at a frantic pace. I'm a licensed clinical social worker and had been working as an administrator in this field for a county health department. I was working at least 50 to 60 hours per week and my job involved a lot of out-of-town travel. It wasn't like I hated my job, but the schedule was just so intense. There was not enough time to take care of my family, let alone myself.
>
> When I got sick, everything had to stop. I was in so much pain and running back and forth to the bathroom that I couldn't continue. I was miserable for almost a year. When I finally got my condition under control, I realized I didn't want to return to the kind of work I was previously doing. I needed to find something that allowed me to still contribute to society, but at a saner pace. I decided that what I really wanted to do was personal coaching. I could use my background as a counselor, help people achieve their personal goals, and still have the time and flexibility to take care of myself. My new career has been very rewarding and I wouldn't trade it for anything. What's funny is that I may not have gotten into this field if it hadn't been for my Crohn's disease.

Stacy had to adjust her career, too:

> I had a career in finance back in the 1980s. I became so ill that for twelve years I couldn't work. It was an extremely difficult period in my life and it's certainly not one I'd like to relive. Fortunately, I finally reached a point when my health improved. It was looking like I could work, and I had to decide what I wanted to do. It was important to me to choose something that enabled me to personally and directly help people. For me, the answer was real estate. It's the most wonderful feeling when I help find someone a home. What's also nice is that this kind of job gives me flexibility to spend time with my children. It comes in handy, too, when I have days I'm not feeling so great. I basically can set my own hours and still earn enough money. If

I never had Crohn's, I'd probably be stuck in some corporate hole crunching numbers and never have enough time to spend with my family. I'm not saying a career in finance couldn't be rewarding for someone else. But in retrospect, I'm glad I had the opportunity to find something different that ended up working better for me. And oddly, I have Crohn's to thank for that.

Sandra's lifelong experience with Crohn's prompted her to become involved with meaningful volunteer work:

I've had Crohn's ever since I was a baby. I know what it's like growing up with a chronic illness. This experience has moved me to help other children with chronic illnesses—and their parents—deal with the emotional impact of it all.

Although I still have health problems myself, I am able to volunteer several hours a month at a local children's hospital. It makes me feel good to be able to give back to the world what I've been given—a lot of love and support. My experience with IBD has equipped me to help children with all different kinds of illnesses cope better. It's difficult to describe in words how rewarding it is when I can do something that makes a sick child happy. But it's truly a blessing and I'm so thankful I have the ability to do it.

Jamie found she could do a lot of good through fundraising:

My experience with Crohn's has prompted me to do what I can to raise money for better treatments and—ultimately—a cure for IBD. Raising money through the CCFA walk-a-thons and bowl-a-thons has been empowering for me because it's something over which I have direct control. I don't know how to find a cure myself, but I can raise money, which enables researchers to make greater progress toward this goal. I feel a lot better doing this than just sitting around and waiting for my next flare.

I'm at a point where I can bring in about $2,000 to $3,000 per event. I'm also on my local CCFA's walk-a-thon committee and teach other people my strategies for fundraising. If we can all bring in a couple of thousand dollars—or even a few hundred—we will greatly diminish the time till we have better treatments and a cure.

Relationships

IBD can affect major relationships for better and for worse (see Chapter 13, *Relationships*). Although not everyone is so lucky, some people have unexpectedly found that IBD led them to new friends and enhanced relationships with loved ones.

Having Crohn's steered Cheryl toward many wonderful people:

> I've had Crohn's for 25 years. It's been a rough road, and I don't think it's one I'd choose to live over again. But I can acknowledge that a number of good things have come out of the whole experience. One of these is some of the people I've gotten to know along the way— including those from my support group. There's a lot of camaraderie in our group. It is so wonderful to actually be able to laugh with others about the horrors of IBD. I feel very connected to these people and I have learned so much from all of them. They're like a database I always have access to and can draw from whenever I need something. What's nice, too, is that my relationships with some of the people go beyond the group. I have made some true friends who I never would have met if I hadn't developed my illness.

Susie's illness experience helped her discover how much she is loved:

> I received an outpouring of love from many different friends and family members. But the support from my husband has just been phenomenal. My illness has been a major stress in our lives, yet he's stayed with me through it all. As a result, our love has grown stronger and stronger.
>
> Let's face it—I got the short stick in life. There's nothing good about IBD. But through even the worst of it, I've still found some good things to be thankful for. My husband is one of them.

Perspective

Sometimes you don't know how good you have it until you don't. This statement basically sums up how many people feel once they are stricken with a chronic illness such as IBD. When a disease robs you of your health, vitality, and ability to do what you wants to do, your perspective on life may change. What used to seem important suddenly doesn't anymore. And the things that used to be taken for granted can quickly become greatly appreciated.

Crohn's gave Stacy a new perspective on life:

> *I think almost anyone with a chronic illness is going to see things a bit differently than the average person. I know for me—after all I've been through—I don't sweat the small stuff anymore. I've been through the big stuff and don't let life's minor problems get to me the way I used to.*
>
> *I think my experience with Crohn's has also enabled me to appreciate things in life more. What kinds of things? Well—for one—a good roll of toilet paper! But seriously, I never take my family, friends, and health for granted. I also greatly appreciate my ability to eat and enjoy food. Another thing I'm thankful for is simply the ability to get out every day and feel like I'm a normal part of the world. Of course, just because you are sick doesn't mean you're not a normal part of the world. But it's different when you are so ill that you are essentially homebound and can't even make it to the mailbox, much less the grocery store. To have the freedom to go out and do what I want is something I never take for granted anymore.*

Larry has learned to better appreciate things, too:

> *Make no mistake, Crohn's is a terrible disease. But I'll admit that it has made me appreciate certain things in life. It's made me realize how valuable time is because I have less of it per week that I can enjoy and use productively. Since my case is severe and I'm frequently in a lot of pain, I maybe have only 20 to 30 hours a week that I can enjoy and use productively. It's frustrating because it used to be at least triple that. However, this limited amount of time really makes me appreciate not only how valuable time itself is, but also the beauty there is in life, such as in art, nature, or simply a comfortable, peaceful moment.*

Cheryl doesn't take much for granted either:

> *I go for a walk every day, and I literally do stop and smell the roses!*

Finding meaning

Some people come to terms with their illness by finding meaning in it. This may seem unusual, because many think of disease as only a physical problem that causes much pain, grief, and suffering. It is true: IBD does cause a lot of problems in people's lives. There's no doubt about that. Over time, however, some people begin to feel their illness has a meaning beyond the physical dysfunction it causes.

If you find meaning in your illness, it is usually very personal and unique. Different people interpret major life events in a variety of ways. This is totally normal, and no single individual's interpretation of her IBD is more right than anyone else's. However, trying to find some sort of purpose to all the suffering helps some people cope more effectively with what would otherwise be a senseless experience.

Brenda feels she learned a lot from her illness:

> I feel I learned some very important lessons through my experience with Crohn's. From a young age, I've been a very driven person. I have a lot of different interests and I've always felt I needed to do, do, do so that I could be as productive as possible. My Crohn's didn't completely wipe me out, but it definitely made me stop and slow down. Previously, I was always tied up in all my different roles—as a wife, a mother, a therapist, or a volunteer for different causes. But when I hit bottom and was hospitalized, I was scooped out from all my different roles. I was just left with being me. That's when I began to realize that my value as a human being is not based on what I do or what I bring to the table. I have value just being me. After all, I'm a human being, not a human doing. Learning this was one of the most freeing experiences for me. I don't know when I would have had time to learn this if the Crohn's hadn't given me the opportunity to stop and discover this.

Craig found symbolism in his illness:

> I don't know why I had to go through all the pain and suffering with the Crohn's for so many years. For a long time, I never even tried to see any meaning in it. Crohn's was just something that kept constantly interfering with everything I wanted to do. However, as my condition worsened despite stronger and stronger medical treatment, I felt I needed to explore as many options as possible. I read many different books, some of which talked about how people have used their illness

experience to learn more about themselves. I wasn't totally comfortable with the concept, but I figured I didn't have much to lose by trying to figure out what meaning my illness might have. I worked with a therapist on this, and also did a lot of work on my own.

As I began exploring this issue, I kept asking myself: of all the different illnesses there are, why did I get this one that essentially cuts me right through the middle of my body? Interestingly, a common theme throughout my life was that I always seemed to be caught in the middle of things. As a born diplomat, I was always trying to create peace and harmony between others around me. I could also always see both sides of any controversial issue and often felt torn right down the middle between which side was the right one. How interesting it was then that I had this illness that was literally eating me up in the middle of my body.

Don't get me wrong—I'm not in any way trying to personality-type people with Crohn's. I'm also not saying that my being caught in the middle of things caused my disease. But by trying to find the symbolism, I learned something about myself that I needed to change—and that was not to let myself get torn apart between opposing people or different viewpoints. Learning this did not cure my disease or even put it in remission. But it helped me live my life in a healthier way—even if didn't make me physically healthier.

Cheryl felt her body was trying to tell her something:

I've spent a lot of time trying to figure out why I have this disease and what it could possibly mean. I can't say I've completely figured it out yet, but I feel I have a much greater understanding than I did many years ago.

I know this might sound strange to some people, but I really feel my illness helped move me to a more appropriate path in life. For years, I was trying to be someone I wasn't. I had a successful career in the business world and I was working toward the goal of becoming the president of a large, successful company. I'm not saying that this couldn't be the right path for someone else. I know many people make valuable contributions to society through the business world. But I had this gut feeling that this was not what I was put on this earth to do. However, I chose to ignore this feeling and just kept along the same track. I also chose to ignore my Crohn's symptoms, such as cramping and diarrhea. After all, I had been dealing with this illness since I was 12, and wasn't going to let it get in the way.

As time went on, though, my symptoms got more and more severe. In fact, they got so severe that I could no longer work. I later realized that it was as if my body was at first giving me gentle messages that something was off. And then when I didn't listen to those signals, the messages had to get louder and louder until I could no longer ignore what my body was trying to tell me. It's interesting, too, how the gut feeling I had about playing a role I wasn't cut out for correlated with where I was having symptoms in my body.

I used to be angry at my body for betraying me and angry at my illness for interfering with what I wanted to do. And I still have days when I'm mad about being sick. However, I no longer blame myself or my body for the disease. I accept that I cannot predict or control my future, and I believe that this is all happening for a reason—so that I can fulfill my true purpose in life.

Karen feels she grew more emotionally resilient as a result of her disease:

I guess it's true that through adversity comes strength. Although it certainly would have been preferable not to go through all the suffering, I have to say that dealing with my IBD was good training ground for general life coping skills—both for helping me and other people. Although nothing can really prepare you for the unexpected loss of a loved one, I felt my illness experience helped me in this area since there are similar stages you go through, such as denial, anger, and acceptance. Additionally, I've had the resources to help others with different chronic illnesses, and this has been quite rewarding. So I definitely believe there was a purpose for my illness since it helped me to help myself and others.

Facing the future

Living with IBD involves living with uncertainty. Of course, everyone faces the unknown whether they have a chronic illness or not. But it's a bit different for people with Crohn's and ulcerative colitis. The capricious nature of these diseases can make it very difficult to predict your state of health—not only next year, but next month or next week. It's not easy living with this kind of uncertainty. It's therefore totally understandable that people with IBD often wonder how they'll live their lives with such a sword dangling above their heads. For example, they wonder whether they can fulfill their dreams and accomplish their goals. They wonder what long-term effects their medications are having on their bodies. They wonder if they'll make it to the bathroom in time. They wonder what the future holds for them. All these concerns and many more are very normal for someone living with Crohn's disease or ulcerative colitis.

No one can predict the course of your illness, and no one can predict the exact timing of better treatments or, ultimately, a cure. However, IBD organizations around the world are raising more money every year for research to discover the cause and cure of Crohn's and colitis. In the meantime, it may not always be easy, but it's still possible to live a meaningful, productive, and enjoyable life despite your IBD.

Carla explains:

> There's not much I can do about having ulcerative colitis. After all, I've had it now for about 35 years. However, I can choose how I react to it. Of course, it's important not to deny negative emotions. But once you acknowledge and express those, it's important to try and move forward with a more positive approach. I've found if I dwell on the negative for too long, I only feel worse. But if I focus more on the positive, such as by trying to figure out what I can learn from the negative experience of IBD, I feel I'm contributing toward my spiritual growth and development.

> Besides, at this point, I've been through so many flares that I know the routine quite well. Every flare passes—it always does. When the next one comes, I'll get through that one, too. I've set my life up such that I have all the resources I need, including my own internal coping skills, my spirituality, loving help from people around me, and a great doctor. I have what I need to get through whatever is coming next.

> I heard a quote once—I can't remember who said it—but it goes like this, "Living well is the best revenge." It's not that I feel I need to take revenge against my illness, but the point is that I'm not going to let this disease get me down or interfere with my life goals. I intend to live well despite it.

Cheryl shares this outlook:

> I used to be so unsure of my future with Crohn's. For a time, I didn't know what to expect from one moment to the next. I found myself trying to prepare for what was around the corner—but that was frustrating because I never really knew what was coming. With the help of surgery and a good therapist, however, I eventually reached a place of peaceful acceptance. Yes, I still have moments when I ask, "Why me?" But I always find my way back to accepting this path that I'm on. It actually feels quite liberating when I do.
>
> I'm going to have this disease for the rest of my life. Fortunately, I can now say that Crohn's and I have learned how to live together. It's part of who I am, but it doesn't control my life. I can face my future, even with Crohn's at my side.

Stacy expresses her views:

> I've had Crohn's for some 25 years. I made up my mind early on that it wasn't going to control my life. I simply didn't want to give up my plans and dreams.
>
> I figured I had two choices. I could lie down and let the disease walk all over me, or I could move forward and find other ways to go on with my life. It's true. It did interfere with a lot of things, but I learned to work around the illness. For example, I really wanted to have children. My case was so severe that the Crohn's physically prevented me from having kids. So I adopted, and I now have two beautiful daughters. I also had to change my career to give myself more flexibility, but that ended up working out for the best, too.
>
> Yeah, facing the future with the burden of IBD is sometimes scary. But I always tell people that if they have a dream, they should just go for it. Sometimes you may have to alter your course, but you can still find ways to make your life work.

Resources

Organizations

IBD

Crohn's and Colitis Foundation of America (CCFA)
386 Park Ave. South
New York, NY 10016-8804
(800) 932-2423 or (212) 685-3440
http://www.ccfa.org/

CCFA's mission is to raise money for research to prevent and cure Crohn's disease and ulcerative colitis. The organization also provides education and support to children and adults affected by these diseases, including support groups, summer camps for kids, seminars, and a variety of books and pamphlets.

Crohn's and Colitis Foundation of Canada (CCFC)
60 St. Clair Ave. East, Suite 600
Toronto, ON, M4T 1N5 Canada
(800) 387-1479 or (416) 920-5035
http://www.ccfc.ca/

This Canadian volunteer organization's mission is to raise money for research in order to find a cure for Crohn's disease and ulcerative colitis. The web site provides detailed information on research, fundraising programs, and volunteer opportunities.

Children with Intestinal and Liver Disorders Foundation (CH.I.L.D Foundation)
1188 West Georgia St., Suite 1150
Vancouver, BC, V6E 4A2, Canada
(877) 672-4453 or (604) 736-0645
http://www.child.ca/

The CH.I.L.D. Foundation is a volunteer-run organization whose goal is to raise money for medical research to find a cure for children with Crohn's disease, ulcerative colitis, and other digestive disorders.

National Association for Colitis and Crohn's Disease (NACC)
4 Beaumont House
Sutton Road
St. Albans, Herts AL1 5HH
United Kingdom
Tel. administration: 011 44 (0) 1727 830038
http://www.nacc.org.uk/

The NACC raises money for IBD research and provides information and support to those with Crohn's and ulcerative colitis.

Australian Crohn's and Colitis Association (ACCA)
P.O. Box 201
Mooroolbark, VIC 3138
Australia
Tel.: 011 61 3 9726 9008
http://www.acca.net.au/

The ACCA's goal is to promote awareness about IBD while providing education to those with the disease. It also financially supports research to help find the cause and cure of Crohn's disease and ulcerative colitis.

Ostomy

International Ostomy Association (IOA)
http://www.ostomyinternational.org/

The IOA's mission is to improve the quality of life for people with ostomies worldwide.

United Ostomy Association (UOA)
19772 MacArthur Blvd., Suite 200
Irvine, CA 92612-2405
(800) 826-0826
http://www.uoa.org/

The UOA is a volunteer-based health organization whose goal is to provide information, education, support, and advocacy to people who have or will have intestinal or urinary diversions.

Children

National Information Center for Children and Youth with Disabilities (NICHCY)
P.O. Box 1492
Washington, DC 20013-1492
(800) 695-0285 or (202) 884-8200
http://www.nichcy.org/

A clearinghouse that provides pamphlets and information on disabilities and the rights of disabled children and their parents.

STARBRIGHT Foundation
11835 West Olympic Blvd., Suite 500
Los Angeles, CA 90064
(310) 479-1212
http://www.starbright.org/

STARBRIGHT is a nonprofit organization that creates and distributes programs for seriously ill children including STARBRIGHT Videos with Attitude, a video series for teens about communicating with healthcare professionals, returning to school, and coping with frequent and prolonged hospitalizations.

Drug reimbursement

Pharmaceutical Research and Manufacturers of America
1100 15th St., NW
Washington DC 20005
(202) 835-3400
http://www.phrma.org/pap/

The directory of patient assistance programs lists companies that provide prescription medicines free of charge to physicians whose patients might not otherwise have access to necessary medicines.

Centers for Medicare & Medicaid Services
Medicare Prescription Drug Assistance Program
7500 Security Blvd.
Baltimore, MD 21244-1850
(410) 786-3000
http://www.medicare.gov/Prescription/Home.asp

Provides information on programs that offer discounts or free medications to individuals in need.

RxHope.com
254 Mountain Ave., Building B., Suite 200
Hackettstown, NJ 07840
(908) 850-8004
http://www.rxhope.com/

Resource for patient assistance programs offered by the pharaceutical industry as well as federal, state, and charitable organizations.

Employment

The Disability Rights Education and Defense Fund (DREDF)
2212 Sixth St.
Berkeley, CA 94710
(800) 348-4232 or (510) 644-2555
http://www.dredf.org/

DREDF's mission is to protect and advance the rights of people with disabilities. They can answer questions about the Americans with Disabilities Act, explain how to file a complaint, and provides dispute resolution. They also provide advocacy, training, and technical assistance to families who have children with disabilities.

Job Accommodation Network (JAN)
P.O. Box 6080
Morgantown, WV 26506-6080
(800) 526-7234
http://www.jan.wvu.edu/

An international consulting service that provides free information about how employers can accommodate people with disabilities. The service also provides information on the Americans with Disabilities Act (ADA). Provides information on starting small businesses to people with disabilities.

Gastroenterology

The following are professional organizations for gastroenterologists. They also provide information to patients as well as professionals.

American College of Gastroenterology (ACG)
4900 B South 31st St.
Arlington, VA 22206-1656
(703) 820-7400
http://www.acg.gi.org/

American Gastroenterological Association (AGA)
4930 Del Ray Ave.
Bethesda, MD 20814
(301) 654-2055
http://www.gastro.org/

North American Society for Pediatric Gastroenterology, Hepatology and Nutrition (NASPGHAN)
P.O. Box 6
Flourtown, PA 19031
(215) 233-0808
http://www.naspghan.org/

Insurance

Patient Advocacy Coalition, Inc.
777 East Girard Ave., Suite 250
Englewood, CO 80110
(303) 744-7667
http://www.patientadvocacy.net/

Helps resolve insurance reimbursement problems.

Patient Advocate Foundation
700 Thimble Shoals Blvd., Suite 200
Newport News, VA 23606
(800) 532-5274 or (757) 873-6668
http://www.patientadvocate.org/

Provides publications, help with insurance problems, and referrals to attorneys.

The National Association of Insurance Commissioners (NAIC)
2301 McGee St., Suite 800
Kansas City, MO 64108-2662
(816) 842-3600
http://www.naic.org/

This is an organization of insurance regulators from the 50 states, the District of Columbia, and the four US territories. The NAIC's web site links to each state's insurance regulator at *http://www.naic.org/1regulator/usamap.htm*

Insure Kids Now!
(877) 543-7669
http://www.insurekidsnow.gov/

The US Department of Health and Human Services began the Insure Kids Now! Program to link the nation's uninsured children with free or low-cost health insurance.

Medical information research (fee-based)

The following companies provide customized research on any medical condition or health topic.

The Health Resource
933 Faulkner
Conway, AR 72034
(800) 949-0090 or (501) 329-5272
http://www.thehealthresource.com/

Mr. Health Search
1141 Catalina Drive, #178
Livermore, California 94550
(800) 794-5015 or (925) 456-2927
http://www.mrhealthsearch.com/

Mind/Body

The Academy for Guided Imagery
P.O. Box 2070
Mill Valley, CA 94942
(800) 726-2070
http://www.interactiveimagery.com/

This organization trains health professionals to use interactive guided imagery with their patients and clients. Self-care books and tapes on guided imagery are available for sale. They can assist in locating a professional in your area to help you learn visualization.

The American Society of Clinical Hypnosis
140 N. Bloomingdale Road
Bloomingdale, IL 60108-1017
(630) 980-4740
http://www.asch.net/

A membership organization for doctors, psychologists, and dentists who use hypnosis in their practices. For referral to a local member, send request with a self-addressed, stamped envelope or visit the web site.

Center for Attitudinal Healing
33 Buchanan Drive
Sausalito, CA 94965
(415) 331-6161
http://www.healingcenter.org/

A nonprofit, nonsectarian group that sponsors local and national workshops for children and adults with chronic and life-threatening diseases. The emphasis is on spiritual and emotional support. They have also published several excellent books and tapes.

Laughter Therapy
P.O. Box 827
Monterey, CA 93942
http://www.candidcamera.com/cc7/cc7.html

Laughter therapy is a nonprofit organization founded by Alan Funt of the *Candid Camera* television series. People with illnesses can borrow *Candid Camera* videotapes.

Other medical organizations

The American Board of Medical Specialties (ABMS)
1007 Church St., Suite 404
Evanston, IL 60201
(866) 275-2267 (Doctor Verification Service)
(847) 491-9091
http://www.abms.org/

The ABMS publishes the *Official ABMS Directory of Board Certified Specialists,* which is found at many libraries. You can use it to check your doctor's credentials.

MedicAlert Foundation International
2323 Colorado Ave.
Turlock, CA 95382
(888) 633-4298 or (209) 668-3333 (from outside the United States)
http://www.medicalert.org/

A nonprofit organization whose mission is to protect and save lives. They provide MedicAlert bracelets and wallet cards. Medical personnel can call the phone number on your bracelet or card to receive your vital medical information when you can't speak for yourself.

National Digestive Diseases Information Clearinghouse (NDDIC)
2 Information Way
Bethesda, MD 20892-3570
(800) 891-5389 or (301) 654-3810
http://www.niddk.nih.gov/health/digest/nddic.htm

The NDDIC is a division of the National Diabetes & Digestive & Kidney Disease (NIDDK). This government organization provides information on digestive diseases to both consumers and professionals.

National Library of Medicine
8600 Rockville Pike
Bethesda, MD 20894
(888) 346-3656
http://www.nlm.nih.gov/

A US government organization providing access to a wealth of health and medical information on just about every topic.

Psychotherapy/Counseling

The following organizations can refer you to a mental healthcare professional in your local area:

The American Association for Marriage and Family Therapy (AAMFT)
112 South Alfred St.
Alexandria, VA 22314-3061
(703) 838-9808
http://www.aamft.org/

The American Psychiatric Association (APA)
1000 Wilson Blvd., Suite 1825
Arlington, VA 22209-3901
(888) 357-7924 or (703) 907-7300
http://www.psych.org/

The American Psychological Association (APA)
750 First St., NE
Washington, DC 20002-4242
(800) 374-2721 or (202) 336-5500
http://www.apa.org/

The National Association of Social Workers (NASW)
750 First St., NE, Suite 700
Washington, DC 20002-4241
(202) 408-8600
http://www.naswdc.org/

Books

IBD

Benirschke, Rolf. *Alive and Kicking.* San Diego, CA: Rolf Benirschke Enterprises, 1999. An inspiring, true-life story of a football star's experience with ulcerative colitis and then later an ostomy.

Benkov, Keith, and Winter, Harland. *Managing Your Child's Crohn's Disease or Ulcerative Colitis.* New York: Mastermedia Limited, 1996. A comprehensive guide for parents who have a child with IBD.

Gottschall, Elaine. *Breaking the Vicious Cycle.* Kirkton, Ontario: The Kirkton Press, 1994. Outlines a diet that may help some people control their Crohn's disease or ulcerative colitis. Includes recipes.

Gomez, Joan. *Positive Options for Crohn's Disease: Self-Help and Treatment.* Alameda, CA: Hunter House, 2000. Written by a doctor, this book provides information on Crohn's disease, with an emphasis on dietary and lifestyle changes to help manage the illness.

Greenwood, Jan. *The IBD Nutrition Book.* New York: Wiley, 1992. Provides nutritional and dietary information for those with IBD. Includes recipes.

Harper, Virginia. *Controlling Crohn's Disease: The Natural Way.* New York: Kensington Publishing, 2002. A woman with a long history of Crohn's shares her path toward health. The focus of the book is on dietary and lifestyles changes to help control the disease.

Kirsner, Joseph B. (ed.) *Inflammatory Bowel Disease.* Philadelphia: Saunders, 2000. Written for healthcare professionals and has 47 chapters covering the latest research on IBD.

Kron, Audrey. *Ask Audrey: The Author's Personal and Professional Experience in the Day-to-Day Living with Inflammatory Bowel Disease.* West Bloomfield, MI: Audrey Kron, 1999. A psychotherapist with Crohn's disease shares her personal story of living with the disease and offers many questions and answers about coping with the emotional impact of IBD. Can be ordered by calling (248) 626-6960 or on the Web at *http://www.chronicillness.com/*

Nielson, Peter. *Will of Iron: A Champion's Journey.* Ann Arbor, MI: Momentum Books, 1992. A fragile Brooklyn teenager with Crohn's disease grows up to become Mr. International Universe. An inspiring, motivational book that includes many health and fitness tips.

Saibil, Fred. *Crohn's Disease and Ulcerative Colitis: Everything You Need to Know.* Buffalo, NY: Firefly Books, 1997. A clear and easy-to-understand patient guide, written by a gastroenterologist.

Scala, James. *The New Eating Right for a Bad Gut.* New York: Plume, 2000. Provides dietary suggestions for helping manage Crohn's disease and ulcerative colitis.

Sklar, Jill. *The First Year—Crohn's Disease and Ulcerative Colitis: An Essential Guide for the Newly Diagnosed.* New York: Marlowe, 2002. A well-written, comprehensive book on IBD for the newly diagnosed. The author is a patient with years of Crohn's experience.

Stein, Stanley, and Rood, Richard (eds.). *Inflammatory Bowel Disease: A Guide for Patients and Their Families.* New York: Lippincott–Raven, 1999. The official patient guide of the Crohn's and Colitis Foundation of America (CCFA).

Steiner-Grossman, Penny, Peter Banks, and Daniel Present. *The New People . . . Not Patients: A Source Book for Living with Inflammatory Bowel Disease.* Dubuque, IA: Kendall-Hunt Publishing, 1997. A great resource book for people with Crohn's disease and ulcerative colitis.

Thompson, Grant. *The Angry Gut: Coping with Colitis & Crohn's Disease.* New York: Plenum Publishing, 1993. Written by a gastroenterologist, this comprehensive book is ideal for those wanting more technical information than is usually covered in most consumer publications.

Trachter, Amy. *Coping with Crohn's Disease.* Oakland, CA: New Harbinger Publications, 2001. Written by a clinical psychologist, this book focuses on the emotional challenges faced by people with Crohn's disease. A practical guide that offers both compassion and support.

Zonderman, Jon, and Vender, Ronald. *Crohn's Disease and Ulcerative Colitis.* Jackson, MS: University Press of Mississippi, 2000. A Crohn's patient and his doctor team up to write a book on IBD.

Children's books

Hautzig, Deborah. *A Visit to the Sesame Street Hospital.* New York: Random House, 1985. Grover, his mother, Ernie, and Bert visit the Sesame Street Hospital in preparation for Grover's upcoming operation.

Peterkin, Allan. *What About Me? When Brothers and Sisters Get Sick.* Washington, DC: Magination Press, 1992. Describes the feelings of siblings whose brother or sister is hospitalized.

Rogers, Fred. *Going to the Hospital.* New York: Putnam's, 1997. With pictures and words, TV's beloved Mr. Rogers helps children ages 3 to 8 learn about hospitals.

Sherkin-Langer, Ferne. *When Mommy Is Sick.* Morton Grove, IL: Albert Witman & Co., 1995. A picture book that helps children who have a parent who is ill or hospitalized. Written by a nurse who is a mother and also has Crohn's disease.

Doctor–Patient Relationship

Keene, Nancy. *Working with Your Doctor: Getting the Healthcare You Deserve.* Sebastopol, CA: O'Reilly, 1998. Contains practical advice to help people take an active role in maintaining health and steps to improve and strengthen the doctor–patient relationship.

Korsch, Barbara, and Harding, Caroline. *The Intelligent Patient's Guide to the Doctor–Patient Relationship: Learning How to Talk So Your Doctor Will Listen.* New York: Oxford University Press, 1998. A book that examines doctor–patient relationships and what can be done to improve communication.

Drugs

Physician's Desk Reference. Oradell, NJ: Medical Economics Data, 2003. Issued yearly, lists authoritative information on all FDA-approved drugs. Technical language. Available at reference desk in most libraries.

Briggs, Gerald, Roger Freeman, and Sumner Yaffe. *Drugs in Pregnancy and Lactation.* Philadelphia: Lippincott Williams & Wilkins, 2001. Reference book that provides useful and comprehensive information to doctors and pregnant women on medications and their effects on a developing fetus and newborn.

Silverman, Harold (ed.) *The Pill Book.* New York: Bantam Books, 2002. Written for the consumer, this book provides information on 1,500 drugs.

USP DI, Vol. 2: *Advice for the Patient: Drug Information in Lay Language.* Greenwood Village, CO: United States Pharmacopeial Convention, 2002. Contains detailed drug information in nonmedical language. Available in most libraries.

Zuckerman, Eugenia, and Ingelfinger, Julie. *Coping with Prednisone.* New York: St. Martin's Griffin, 1997. A patient with a rare lung disease teams up with her sister, a physician, to write a book offering guidance to those living with the side effects of prednisone and other cortisone-like medicines.

General digestive health

Aron, Jeffrey M., and Aron, Harriett E. *Gut-Check: Your Prime Source for Bowel Health and Colon Cancer Prevention.* Bloomington, IN: 1st Books Library, 2001. Written by a gastroenterologist, this book is a comprehensive and user-friendly guide for bowel care. See Dr. Aron's web site at *http://www.gut-check.com/*

Lipsky, Elizabeth. *Digestive Wellness.* Los Angeles: Keats Publishing, 2000. A clinical nutritionist provides suggestions and advice for achieving health through digestive wellness.

General natural health

Murray, Michael. *The Pill Book: Guide to Natural Medicines.* New York: Bantam Books, 2002. Describes safety and effectiveness of 250 of the most popular natural health supplements. Also includes side effects, drug/food interactions, and cautions/warnings.

Murray, Michael, and Pizzorno, Joseph. *Encyclopedia of Natural Medicine.* Rocklin, CA: Prima Publishing, 1998. A great complementary health resource for any household. In addition to tips on general health, it provides natural health suggestions for many illnesses from A to Z, including IBD.

Weil, Andrew. *8 Weeks to Optimum Health.* New York: Fawcett Books, 1998. This well-known physician specializing in integrative medicine shares his tips for healthy living.

Hospitalization

Inlander, Charles, and Weiner, Ed. *Take This Book to the Hospital with You: A Consumer Guide to Surviving Your Hospital Stay.* New York: St. Martins, 1997. Provides practical advice for hospital stays, including getting the treatment you need and scrutinizing hospital bills.

Keene, Nancy. *Your Child in the Hospital: A Practical Guide for Parents.* 2nd edition. Sebastopol, CA: O'Reilly, 1999. A pocket guide full of parent stories to help parents prepare their child physically and emotionally for hospitalizations. Also available in Spanish.

Ostomy

Benirschke, Rolf. *Great Comebacks from Ostomy Surgery*. San Diego, CA: Rolf Benirschke Enterprises, 2002. An inspiring book featuring the stories of fifteen people who have undergone ostomy surgery.

Barrie, Barbara. *Don't Die of Embarrassment: Life After Colostomy and Other Adventures*. New York: Fireside, 1997. Actress Barbara Barrie tells her story of overcoming colon cancer and living with a colostomy.

Kupfer, Barbara, et al. *Yes We Can: Advice on Traveling with an Ostomy and Tips for Everyday Living*. Lanham, MD: Chandler House Press, 2000. Book features stories and tips of people traveling the world with their ostomies. Provides extensive listings of resources for people with ostomies traveling abroad.

Mullen, Barbara, and Mcginn, Kerry. *The Ostomy Book*. Palo Alto, CA: Bull Publishing, 1992. A comprehensive book about living with a colostomy, ileostomy, or urostomy.

White, Craig. *Positive Options for Living with Your Ostomy*. Alameda, CA: Hunter House, 2002. Written by a psychologist, this book provides emotional support and advice for those living with ostomies.

Other health/medical

Case, Shelley. *Gluten-Free Diet: A Comprehensive Resource Guide*. Regina, Saskatchewan: Case Nutrition Consulting, 2002. A well-researched guide that's ideal for both patients and professionals who deal with gluten-restricted diets.

Oster, Nancy, Lucy Thomas, and Darol Joseff. *Making Informed Medical Decisions*. Sebastopol, CA: O'Reilly, 2000. This clear and easy-to-understand book provides many resources for those seeking medical information for themselves or loved ones.

Psychology, coping, and mind–body healing

Benson, Herbert, MD. *The Relaxation Response*. New York: Avon Books, 1990. This is an excellent resource for the relaxation method of pain relief.

Brigham, Deirdre. *Imagery for Getting Well*. New York: Norton, 1996. A comprehensive resource on mind–body therapies that includes imagery exercises for specific illnesses, including IBD.

Corsini, Raymond, and Wedding, Danny. *Current Psychotherapies*. Itasca, IL: Peacock Publishers, 2000. Provides extensive information on fifteen different psychotherapeutic approaches.

Donaghue, Paul, and Siegel, Mary. *Sick and Tired of Feeling Sick and Tired: Living with Invisible Chronic Illness*. New York: Norton, 2000. Written by two psychologists, this book provides support and guidance for those living with chronic diseases that aren't always apparent to others.

Farhi, Donna. *The Breathing Book: Good Health and Vitality Through Essential Breath Work*. New York: Holt, 1996. Written by a yoga instructor, this book is a practical guide for breathing techniques that may help improve your physical and mental health.

Gurman, S. Alan, and Messer, Stanley (eds.). *Essential Psychotherapies*. New York: Guilford Press, 1997. Provides extensive coverage of twelve different types of psychotherapy.

Kron, Audrey. *Meeting the Challenge: Living with Chronic Illness*. West Bloomfield, MI: Audrey Kron, 1996. Provides practical advice and guidance for those living with a chronic illness. Written by a psychotherapist with a long history of Crohn's disease. Can be ordered by calling (248) 626-6960 or on the Web at *http://www.chronicillness.com/*

LeShan, Lawrence. *How to Meditate: A Guide to Self-Discovery.* Boston: Little Brown, 1999. Originally published in 1974, this classic can help you learn the art of meditation.

Lewis, Sheldon, and Sheila Lewis. *Stress-Proofing Your Child: Mind–Body Exercises to Enhance Your Child's Health.* New York: Bantam Books, 1996. This book is highly recommended for all parents. It clearly explains easy ways to teach children techniques such as guided imagery, deep breathing, and meditation to decrease stress, increase a child's sense of control, and boost children's confidence. A wonderful, practical book.

McCue, Kathleen, and Bonn, Ron. *How to Help Children Through a Parent's Serious Illness.* New York: St. Martin's, 1996. This book offers practical advice and guidance from a child-life specialist.

Register, Cheri. *The Chronic Illness Experience: Embracing the Imperfect Life.* Center City, MN: Hazelden Information Education, 1999. Written by an author with a rare chronic illness, this book shows how people with chronic illness can still live meaningful lives.

Rossman, Martin. *Guided Imagery for Self-Healing.* Tiburon, CA: Kramer, 2000. A comprehensive guide for people interested in learning how to use guided imagery to improve the quality of their lives.

Brochures

The Crohn's and Colitis Foundation of America (CCFA) publishes many different brochures on topics related to IBD. Call the CCFA national office at (800) 932-2423, ext. 212, to receive free copies. All the brochures are also available online at the CCFA web site in PDF format: *http://www.ccfa.org/brochures/*

Here are the various brochures available on IBD: *About Crohn's Disease; About Ulcerative Colitis; Medications; Maintenance Therapy; Diet and Nutrition; Emotional Factors; Complications; Understanding Colorectal Cancer; Surgery; Women's Issues; A Parent's Guide; A Teacher's Guide; A Guide for Children and Teenagers.*

Audiotapes

Feldman-Saylor, Nancy. *Healing Journey for Crohn's and Colitis.* InnerVision Studio Wellness Series, 1994. Cooling imagery assists listeners in working with their immune system to create a more comfortable internal environment. To order, contact InnerVision Studio: 7451 West Mercada Way, Delray Beach, FL 33446; (561) 499-3601; *http://www.innervisionstudioinc.com/*

Naparstek, Belleruth. *Successful Surgery.* Health Journeys, 2002. Tapes provide imagery and affirmations for a successful surgery and recovery. To order, contact Health Journeys at (800) 800-8661 or go to *http://www.healthjourneys.com/.*

Siegel, Bernie. *Healing Meditations: Enhance Your Immune System and Find the Key to Good Health.* Hay House, 2000. In his own voice, this well-known author and surgeon shares how you can enhance your immune system and general health through a combination of guided imagery and self-hypnosis. Can be ordered by calling (800) 654-5126. Can also be purchased on the Web at *http://www.hayhouse.com/* or *http://www.amazon.com/.*

Siegel, Bernie. *Humor and Healing*. Sounds True, 1994. Dr. Siegel discusses how humor and positive thinking can aid in the healing process. Can be ordered by calling (800) 333-9185. Can also be purchased over the Internet at *http://www.soundstrue.com/* or *http://www.amazon.com/*.

Web sites

IBD

Crohn's and Colitis Foundation of America (CCFA)
http://www.ccfa.org/

Contains a wealth of information on every aspect of Crohn's and colitis from the leading IBD organization in the world.

Crohn's Disease, Ulcerative Colitis, Inflammatory Bowel Disease Pages
http://qurlyjoe.bu.edu/

A patient's web site containing many links to a variety of resources for people with IBD.

Crohn's Disease Resource Center
http://www.healingwell.com/ibd/

A web site containing a wealth of information on both Crohn's and ulcerative colitis, including resources, articles, and book reviews.

David's Crohn's and Colitis Web Page
http://www.geocities.com/HotSprings/Falls/4809/

This web site, founded by a man with ulcerative colitis, contains lots of information of interest to people with IBD.

IBD Humor Page
http://www.calweb.com/~rvincent/ibdhumor.html

A great web site for IBD patients when they need a laugh. Contains many stories.

IBD Patient Community
http://www.ibd.patientcommunity.com/

A very well organized, comprehensive web site providing a wide variety of information for people with IBD.

IBD Sucks
http://www.ibdsucks.com

A message board for people with IBD.

KidsWithIBD.org

http://www.kidswithibd.org/

This web site's purpose is to help promote advocacy and awareness of IBD in children. The web site has many stories of children with IBD and encourages visitors to write to governmental agencies or the media.

Support for Parents with IBDers Message Board

http://www.dragonpack.com/forums/ibdboard/

A message board for parents who have a child with IBD.

Teens with Crohn's Disease web site

http://pages.prodigy.net/mattgreen/

A web site dedicated to teens with Crohn's. Has stories, experience, advice, links, and recipes.

Complementary medicine

Alternative Health News Online

http://www.altmedicine.com/

Web site contains latest research news from both conventional and complementary medicine.

DrWeil.com

http://www.drweil.com/

A comprehensive web site dedicated to integrative medicine.

General health and medical

MayoClinic.com

http://www.mayoclinic.com/

A health and medical web site for consumers. Contains information on diseases and conditions, drugs, healthy living, and more.

MEDLINEplus

http://www.nlm.nih.gov/medlineplus/

A large, consumer-friendly health database, produced by the National Library of Medicine. Includes drug information, a medical encyclopedia, information on illnesses, and much more.

PubMed

http://www.ncbi.nlm.nih.gov/PubMed/

The National Library of Medicine's free search service provides access to more than nine million citations in MEDLINE and PREMEDLINE (with links to participating online journals), and other related databases. Also includes FAQs (frequently asked questions, and answers), news, and clinical alerts.

Rx List—The Internet Drug Index
http://www.rxlist.com/

Information on over 4,500 drugs in both Spanish and English. Also contains a medical dictionary.

Ostomy

The J-pouch Group
http://www.jpouch.org/

A comprehensive web site for people who've had J-pouch surgery. The site includes a discussion board and chat room.

Shaz's Ostomy Pages
http://www.ostomates.org/

An ostomate's comprehensive web site.

United Ostomy Association (UOA)
http://www.uoa.org/

A wealth of information for people with ostomies.

Notes

Chapter 1: Introduction to IBD

1. E. Kangas, M. Matikainen, and J. Mattila, "Is 'Indeterminate Colitis' Crohn's Disease in the Long-Term Follow-Up?" *International Surgery* 79, no. 2 (April–June 1994): 120–23.

2. J. H. Baron, "Inflammatory Bowel Disease up to 1932," *Mt. Sinai Journal of Medicine* 67, no. 3 (May 2000): 174–89.

3. Crohn's & Colitis Foundation of America, Questions and answers about ulcerative colitis, "How Common Is Ulcerative Colitis?" available on the Web at *http://www.ccfa.org/brochures/aboutuc.pdf*.

4. National Institute of Diabetes & Digestive & Kidney Diseases (NIDDK), Digestive Disease Statistics, Inflammatory Bowel Disease, available on the Web at *http://www.niddk.nih.gov/health/digest/pubs/ddstats/ddstats.htm*.

5. R. S. Sandler and G. M. Eisen, "Epidemiology of Inflammatory Bowel Disease," in J. B. Kirsner's *Inflammatory Bowel Disease*, 5th edition (Philadelphia: Saunders, 2000), 89–112.

6. T. Matsumoto and M. Fujishima, "Epidemiologic Aspects of Ulcerative Colitis in Japan—Comparison with Other Countries," *Nippon Rinsho* 57, no. 11 (Nov 1999): 2443–48.

7. S. K. Yang et al., "Incidence and Prevalence of Ulcerative Colitis in Songpa-Kangdong District, Seoul, Korea, 1986–1997," *Journal of Gastroenterology and Hepatology* 15, no. 9 (Sept 2000): 1037–42.

8. E. V. Loftus et al., "Crohn's Disease in Olmsted County, Minnesota, 1940–1993: Incidence, Prevalence, and Survival," *Gastroenterology* 114, no. 6 (June 1998): 1161–68.

9. E. V. Loftus et al., "Ulcerative Colitis in Olmsted County, Minnesota, 1940–1993: Incidence, Prevalence, and Survival," *Gut* 46, no. 3 (March 2000): 336–43.

10. Sandler and Eisen, "Epidemiology of Inflammatory Bowel Disease," 89–112.

11. Y. Niv, G. Abuksis, and G. M. Fraser, "Epidemiology of Crohn's in Israel: A Survey of Israeli Kibbutz Settlements," *American Journal of Gastroenterology* 94, no. 10 (Oct 1999): 2961–65.

12. Matsumoto and Fujishima, "Ulcerative Colitis in Japan," 2443–48.

13. Sandler and Eisen, "Epidemiology of Inflammatory Bowel Disease," 89–112.

14. Sandler and Eisen, "Epidemiology of Inflammatory Bowel Disease," 89–112.

15. J. H. Kurata et al., "Crohn's Disease Among Ethnic Groups in a Large Health Maintenance Organization," *Gastroenterology* 102, no. 6 (June 1992): 1940–48.

16. R. A. Hiatt and L. Kaufman, "Epidemiology of Inflammatory Bowel Disease in a Defined Northern California Population," *Western Journal of Medicine* 149, no. 5 (Nov 1988): 541–46.

17. Kurata et al., "Crohn's Disease Among Ethnic Groups," 1940–48.

18. Y. Niv, G. Abuksis, and G. M. Fraser, "Epidemiology of Ulcerative Colitis in Israel: A Survey of Israeli Kibbutz Settlements," *American Journal of Gastroenterology* 95, no. 3 (March 2000): 693–98.

19. A. Sonnenberg, D. J. McCarty, and S. J. Jacobsen, "Geographic Variation of Inflammatory Bowel Disease Within the United States," *Gastroenterology* 100, no. 1 (Jan 1991): 143–49.

20. S. Shivananda et al., "Incidence of Inflammatory Bowel Disease Across Europe: Is There a Difference Between North and South? Results of the European Collaborative Study on Inflammatory Bowel Disease (EC-IBD)" *Gut* 39, no. 5 (Nov 1996): 690–97.

21. G. A. Thomas et al., "Role of Smoking in Inflammatory Bowel Disease: Implications for Therapy," *Postgraduate Medical Journal* 76, no. 895 (May 2000): 273–79.

22. Sandler and Eisen, "Epidemiology of Inflammatory Bowel Disease," 89–112.

23. M. Orholm et al., "Concordance of Inflammatory Bowel Disease Among Danish Twins: Results of a Nationwide Study," *Scandinavian Journal of Gastroenterology* 35, no. 10 (Oct 2000): 1075–81.

24. V. Binder, "Genetic Epidemiology in Inflammatory Bowel Disease," *Digestive Diseases* 16, no. 6 (Nov–Dec 1998): 351–55.

25. T. Ahmad et al., "Review Article: The Genetics of Inflammatory Bowel Disease," *Alimentary Pharmacology and Therapeutics* 15, no. 6 (June 2001): 731–48.

26. Crohn's and Colitis Foundation of America, "Researchers Find First Gene for Crohn's Disease," available on the Web at *http://www.ccfa.org/news/previous/firstgene.htm.*

27. R. B. Sartor, "Microbial Factors in the Pathogenesis of Crohn's Disease, Ulcerative Colitis, and Experimental Intestinal Inflammation," in J. B. Kirsner's *Inflammatory Bowel Disease,* 5th edition (Philadelphia: Saunders, 2000): 153–78.

28. K. Hulten et al., "Antibacterial Therapy for Crohn's Disease: A Review Emphasizing Therapy Directed Against Mycobacteria," *Digestive Diseases and Sciences* 45, no. 3 (March 2000): 445–56.

29. A. Ekbom et al., "Perinatal Measles Infection and Subsequent Crohn's Disease," *The Lancet* 344, no. 8921 (Aug 1994): 508–10.

30. N. C. Fisher et al., "Measles Virus Serology in Crohn's Disease." *Gut* 41, no. 1 (July 1997): 66–9.

31. T. Y. Ma, "Intestinal Epithelial Barrier Dysfunction in Crohn's Disease," *Proceedings of the Society for Experimental Biology and Medicine* 214, no. 4 (April 1997): 318–27.

32. R. D'Inca, "Intestinal Permeability Test as a Predictor of Clinical Course in Crohn's Disease," *American Journal of Gastroenterology* 94, no. 10 (Oct 1999): 2956–60.

33. F. P. Ryan, A. M. Ward, and C. D. Holdsworth, "Autoimmunity, Inflammatory Bowel Disease, and Hyposplenism," *The Quarterly Journal of Medicine* 78, no. 285 (Jan 1991): 59–63.

34. M. R. Capobianchi et al., "Absence of Circulating Interferon in Patients with Inflammatory Bowel Disease: Suggestions Against Autoimmune Etiology," *Clinical and Experimental Immunology* 90, no. 1 (Oct 1992): 85–7.

35. C. S. North et al., "The Relation of Ulcerative Colitis to Psychiatric Factors: A Review of the Literature," *American Journal of Psychiatry* 147, no. 8 (Aug 1990): 974–81.

36. Sandler and Eisen, "Epidemiology of Inflammatory Bowel Disease," 89–112.

Chapter 3: Diagnostic Procedures

1. The American Nuclear Society, "Estimate Your Personal Annual Radiation Dose," available on the Web at *http://www.ans.org/pi/raddosechart/pdfs/raddosechart.*

2. Health Physics Society, "Measuring Radioactivity," available on the Web at *http://www.hps.org/documents/measuringradioactivity.pdf.*

3. T. Vehmas et al., "Factors Influencing Patient Radiation Doses from Barium Enema Examinations," *Acta Radiologica* 41, no. 2 (March 2000): 167–71.

4. T. Vehmas, "Hawthorne Effect: Shortening of Fluoroscopy Times During Radiation Measurement Studies," *British Journal of Radiology* 70, no. 838 (Oct 1997): 1053–55.

Chapter 4: Complications

1. G. R. Kirk and W. D. Clements, "Crohn's Disease and Colorectal Malignancy," *International Journal of Clinical Practice* 53, no. 4 (June 1999): 314–15.

2. Crohn's and Colitis Foundation of America, "Cancer," available on the Web at *http://www.ccfa.org/medcentral/library/compl/cancer2.htm.*

3. C. D. Gillen et al., "Ulcerative Colitis and Crohn's Disease: A Comparison of the Colorectal Cancer Risk in Extensive Colitis," *Gut* 35, no. 11 (Nov 1994): 590–92.

4. A. Ekbom et al., "Ulcerative Colitis and Colorectal Cancer: A Population-Based Study," *New England Journal of Medicine* 323, no. 18 (1 Nov 1990): 1228–33.

5. Dennis J. Ahnen, MD, "Gastrointestinal Malignancies in Inflammatory Bowel Disease," in J. B. Kirsner's *Inflammatory Bowel Disease,* 5th edition (Philadelphia: Saunders, 2000), 379–96.

6. S. R. Gorfine et al., "Dysplasia Complicating Chronic Ulcerative Colitis: Is Immediate Colectomy Warranted?" *Diseases of the Colon and Rectum* 43, no. 11 (Nov 2000): 1575–81.

7. J. Eaden et al., "Colorectal Cancer Prevention in Ulcerative Colitis: A Case Control Study," *Alimentary Pharmacology & Therapeutics* 14, no. 2 (Feb 2000): 145–53.

8. D. Pinczowski et al., "Risk Factors for Colorectal Cancer in Patients with Ulcerative Colitis: A Case-Control Study," *Gastroenterology* 107, no. 1 (July 1994): 117–20.

9. B. A. Lashner et al., "Effect of Folate Supplementation on the Incidence of Dysplasia and Cancer in Chronic Ulcerative Colitis: A Case-Control Study," *Gastroenterology* 97, no. 2 (Aug 1989): 255–59.

10. L. Krahenbuhl and M. W. Buchler, "Pathophysiology, Clinical Aspects and Therapy of Short Bowel Syndrome," *Der Chirurg* 68, no. 6 (June 1997): 559–67.

11. A. J. Greenstein et al., "Outcome of Toxic Dilatation in Ulcerative and Crohn's Colitis," *Journal of Clinical Gastroenterology* 7, no. 2 (April 1985): 137–43.

12. K. Forssmann and M. V. Singer, "Therapy of Crohn's Disease in Internal Medicine: Short Bowel Syndrome and Toxic Megacolon," *Schweizerische Rundschau fur Medizin Praxis* 87, no. 48 (Nov 26, 1998): 1652–56.

13. C. D. Levine, "Toxic Megacolon: Diagnosis and Treatment Challenges," *AACN Clinical Issues* 10, no. 4 (Nov 1999): 492–99.

14. K. M. Das, "Relationship of Extraintestinal Involvements in Inflammatory Bowel Disease: New Insights into Autoimmune Pathogenesis," *Digestive Disease Science* 44, no. 1 (Jan 1999): 1–13.

15. S. P. Schuettenberg, "Nodular Scleritis, Episcleritis, and Anterior Uveitis as Ocular Complications of Crohn's Disease," *Journal of the American Optometric Association* 62, no. 5 (May 1991): 377–81.

16. J. B. Levine, MD, "Extraintestinal Manifestations of Inflammatory Bowel Disease," in J. B. Kirsner's *Inflammatory Bowel Disease,* 5th edition (Philadelphia: Saunders, 2000), 397–409.

17. Levine, "Extraintestinal Manifestations of Inflammatory Bowel Disease." 397–409.

18. D. Bjorkman, "Nonsteroidal Anti-inflammatory Drug-Associated Toxicity of the Liver, Lower Gastrointestinal Tract, and Esophagus," *American Journal of Medicine* 105, no. 5A (2 Nov 1998): 17S–21S.

19. U. Mahadevan et al., "Safety of Selective Cyclooxygenase-2 Inhibitors in Inflammatory Bowel Disease," *American Journal of Gastroenterology* 97, no. 4 (April 2002): 783–85.

20. M. I. Memon, B. Memon, and M. A. Memon, "Hepatobiliary Manifestations of Inflammatory Bowel Disease," *HPB Surgery: A World Journal of Hepatic, Pancreatic, and Biliary Surgery* 11, no. 6 (Aug 2000): 363–71.

21. V. Raj and D. R. Lichtenstein, "Hepatobiliary Manifestations of Inflammatory Bowel Disease," *Gastroenterology Clinics of North America* 28, no. 2 (June 1999): 491–513.

22. S. A. Mitchell et al., "A Preliminary Trial of High Dose Ursodeoxycholic Acid in Primary Sclerosing Cholangitis," *Gastroenterologyy* 121, no. 4 (Oct 2001): 900–07.

23. R. Caudarella et al., "Renal Stone Formation in Patients with Inflammatory Bowel Disease," *Scanning Microscopy* 7, no. 1 (March 1993): 371–79.

24. P. Barcelo et al., "Randomized Double–Blind Study of Potassium Citrate in Idiopathic Hypocitraturic Calcium Nephrolithiasis," *Journal of Urology* 150, no. 6 (Dec 1993): 1761–64.

25. M. A. Seltzer et al., "Dietary Manipulation with Lemonade to Treat Hypocitraturic Calcium Nephrolithiasis," *Journal of Urology* 156, no. 3 (Sept 1996): 907–09.

26. G. Johansson et al., "Effects of Magnesium Hydroxide in Renal Stone Disease," *Journal of the American College of Nutrition* 1, no. 2 (1982): 179–85.

27. L. K. Massey, H. Roman-Smith, R. A. Sutton, "Effect of Dietary Oxalate and Calcium on Urinary Oxalate and Risk of Calcium Oxalate Stones," *Journal of the American Dietetic Association* 93, no. 8 (Aug 1993): 901–06.

28. B. D. Greenwald, "Skin Disorders in IBD," Crohn's and Colitis Foundation of America, available on the Web at *http://www.ccfa.org/medcentral/library/compl/skin.htm.*

29. Greenwald, "Skin Disorders in IBD."

Chapter 5: Medications

1. W. J. Tremaine et al., "Budesonide CIR Capsules (Once or Twice Daily Divided Dose) in Active Crohn's Disease: A Randomized Placebo-Controlled Study in the United States," *American Journal of Gastroenterology* 97, no. 7 (July 2002): 1748–54.

2. A. Cortot et al., "Switch from Systemic Steroids to Budesonide in Steroid Dependent Patients with Inactive Crohn's Disease," *Gut* 48, no. 2 (Feb 2001): 186–90.

3. G. A. Dayharsh et al., "Epstein-Barr Virus–Positive Lymphoma in Patients with Inflammatory Bowel Disease Treated with Azathioprine or 6-Mercaptopurine," *Gastroenterology* 122, no. 1 (Jan 2002): 72–77.

4. A. Francella et al., "The Safety of 6-Mercaptopurine for Childbearing Patients with Inflammatory Bowel Disease: A Retrospective Cohort Study," *Gastroenterology* 124, no. 1 (Jan 2003): 9–17.

5. A. G. Fraser et al., "The Efficacy of Methotrexate for Maintaining Remission in Inflammatory Bowel Disease," *Alimentary Pharmacology and Therapeutics* 16, no. 4 (April 2002): 693–97.

6. W. J. Sanborn, "Cyclosporine in Ulcerative Colitis: State of the Art," *Acta Gastro-Enterologica Belgica* 64, no. 2 (April–June 2001): 201–04.

7. C. Hermida-Rodriguez et al., "High-Dose Intravenous Cyclosporine in Steroid Refractory Attacks of Inflammatory Bowel Disease," *Hepatogastroenterology* 46, no. 28 (July–Aug 1999): 2265–68.

8. I. T. Cockburn and P. Krupp, "The Risk of Neoplasms in Patients Treated with Cyclosporine A," *Journal of Autoimmunity* 2, no. 5 (Oct 1989): 723–31.

9. P. Rutgeerts et al., "Controlled Trial of Metronidazole Treatment for Prevention of Crohn's Recurrence After Ileal Resection," *Gastroenterology* 108, no. 6 (June 1995): 1617–21.

10. T. E. Madiba and D. C. Bartolo, "Pouchitis Following Restorative Proctocolectomy for Ulcerative Colitis: Incidence and Therapeutic Outcome," *Journal of the Royal College of Surgeons of Edinburgh* 46, no. 6 (Dec 2001): 334–37.

11. U. M. Turunen et al., "Long-Term Treatment of Ulcerative Colitis with Ciprofloxacin: A Prospective, Double-Blind, Placebo-Controlled Study." *Gastroenterology* 115, no. 5 (Nov 1998): 1072–78.

12. G. L. Arnold et al., "Preliminary study of Ciprofloxacin in Active Crohn's Disease," *Inflammatory Bowel Diseases* 8, no. 1 (Jan 2002): 10–15.

13. B. Shen et al., "A Randomized Trial of Ciprofloxacin and Metronidazole to Treat Acute Pouchitis," *Inflammatory Bowel Diseases* 7, no. 4 (Nov 2001): 301–05.

14. K. Leiper, A. I. Morris, and J. M Rhodes, "Open Label Trial of Oral Clarithromycin in Active Crohn's," *Alimentary Pharmacology and Therapeutics* 14, no. 6 (June 2000): 801–06.

15. R. W. Goodgame et al., "Randomized Controlled Trial of Clarithromycin and Ethambutol in the Treatment of Crohn's Disease," *Alimentary Pharmacology and Therapeutics* 15, no. 12 (Dec 2001): 1861–66.

16. S. B. Hanauer et al., "Maintenance Infliximab for Crohn's Disease: The ACCENT I Randomized Trial," *The Lancet* 359, no. 9317 (May 2002): 1541–49.

17. D. H. Present et al., "Infliximab for the Treatment of Fistulas in Patients with Crohn's Disease," *New England Journal of Medicine* 340, no. 18 (6 May 1999): 1398–405.

18. W. Y. Chey et al., "Infliximab for Refractory Ulcerative Colitis," *American Journal of Gastroenterology* 96, no. 8 (Aug 2001): 2373–81.

19. J. Keane et al., "Tuberculosis Associated with Infliximab, a Tumor Necrosis Factor Alpha-Neutralizing Agent," *New England Journal of Medicine* 345, no. 15 (11 Oct 2001): 1098–104.

20. S. Ghosh et al., "Natalizumab for Active Crohn's Disease," *New England Journal of Medicine* 348, no. 1 (2 Jan 2003): 24–32.

21. P. Rutgeerts et al., "Treatment of Active Crohn's Disease with Onercept (Recombinant Human Soluble *p55* Tumour Necrosis Factor Receptor): Results of a Randomized, Open Label, Pilot Study," *Alimentary Pharmacology and Therapeutics* 17, no. 2 (Jan 2003): 185–92.

22. A. Bousvaros and B. Mueller, "Thalidomide in Gastrointestinal Disorders," *Drugs* 61, no. 6 (2001): 777–87.

23. K. Fellerman et al., "Steroid-Unresponsive Acute Attacks of Inflammatory Bowel Disease: Immunomodulation by Tacrolimus (FK506)," *American Journal of Gastroenterology* 93, no. 10 (Oct 1998): 1860–66.

24. T. Orth et al., "Mycophenolate Mofetil versus Azathioprine in Patients with Chronic Active Ulcerative Colitis: A 12-Month Study," *American Journal of Gastroenterology* 95, no. 5 (May 2000): 1201–07.

25. W. J. Sandborn et al., "Transdermal Nicotine for Mildly to Moderately Active Ulcerative Colitis: A Randomized, Double-Blind, Placebo-Controlled Trial," *Annals of Internal Medicine* 126, no. 5 (1 March 1997): 364–71.

26. G. A. Thomas et al., "Transdermal Nicotine as Maintenance Therapy for Ulcerative Colitis," *New England Journal of Medicine* 332, no. 15 (13 April 1995): 988–92.

27. J. T. Green et al., "Nicotine Enemas for Active Ulcerative Colitis—A Pilot Study," *Alimentary Pharmacology and Therapeutics* 11, no. 5 (Oct 1997): 859–63.

28. D. E. Elliott et al., "Does the Failure to Acquire Helminthic Parasites Predispose to Crohn's Disease?" *The FASEB Journal: Official Publication of the Federation of American Societies for Experimental Biology* 14, no. 12 (Sept 2000): 1848–55.

Chapter 6: Surgical Treatments

1. P. Gionchetti et al., "Oral Bacteriotherapy as Maintenance Treatment in Patients with Chronic Pouchitis: A Double-Blind, Placebo-Controlled Trial," *Gastroenterology* 119, no. 2 (Aug 2000): 584–87.

2. L.W. Kohler et al., "Quality of Life After Proctocolectomy: A Comparison of Brooke Ileostomy, Kock Pouch, and Ileal Pouch-Anal Anastomosis," *Gastroenterology* 101, no. 3 (Sept 1991): 679–84.

3. A. P. Meagher et al., "J Ileal Pouch-Anal Anastomosis for Chronic Ulcerative Colitis: Complications and Long-Term Outcome in 1310 Patients," *British Journal of Surgery* 85, no. 6 (June 1998): 800–03.

4. R. R. Dozois et al., "Improved Results with Continent Ileostomy," *Annals of Surgery* 192, no. 3 (Sept 1980): 319–24.

5. V. R. Litle et al., "The Continent Ileostomy: Long-Term Durability and Patient Satisfaction," *Journal of Gastrointestinal Surgery* 3, no. 6 (Nov–Dec 1999): 625–32.

6. O. Bernell, A. Lapidus, and G. Hellers, "Risk Factors for Surgery and Postoperative Recurrence in Crohn's Disease," *Annals of Surgery* 231, no. 1 (Jan 2000): 38–45.

7. A. J. Kroesen and H. J. Buhr, "New Aspects of Surgical Therapy of Recurrent Crohn's Disease," *Yonsei Medical Journal* 41, no. 1 (Feb 2000): 1–7.

8. J. C. Goligher, "The Long-Term Results of Excisional Surgery for Primary and Recurrent Crohn's Disease of the Large Intestine," *Diseases of the Colon and Rectum* 28, no. 1 (Jan 1985): 51–5.

9. S. Strong and V. W. Fazio, "The Surgical Management of Crohn's Disease," in J. B. Kirsner's *Inflammmatory Bowel Disease,* 5th edition (Philadelphia: Saunders, 2000), 658–709.

10. M. Cottone et al., "Smoking Habits and Recurrence in Crohn's Disease," *Gastroenterology* 106, no. 3 (March 1994): 643–48.

11. A. J. Greenstein et al., "Surgery and Its Sequelae in Crohn's Colitis and Ileocolitis," *Archives of Surgery* 116, no. 3 (March 1981): 285–88.

12. Meagher, "J Ileal Pouch-Anal Anastomosis for Chronic Ulcerative Colitis," 800–03.

13. Greenstein, "Surgery and Its Sequelae in Crohn's Colitis and Ileocolitis," 285–88.

14. A. R. MacLean et al., "Risk of Small Bowel Obstruction After the Ileal Pouch–Anal Anastomosis," *Annals of Surgery* 235, no. 2 (Feb 2002): 200–06.

Chapter 7: Diet and Complementary Medicine

1. J. K. Ritchie et al., "Controlled Multicentre Therapeutic Trial of an Unrefined Carbohydrate, Fibre Rich Diet in Crohn's Disease," *British Medical Journal* 295, no. 6597 (29 Aug 1987): 517–20.

2. A. M. Riordan, C. H. Ruxton, and J. O. Hunter, "A Review of Associations Between Crohn's Disease and Consumption of Sugars," *European Journal of Clinical Nutrition* 52, no. 4 (April 1998): 229–38.

3. S. Endres, R. Lorenz, and K. Loeschke, "Lipid Treatment of Inflammatory Bowel Disease," *Current Opinion in Clinical Nutrition and Metabolic Care* 2, no. 2 (March 1999): 117–20.

4. A. K. Akobeng et al., "Double-Blind Randomized Controlled Trial of Glutamine-Enriched Polymeric Diet in Treatment of Active Crohn's Disease," *Journal of Pediatric Gastroenterology and Nutrition* 30, no. 1 (Jan 2000): 78–84.

5. E. Den Hond et al., "Effect of Long-Term Oral Glutamine Supplements on Small Intestinal Permeability in Patients with Crohn's Disease," *Journal of Parenteral and Enteral Nutrition* 23, no. 1 (Jan–Feb 1999): 7–11.

6. K. L. Madsen, "The Use of Probiotics in Gastrointestinal Disease," *Canadian Journal of Gastroenterology* 15, no. 12 (Dec 2001): 817–22.

7. P. Rawsthorne et al., "An International Survey of the Use and Attitudes Regarding Alternative Medicine by Patients with Inflammatory Bowel Disease," *American Journal of Gastroenterology* 94, no. 5 (May 1999): 1298–303.

8. R. Heuschkel et al., "Complementary Medicine Use in Children and Young Adults with Inflammatory Bowel Disease," *American Journal of Gastroenterology* 97, no. 2 (Feb 2002): 382–88.

9. C. Yang and H. Yan, "Observation of the Efficacy of Acupuncture and Moxibustion in 62 Cases of Chronic Colitis," *Journal of Traditional Chinese Medicine* 19, no. 2 (June 1999): 111–14.

10. J. Ezzo et al., "Is Acupuncture Effective for the Treatment of Chronic Pain? A Systematic Review," *Pain* 86, no. 3 (June 2000): 217–25.

11. M. H. Pittler and E. Ernst, "Peppermint Oil for Irritable Bowel Syndrome: A Critical Review and Meta-analysis," *American Journal of Gastorenterology* 93, no. 7 (July 1998): 1131–35.

12. R. M. Kline et al., "Enteric-Coated, Ph-Dependent Peppermint Oil Capsules for the Treatment of Irritable Bowel Syndrome in Children," *Journal of Pediatrics* 138, no. 1 (Jan 2001): 125–28.

Chapter 8: Alternative Forms of Feeding

1. S. Verma et al., "Polymeric versus Elemental Diet as Primary Treatment in Active Crohn's Disease: A Randomized, Double-Blind Trial," *American Journal of Gastroenterology* 95, no. 3 (March 2000): 735–39.

2. R. Meier, "Chronic Inflammatory Bowel Disease and Nutrition," *Schweizerische Medizinische Wochenschrift,* Supplementum 79 (1996): 14S–24S.

3. Y. Le Quintrec et al., "Exclusive Elemental Enteral Diet in Cortico-resistant and Cortico-dependent Forms of Crohn's Disease," *Gastroeneterologie Clininque et Biologique* 11, no. 6–7 (June–July 1987): 477–82.

4. R. M. Beattie, B. S. Bentsen, and T. T. MacDonald, "Childhood Crohn's Disease and the Efficacy of Enteral Diets," *Nutrition* 14, no. 4 (April 1998): 345–50.

5. D. Schwab, M. Raithel, and E. G. Hahn, "Enteral Nutrition in Acute Crohn's Disease," *Zeitschrift für Gastroenterologie* 36, no. 11 (Nov 1998): 983–95.

6. R. Meier, "Chronic Inflammatory Bowel Disease and Nutrition," 14S–24S.

7. A. M. Griffiths et al., "Meta-analysis of Enteral Nutrition as a Primary Treatment of Active Crohn's Disease," *Gastroenterology* 108, no. 4 (April 1995): 1056–67.

8. M. Wilschanski et al., "Supplementary Elemental Nutrition Maintains Remission in Pediatric Crohn's Disease," *Gut* 38, no. 4 (April 1996): 543–48.

9. S. Verma et al., "Polymeric versus Elemental Diet as Primary Treatment in Active Crohn's Disease," 735–39.

10. D. Rigaud et al., "Controlled Trial Comparing Two Types of Enteral Nutrition in Treatment of Active Crohn's Disease: Elemental versus Polymeric Diet," *Gut* 32, no. 12 (Dec 1991): 1492–97.

11. M. H. Giaffer, G. North, and C. D. Holdworth, "Controlled Trial of Polymeric versus Elemental Diet in Treatment of Active Crohn's Disease," *The Lancet* 335, no. 8693 (7 April 1990): 816–19.

12. M. Seo et al., "The Role of Total Parenteral Nutrition in the Management of Patients with Acute Attacks of Inflammatory Bowel Disease," *Journal of Clinical Gastroenterology* 29, no. 3 (Oct 1999): 270–75.

13. Y. Yamazaki et al., "The Medical, Nutritional and Surgical Treatment of Fistulae in Crohn's Disease," *Japanese Journal of Surgery* 20, no. 4 (July 1990): 376–83.

Chapter 10: Going to the Hospital

1. W. R. Jarvis. "Selected Aspects of the Socio-economic Impact of Nosocomial Infections: Morbidity, Mortality, Cost, and Prevention," *Infection Control and Hospital Epidemiology* 17, no. 8 (Aug 1996): 552–57.

2. National Nosocomial Infections Surveillance (NNIS), Dec 1999 report, available on the Web at *http://www.cdc.gov/ncidod/hip/surveill/nnis.htm.*

3. J. Lazarou et al., "Incidence of Adverse Drug Reactions in Hospitalized Patients: A Meta-analysis of Prospective Studies," *Journal of the American Medical Association* 279, no. 15 (15 April 1998): 1200–05.

Chapter 12: Coping with Prednisone

1. K. L. Tucker, M. T. Hannan, and D. P. Kiel, "The Acid–Base Hypothesis: Diet and Bone in the Farmington Osteoporosis Study," *European Journal of Nutrition* 40, no. 5 (Oct 2001): 231–37.

2. J. Homik et al., "Calcium and Vitamin D for Corticosteroid-Induced Osteoporosis," *Conchrane Database of Systematic Reviews* 2 (2000): CD000952.

3. J. E. Sojka and C. M. Weaver, "Magnesium Supplementation and Osteoporosis," *Nutrition Reviews* 53, no. 3 (March 1995): 71–4.

4. H. Glerup et al., "Commonly Recommended Daily Intake of Vitamin D is Not Sufficient if Sunlight Exposure is Limited," *Journal of Internal Medicine* 247, no. 2 (Feb 2000): 260–68.

5. C. R. Kessenich and C. J. Rosen, "Vitamin D and Bone Status in Elderly Women," *Orthopaedic Nursing* 15, no. 3 (May–June 1996): 67–71.

6. S. M. Moeller, P. F. Jacques, and J. B. Blumberg, "The Potential Role of Dietary Xanthophylls in Cataract and Age-Related Macular Degeneration," *Journal of the American College of Nutrition* 19, no. 5 Suppl (Oct 2000): 522S–527S.

7. S. Zigman, "The Role of Sunlight in Human Cataract Formation," *Survey of Ophthalmology* 27, no. 5 (March–April 1983): 317–25.

8. J. M. Weintraub et al., "Smoking Cessation and Risk of Cataract Extraction Among US Women and Men," *American Journal of Epidemiology* 155, no. 1 (Jan 2002): 72–9.

9. B. Dreno et al., "Multicenter Randomized Comparative Double-Blind Controlled Clinical Trial of the Safety and Efficacy of Zinc Gluconate versus Minocycline Hydrochloride in the Treatment of Inflammatory Acne Vulgaris," *Dermatology* 203, no. 2 (2001): 135–40.

Chapter 13: Relationships

1. R. Burakoff, "Fertility and Pregnancy in Inflammatory Bowel Disease," in J. B. Kirsner's *Inflammmatory Bowel Disease,* 5th edition (Philadelphia: Saunders, 2000): 372–78.

2. H. Masui et al., "Male Sexual Function After Autonomic Nerve-Preserving Operation for Rectal Cancer," *Diseases of the Colon and Rectum* 39, no. 10 (Oct 1996): 1140–45.

Chapter 14: Fertility and Pregnancy

1. C. O'Morain et al., "Reversible Male Infertility Due to Sulphasalazine: Studies in Man and Rat," *Gut* 25, no. 10 (Oct 1984): 1078–84.

2. K. Ording Olsen et al., "Ulcerative Colitis: Female Fecundity Before Diagnosis, During Disease, and After Surgery Compared with a Population Sample," *Gastroenterology* 122, no. 1 (Jan 2002): 15–19.

3. M. Hudson et al., "Fertility and Pregnancy in Inflammatory Bowel Disease," *International Journal of Gynaecology and Obstetrics* 58, no. 2 (Aug 1997): 229–37.

4. M. Mogadam et al., "The Course of Inflammatory Bowel Disease During Pregnancy and the Postpartum," *American Journal of Gastroenterology* 75, no. 4 (April 1981): 265–69.

5. Mogadam et al., "The Course of Inflammatory Bowel Disease During Pregnancy and the Postpartum," 265–69.

6. M. R. Morton, "Inflammatory Bowel Disease Presenting in Pregnancy," *The Australian and New Zealand Journal of Obstetrics & Gynaecology* 32, no. 1 (Feb 1992): 40–42.

7. D. D. Moeller, "Crohn's Disease Beginning During Pregnancy," *Southern Medical Journal* 81, no. 8 (Aug 1988): 1067.

8. J. A. Dominitz, J. C. Young, and E. J. Boyko, "Outcome of Infants Born to Mothers with Inflammatory Bowel Disease: A Population-Based Cohort Study," *American Journal of Gastroenterology* 97, no. 3 (March 2002): 641–48.

9. R. Burakoff, "Fertility and Pregnancy in Inflammatory Bowel Disease," in J. B. Kirsner's *Inflammatory Bowel Disease,* 5th edition (Philadelphia: Saunders, 2000), 372–78.

10. M. Mogadam et al., "Pregnancy in Inflammatory Bowel Disease: Effect of Sulfasalazine and Corticosteroids on Fetal Outcome," *Gastroenterology* 80, no. 1 (Jan 1981): 72–76.

11. P. Marteau et al., "Foetal Outcome in Women with Inflammatory Bowel Disease Treated During Pregnancy with Oral Mesalazine Microgranules," *Alimentary Pharmacology & Therapeutics* 12, no. 11 (Nov 1998): 1101–08.

12. Burakoff, "Fertility and Pregnancy in Inflammatory Bowel Disease," 372–78.

13. W. Connell and A. Miller, "Treating Inflammatory Bowel Disease During Pregnancy: Risks and Safety of Drug Therapy," *Drug Safety: An International Journal of Medical Toxicology and Drug Experience* 21, no. 4 (Oct 1999): 311–23.

14. E. M. Alstead et al., "Safety of Azathioprine in Pregnancy in Inflammatory Bowel Disease," *Gastroenterology* 99, no. 2 (Aug 1990): 443–46.

15. A. Francella et al., "The Safety of 6-Mercaptopurine for Childbearing Patients with Inflammatory Bowel Disease: A Retrospective Cohort Study," *Gastroenterology* 124, no. 1 (Jan 2003): 9–17.

16. R. O. Rajapaske et al., "Outcome of Pregnancies When Fathers Are Treated with 6-Mercaptopurine for Inflammatory Bowel Disease," *American Journal of Gastroenterology* 95, no. 3 (March 2000): 684–88.

17. Burakoff, "Fertility and Pregnancy in Inflammatory Bowel Disease," 372–78.

18. A. Einarson et al., "Prospective, Controlled, Multicentre Study of Loperamide in Pregnancy," *Canadian Journal of Gastroenterology* 14, no. 3 (March 2000): 185–87.

19. B. Bar Oz et al., "Pregnancy Outcome After Cyclosporine Therapy During Pregnancy," *Transplantation* 71, no. 8 (April 2001): 1051–55.

20. D. B. Sachar, "The Safety of Sulfasalazine: The Gastroenterologists' Experience," *Journal of Rheumatology,* Suppl 16 (Sept 1988): 14–16.

21. J. B. Anderson, G. M. Turner, and R. C. Williamson, "Fulminant Ulcerative Colitis in Late Pregnancy and the Puerperium," *Journal of the Royal Society of Medicine* 80, no. 8 (Aug 1987): 492–94.

22. K. Teahon et al., "Elemental Diet in the Management of Crohn's Disease During Pregnancy," *Gut* 32, no. 9 (Sept 1991): 1079–81.

23. V. Binder, "Genetic Epidemiology in Inflammatory Bowel Disease," *Digestive Diseases* 16, no. 6 (Nov 1998): 351–55.

24. M. P. Roth et al., "Familial Empiric Risk Estimates of Inflammatory Bowel Disease in Ashkenazi Jews," *Gastroenterology* 96, no. 4 (April 1989): 1016–20.

25. R. A. Bennett, P. H. Rubin, and D. H. Present, "Frequency of Inflammatory Bowel Disease in Offspring of Couples Both Presenting with Inflammatory Bowel Disease," *Gastroenterology* 100, no. 6 (June 1991): 1638–43.

Chapter 15: Children and Teens

1. Crohn's & Colitis Foundation of America, "Crohn's Disease and Ulcerative Colitis: A Parent's Guide," available on the Web at *http://www.ccfa .org/brochures/parents.pdf.*

2. R. M. Beattie, B. S. Bentsen, and T. T. MacDonald, "Childhood Crohn's Disease and the Efficacy of Enteral Diets," *Nutrition* 14, no. 4 (April 1998): 345–50.

3. A. M. Griffiths et al., "Meta-analysis of Enteral Nutrition as a Primary Treatment of Active Crohn's Disease," *Gastroenterology* 108, no. 4 (April 1995): 1056–67.

Chapter 16: Record-Keeping, Insurance, Employment, and Disability

1. Social Security Administration, "Flow of Cases Through the Disability Process," 20 June 2002, available on the Web at *http://www.ssa.gov/ disability/disability_process_welcome.htm.*

Chapter 17: Emotions and Coping

1. P. Salmon, "Effects of Exercise on Anxiety, Depression, and Sensitivity to Stress: A Unifying Theory," *Clinical Psychology Review* 21, no. 1 (Feb 2001): 33–61.

2. B. Nemets, Z. Stahl, and R. H. Belmaker, "Addition of Omega-3 Fatty Acid to Maintenance Medication Treatment for Recurrent Unipolar Depressive Disorder," *American Journal of Psychiatry* 159, no. 3 (March 2002): 477–79.

3. J. B. Meisholder and E. N. Chandler, "Prayer and Health Outcomes in Church Members," *Alternative Therapies in Health and Medicine* 6, no. 4 (July 2000): 56–60.

4. "Digital Divide Still an Issue, Consumer Groups Say," *The Mercury News,* 30 May 2002, available on the Web at *http://www.siliconvalley.com/mld/ siliconvalley/news/editorial/3368030.htm.*

5. "One Out of Five Americans Find Internet Essential," MacCentral Online, 9 Sept 2002, available on the Web at *http://www.creativepro.com/story/ news/17582.html.*

6. K. Allen, B. E. Shykoff, and J. L. Izzo, "Pet Ownership, But Not Ace Inhibitor Therapy, Blunts Home Blood Pressure Responses to Mental Stress," *Hypertension* 38, no. 4 (Oct 2001): 815–20.

Index

A

Abscesses, 56–57
  emergency surgery for, 93, 108
  perforations and, 94
Academy for Guided Imagery, 303, 372, 396
Acetaminophen with codeine, 87
Acne and prednisone, 240
Acupuncture, 140–141
Address books for hospitalizations, 186
Adhesions. *See also* Small-bowel obstructions
  scar tissue and, 64
Adolescents. *See* Children and teenagers
Adrenal glands and prednisone, 248
Advocacy
  for children, 310
  hospital nurses and, 193–194
Africa, IBD in, 11
African Americans, 12–13
  osteoporosis risk and, 236
Age
  cancer risk and age of IBD diagnosis, 58–59
  inflammatory bowel disease (IBD) and, 12
  recurrence after surgery and, 113
  as risk factor, 10
Alcohol use, Flagyl and, 82
Alimentary tract, 1–2, 3
Allergic reactions
  food allergies, 306
  to infliximab, 85–86
  of peristomal skin, 217–218
  to sulfasalazine, 73
  surgery and, 115
Allopathic medicine. *See* Complementary therapies
Almond flours, 132
Aloe vera, 141–142
Alpha-4 integren, 89
Amebic dysentery, 38
American Association for Marriage and Family
    Therapy (AAMFT), 376, 397
American Board of Internal Medicine (ABIM), 170

American Board of Medical Specialties (ABMS), 396
  credential information from, 168–169, 170
American College of Gastroenterology (ACG), 394
American Gastroenterological Association (AGA), 394
American Medical Association (AMA), Physician
    Select Web site, 169, 170
American Medical Association Directory of Physicians in
    the US, 170
American Nuclear Society (ANS), 45
American Psychiatric Association (APA), 397
American Psychological Association (APA), 376, 398
The American Society of Clinical Hypnosis, 396
Americans with Disabilities Act (ADA), 345–348
  exhaustion of administrative remedies, 347
  violations, dealing with, 347–348
Anaerobic intestinal bacteria, Flagyl for, 81
Anal anastomosis, Flagyl and, 82
Anatomy of an Illness (Cousins), 370
Androgen hormones, 232, 233
Anemia
  as Crohn's disease symptom, 27–28
  as ulcerative colitis symptom, 23–24
Anesthesiologists, 117
Anger
  of children, 323–324
  dealing with, 357–359
  of parents, 298
Animals, support from, 374
Ankylosing spondylitis, 66
Antegren, 89
Antibiotics, 81–83. *See also* specific types
  breastfeeding and, 286
  for fistulas, 57
  for pouchitis, 102–103
  pregnancy and, 283
  preoperative antibiotics, 116
Antidepressant drugs, 361
Antidiarrheal drugs, 86–87
  pregnancy and, 283
Antispasmodic drugs, 88
Antituberculosis drugs, 83–84

415

C

CADD-TPN pump, 157
Calcitonin, 236
   nasal spray, 234
Calcium
   osteoporosis, prevention of, 235
   in vegan diet, 134
Calcium oxalate, 68
Calendar and medical records, 331
Campylobacter, 38
Canasa, 75
Cancer, 58–61
   azathioprine and, 79
   colectomy and, 60
   cyclosporine and, 81
   duration of IBD and, 59
   dysplasia and, 59–60
   emergency surgery for, 93
   5-aminosalicylic acid (5-ASA) drugs and, 60–61
   folic acid and, 61
   J-pouch surgery and, 100–101
   mandatory ostomies, 212–213
   methotrexate and, 79
   6-MP and, 79
Candida albicans infection, 39
Carbohydrates, insomnia and, 246
CARD15 gene, 15
Carotenoids, 238
Case, Shelley, 130
Cataracts and prednisone, 237–238
Cats, support from, 374
Caucasians, 12–13
   osteoporosis risk and, 236
Cecum, 2
Celebrex, 67
Celecoxib, 67
Cellcept, 90
Center for Attitudinal Healing, 396
The Centers for Medicare and Medicaid Services, 336, 339
   free medication information, 393
Cesarean sections, 277–278
Chambers of commerce, health insurance through, 336
Changing physicians, 178–180
Charged coupled device (CCD) chips, 46
Child life programs, 294
   for surgery, 307–308
Children and teenagers, 291–334. *See also* Growth issues; Hospitals; School issues
   blaming of parents by, 363
   blood tests for, 292–293
   books, list of, 399
   comfort objects for, 296

communication in parent-child relationship, 323–324
   coping with tests and procedures, 294–297
   endoscopic procedures for, 293
   enteral feeding and, 145
   Family and Medical Leave Act (FMLA) and care for, 348–349
   friends and, 317–319
   guided imagery, using, 303
   helping children cope, tips for, 255–256
   heredity and IBD, 289–290
   imaging procedures for, 293–294
   medications for, 302–305
   nutritional therapy, 305–306
   onset with, 291–292
   organizations for children, list of, 392–393
   ostomy support for, 226–227
   pain of procedures, reducing, 295–297
   preparing children, 295
   puberty delays, 312
   reactions of, 297–300
   relationships with, 253–256
   responsibility for medications, 304–305
   rewards after procedures, 296–297
   schedules for medication, 303
   sharing information with, 300–302
   siblings, relationships with, 321–323
   summer camps for, 318–319
   support groups for, 318
   surgery for, 307–308
   symptoms of, 291–292
   tips for parents, 319–321
   treatment of children, 302–311
   Web sites, list of, 405
Children with Intestinal and Liver Disorders Foundation (CH.I.L.D Foundation), 391
Chiropractic, 141
Chloraseptic for feeding tube irrigation, 151
Cholesterol and gallstones, 67–68
Chromosomes, research on, 15
Chronic fatigue syndrome (CFS), 39
Church community, support from, 369–370
Ciprofloxacin (Cipro), 83
   breastfeeding and, 286
   for pouchitis, 102–103
   pregnancy and, 283
Cirrhosis, 68
Citrates and kidney stones, 69
Clarithromycin, 83–84
Clear liquid diet, 127–128
   postoperative diet, 121
Closed pouches, 216
Clostridium, 38
Clothing for hospitalizations, 186

National Library of Medicine, 397
Nausea
    antidiarrheal drugs and, 87
    ciprofloxacin and, 83
    clarithromycin and, 84
    as Crohn's disease symptom, 29
    cyclosporine and, 81
    Flagyl and, 82
    infliximab and, 85
    methotrexate and, 80
    pain medications and, 87
    from 6-MP, 78
    strictures and, 63
    sulfasalazine causing, 73, 74
Needle sticks, 295
Neoral. *See* Cyclosporine
Nicotine and IBD, 90
NOD2 gene, 15
North American Society for Pediatric
        Gastroenterology, Hepatology and
        Nutrition (NASPGHAN), 394
NSAIDs (nonsteroidal anti-inflammatory drugs), 66
NuLytely, 52
Numbness, Flagyl and, 83
Nurses. *See also* Enterostomal therapy (ET) nurses
    home health nurses on discharge from hospital,
        206
    hospital nurses, working with, 193–194
    referrals to physicians, 166
Nursing women, 284–286
Nut flours, 132
Nutritional therapy. *See also* Enteral feeding
    for children and teenagers, 305–306
    growth issues and, 312
    parenteral feeding, 152–159
    partial parenteral nutrition (PPN), 154
Nuts as irritant, 19

O

Oat-free diet, 130–131
Obsessive thinking and prednisone, 246–247
Obstructions, 63–64. *See also* Small-bowel
        obstructions
    emergency surgery for, 94
    pregnancy and, 277, 287
    total parental nutrition (TPN) and, 155
Occult blood tests, 37–38
Occupation as risk factor, 10
*Official ABMS Directory of Board Certified Medical
        Specialists,* 170
Olsalazine, 74
    pregnancy and, 279–280
Omega-3 fatty acids, 135–136
One-piece pouching systems, 216–217
Onercept, 89

Online support, 373–374
Operations. *See* Surgery
Optimental, 146
Organizations, list of, 391–398
Organ transplants, cyclosporine and, 80
Osteoporosis, prednisone and, 234–236
Ostomies, x, 208–230, 209. *See also* Stomas
    activities with, 223–224
    attitude and coping with, 228–230
    books on, 401
    Brooke ileostomy, 97–99
    changing appliances, 218, 220–221
    cleanliness and, 218
    coping with, 226–230
    deodorant products, 221
    elective ostomies, 213–214
    emptying pouches, 219–220
    gas, dealing with, 222–223
    living with, 99
    loop ostomy, 100
    mandatory ostomies, 212–213
    odor control, 221–222
    one-piece pouching systems, 216–217
    organizations, list of, 392392
    personal relationships and, 224–225
    perspective, maintaining, 229–230
    pouching systems, 215–217
    psychotherapy support and, 227–228
    skin care with, 217–219
    two-piece pouching systems, 215–216
    types of, 208–212
    ureostomies, 211–212
    Web sites, list of, 405
Ostomy belts, 224
Oxalates, 69
Oxygen, hemoglobin and, 34–35

P

Pain. *See also* Cramping
    children and teenagers, reducing pain for,
        295–297
    coping with, 365–367
    as Crohn's disease symptom, 28–29
    postoperative pain, 119, 120–121
    types of, 365–366
    as ulcerative colitis symptom, 25
Pain medications, 87–88
    patient-controlled analgesia (PCA), 120–121
    for postoperative pain, 119–120
Pajamas for hospitalizations, 186
Pancolitis, 8, 9
    cancer risk and, 59
Pancreas
    azathioprine and inflammation of, 78
    6-MP and inflammation of, 78

About the Author

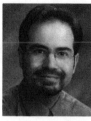 AUTHOR CLIFF KALIBJIAN was diagnosed with IBD over 20 years ago at the age of 13. He obtained a BA in psychology from University of California at Berkeley, and owns a medical information research business that provides customized research on any medical condition or health topic to consumers and professionals. Over the years, Cliff has been involved with volunteer activities to help those with IBD, including his roles as a support group facilitator, a fund raiser for many walk-a-thons and bowl-a-thons, and a camp counselor for children with IBD. He also works as a health and safety analyst at a large company.

Colophon

Patient-Centered Guides are about the experience of illness. They contain personal stories as well as a combination of practical and medical information.

The cover of *Straight from the Gut* was designed by Kristen Throop of Combustion Creative. The warm colors and quilt-like patterns are intended to convey a sense of comfort. The layout was created on a Macintosh using Quark 5.0. Fonts in the design are: Berkeley, Coronet, GillSans, Minion Ornaments, Throhand, and Univers Ultra Condensed. The design was built with tints of three PMS colors.

Rad Proctor designed the interior layout for the book based on a series design by Nancy Priest and Edie Freedman. The interior fonts are Berkeley and Franklin Gothic. The text was prepared using FrameMaker.

The book was copyedited by Paulette Miley and proofread by Marianne Rogoff. Tom Dorsaneo, Marianne Rogoff, and Katherine Stimson conducted quality assurance checks. Katherine Stimson wrote the index. The illustrations that appear in this book were produced by Rob Romano. Interior composition was done by Rad Proctor and Tom Dorsaneo.